Innovation in Health Informatics: Smart Health Care

Innovation in Health Informatics: Smart Health Care

Editor: Jett Jacob

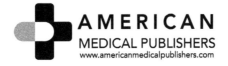

AMERICAN
MEDICAL PUBLISHERS
www.americanmedicalpublishers.com

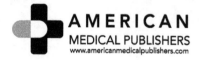

Cataloging-in-Publication Data

Innovation in health informatics : smart health care / edited by Jett Jacob.
   p. cm.
Includes bibliographical references and index.
ISBN 978-1-63927-699-8
1. Medical informatics. 2. Medical care--Technological innovations. 3. Medicine--Data processing.
4. Information storage and retrieval systems--Medicine. 5. Medical innovations. 6. Medical technology.
7. Artificial intelligence--Medical applications. I. Jacob, Jett.
R858 .I56 2023
610.285--dc23

American Medical Publishers,
41 Flatbush Avenue,
1st Floor, New York,
NY 11217, USA

ISBN 978-1-63927-699-8 (Hardback)

Contents

Preface

Every book is initially just a concept; it takes months of research and hard work to give it the final shape in which the readers receive it. In its early stages, this book also went through rigorous reviewing. The notable contributions made by experts from across the globe were first molded into patterned chapters and then arranged in a sensibly sequential manner to bring out the best results.

Health informatics, also called medical informatics, refers to the field of study that draws from three main subjects, namely, information science, computer science and health care. It involves the use of resources, devices and methods for acquiring, storing, retrieving and using information for health and biomedicine. In the last few decades, there has been a remarkable progress in information and communication technologies (ICT), which have laid the foundation for innovations in healthcare. The healthcare facilities primarily focus on delivering efficient, patient-centered and sustainable healthcare systems. This has been made possible by extensive use of technologies such as big data, medical data analytics, artificial intelligence, machine learning, virtual reality, augmented reality, 5G, internet of things (IOT), nanotechnologies and biotechnologies. Some of the important innovations that have dramatically changed health care and informatics include apps that enable communication with healthcare providers, telemedicine, electronic health records, wearable technology, 3-D bioprinting, etc. This book is compiled in such a manner, that it will provide in-depth knowledge about the concept of smart health care that includes widespread use of health informatics. Its aim is to present researches that have transformed this discipline and aided its advancement. The book will serve as a reference to a broad spectrum of readers.

It has been my immense pleasure to be a part of this project and to contribute my years of learning in such a meaningful form. I would like to take this opportunity to thank all the people who have been associated with the completion of this book at any step.

Editor

Portable Sleep Apnea Syndrome Screening and Event Detection Using Long Short-Term Memory Recurrent Neural Network

Hung-Chi Chang [1], Hau-Tieng Wu [2], Po-Chiun Huang [1], Hsi-Pin Ma [1], Yu-Lun Lo [3,*] and Yuan-Hao Huang [1,*]

[1] Department of Electrical Engineering, National Tsing Hua University, Hsinchu 30013, Taiwan; Scott_Chang@asus.com (H.-C.C.); pchuang@ee.nthu.edu.tw (P.-C.H.); hp@ee.nthu.edu.tw (H.-P.M.)

[2] Department of Mathematics and Department of Statistical Science, Duke University, Durham, NC 27708, USA; hauwu@math.duke.edu

[3] Department of Thoracic Medicine, Healthcare Center, Chang Gung Memorial Hospital, School of Medicine, Chang Gung University, Taipei 33302, Taiwan

*   Correspondence: lo3043@cgmh.org.tw (Y.-L.L.); yhhuang@ee.nthu.edu.tw (Y.-H.H.)

Abstract: Obstructive sleep apnea/hypopnea syndrome (OSAHS) is characterized by repeated airflow partial reduction or complete cessation due to upper airway collapse during sleep. OSAHS can induce frequent awake and intermittent hypoxia that is associated with hypertension and cardiovascular events. Full-channel Polysomnography (PSG) is the gold standard for diagnosing OSAHS; however, this PSG evaluation process is unsuitable for home screening. To solve this problem, a measuring module integrating abdominal and thoracic triaxial accelerometers, a pulsed oximeter (SpO_2) and an electrocardiogram sensor was devised in this study. Moreover, a long short-term memory recurrent neural network model is proposed to classify four types of sleep breathing patterns, namely obstructive sleep apnea (OSA), central sleep apnea (CSA), hypopnea (HYP) events and normal breathing (NOR). The proposed algorithm not only reports the apnea-hypopnea index (AHI) through the acquired overnight signals but also identifies the occurrences of OSA, CSA, HYP and NOR, which assists in OSAHS diagnosis. In the clinical experiment with 115 participants, the performances of the proposed system and algorithm were compared with those of traditional expert interpretation based on PSG signals. The accuracy of AHI severity group classification was 89.3%, and the AHI difference for PSG expert interpretation was 5.0 ± 4.5. The overall accuracy of detecting abnormal OSA, CSA and HYP events was 92.3%.

Keywords: abdominal movement signal; hypopnea; LSTM-RNN; neural network; oxygen saturation; sleep apnea syndrome; sleep–wake detection; synchrosqueezing transform; triaxial accelerometer; thoracic movement signal

1. Introduction

According to a recent report [1], 13% men and 6% women between the ages of 30 and 70 years are affected by obstructive sleep apnea-hypopnea syndrome (OSAHS). Patients suffering from OSAHS have symptoms such as excessive daytime sleepiness, morning headache, hypertension and decreased libido [2]. However, people are often unaware of OSAHS because apnea/hypopnea events only occur during sleep. According to the American Academy of Sleep Medicine scoring manual [3], an apnea event is identified when a drop of 90% respiratory airflow lasts for at least 10 s. Moreover, a hypopnea event is defined when a drop of over 30% respiratory airflow lasts for at least 10 s with at least 3% associated decrease in oxygen saturation (SpO_2) or arousal from sleep. The apnea-hypopnea index (AHI), which is defined as the total number of apnea and hypopnea events per hour of sleep, is a vital metric to quantize the severity of sleep breathing disorder. Although AHI is recently criticized and other phenotype information of sleep breathing problems should be considered in clinical diagnosis [4], it still is a reliable metric for SDB screening at home before the patients are recommended for other decent testing or diagnosis in hospital. Full-channel polysomnography (PSG) is the traditional method of diagnosing OSAHS. In PSG, various physical and biological signals containing sleep information are comprehensively recorded. Although PSG is the standard for diagnosing OSAHS, it has several drawbacks. Subjects are required to wear numerous sensors (more than 20 channels) for monitoring the condition of the body during sleep. The PSG examination can be performed only in the hospital and the sleep quality of the patients can be influenced by several external constraints. Moreover, to diagnose an OSAHS patient, it usually requires more than 6 h for a doctor or sleep technician to observe multichannel and overnight PSG signals and to label the sleep breathing events accordingly. Therefore, PSG measurement and diagnosis are expensive, time consuming and unsuitable for large-scale home-based screening. Several solutions have been proposed to alleviate this difficulty. A common solution is reducing the number of sensors. Several issues on the ambulatory monitoring for obstructive sleep apnea syndrome were raised by [5], and guidelines of using critical channels were also provided for sleep disorder diagnosis and management. In general, these solutions are classified into four classes [6]. A Level-III or Level-IV solution is considered in this paper.

In the past decade, several reduced-channel technologies have been developed to evaluate OSAHS severity. Multiple biological signals, such as electrocardiogram (ECG) [7], ballistocardiography [8], SpO_2 [9], respiratory efforts [10] and snoring sounds [11], have been used to derive statistical or instantaneous signal features that are highly related with apnea events for sleep event identification. With the derived features from the selected sensors, various automatic annotation algorithms have been developed for sleep apnea events. Classification levels are of two types—the AHI level and event level. At the AHI level, the AHI of the whole night sleep is estimated for diagnosis. At the event level, each single apnea and hypopnea event is identified and classified and hence the AHI is accordingly calculated for the diagnosis. For the classification, various machine learning techniques such as support vector machine (SVM) [12], ensemble classifiers [13], and Bayesian network-based classifier [14] have been used to identify the sleep apnea events. Recently, a convolutional-neural-network-based deep learning framework [15] was proposed to detect obstructive sleep apnea events. In another study [7], the hidden-Markov-model-based deep neural network was used for detecting sleep apnea based on ECG signals. Raw biological signals without feature extraction have been used in several studies for detecting sleep apnea events through deep learning [9]. Quiceno-Manrique [16], Mendez [17], De Chazal [13] and Novak [18] used ECG signal for diagnosing OSAHS. In [10,19], abdominal (ABD) and thoracic (THO) movements were proven to be excellent parameters for diagnosing OSA occurrence. In [20], multiple channels, SpO_2 and photoplethysmography (PPG) were used to estimate the blood volume changes for OSA prediction. For other literature works, refer to [21,22]. The primary differences and contributions of this study are presented as follows:

- This study is the first work to apply two triaxial accelerometers, a single-lead ECG and a finger oximeter for portable sleep apnea syndrome screening. The clinic experiments were performed by recording overnight signals of suspected patients under the approval of Institutional Review Board of hospital. Most works designed new sensing devices without clinic experiments or developed new detection algorithms by using public database.

- This work proposes a complete systematic framework of sensing devices and algorithms to detect and identify OSA, central sleep apnea (CSA) and hypopnea (HYP) events. This system can not only evaluate AHI values but also provide reliable event-level classification results of various sleep apnea events. Except our previous work [23] based on piezo-electronic bands, most works can only detect OSA events and evaluate AHI only.

In this study, a hardware solution was combined with a novel neural-network-based classification technique for identifying OSA, CSA and HYP events and NOR breathing by using two triaxial accelerometers (TAA), a pulsed oximeter and ECG. The proposed classification algorithm performs event level prediction but not the AHI level prediction. The features of the abdominal TAA (ABD-TAA), thoracic TAA (THO-TAA) and SpO_2 signals were extracted from the recorded signals. Then, a modified long short-term memory recurrent neural network (LSTM-RNN) was proposed to classify the OSA, CSA and HYP events and NOR breathing in the overnight recorded signals. To avoid underestimation of the AHI from the predicted apnea and hypopnea events, the sleep–wake status was predicted by analyzing the ECG signal with a CNN classifier. The AHI severity group classification, AHI difference and OSA/CSA/HYP event and normal breathing classification were also analyzed to demonstrate the superiority of the proposed OSAHS screening system.

This study aimed to develop an unattended sleep apnea screening system that can be incorporated in the personal healthcare services with less labeling labor. The proposed screening system can be applied to evaluate the long-term sleep breathing performance of the potential subjects. These devices should be used in patients with a high pretest probability for obstructive sleep apnea/hypopnea syndrome according to 2007 AASM guideline (Reference 4) for the home-base diagnosis test. Patients suspected with respiratory, cardiologic and neurologic disorders should be excluded in this test. Primary care physician or sleep specialist would be the one who arranges this test.

2. Material and Methods

2.1. Material

The THO and ABD movements were recorded using piezo-electric bands at a sampling rate of 100 Hz on the Alice 5 PSG acquisition system (Philips Respironics, Murrysville, PA, USA). The SpO_2 signals were also recorded at a sampling rate of 1 Hz in the PSG signals. The OSA, CSA and HYP events and NOR breathing were identified and labeled by sleep experts in the PSG signals as the reference classifier. At the same time as the PSG recoding process, the proposed THO-TAA, ABD-TAA and ECG sensing devices were also attached to the chest and abdomen of the participant for capturing the signals required for the proposed AHI evaluation system. Polysomnography (Alice 5, Respironics) was performed on all patients using standard techniques. Sleep stages and arousals were scored according to the AASM criteria [3]. Respiratory efforts were measured by piezo-electric bands, and arterial oxygen saturation was measured by pulse oximetry.

Established criteria were used to score respiratory events such as hypopnea, obstructive apnea, central apnea and mixed type apnea [3] during sleeping time. Apnea was defined as nasal flow cessation for more than 10 s. It was scored as obstructive (OSA) if the paradoxical respiratory and abdominal efforts were observed. It was scored as central (CSA) if none of these excursions were observed. It was scored as mixed if this effort is resumed toward the end of the period of apnea. The mixed type apnea was classified as OSA in this work because of its similar contribution factors to OSA. Hypopnea (HYP) was defined as a 30% reduction in nasal pressure transducer followed by an arousal or more than 3% decrease in SpO_2. In this work, a segment signal was scored as normal if none of the above-mentioned events was identified.

2.2. Integrated Sensing System

Figure 1a depicts the proposed integrated sensing system that captures biomedical signals for sleep event detection/classification and AHI evaluation. A 27-g sensing device was devised and fabricated with a nine-axis accelerometer, an ECG sensor, a Bluetooth module and a microcontroller (Figure 1b). The sensing device included an ultra-low-power microcontroller (MSP430) that controlled MPU9250 to capture TAA signals, which were then delivered to a mobile device, such as smartphone or tablet, through Bluetooth module CC2541. The integrated sensing system could continuously sense and record signals for 34 h with a 300 mAh battery. The signal word-length and sampling rate are 12 bits/500 Hz and 16 bits/50 Hz for the ECG and accelerator, respectively. The transmission baud rate from a sensor device to iOS device is 115,200 bps. The bandwidth and reliability was verified to be sufficient for continuous transmission of the overnight ECG and acceleration signals. The reconnection procedure was also implemented in the Bluetooth link in case that patients might wake up and leave the transmission coverage, for example to go to restroom at night.

In the clinical experiment, two integrated TAA/ECG sensing devices were attached on the chest and abdomen of the participants and the ECG electrode was attached to the chest (Figure 1c). To record respiratory information, one sensing device was placed from the left parasternal line, 4th or 5th intercostal space to the mid-clavicle line to measure the maximal thoracic movement. The other sensing device was placed from the left subcostal anterior axillary line to the umbilical area to measure the maximal abdomen movement. In this way, we not only obtained strong thoracic and abdomen movement signal but also strong EKG signal. In the proposed recording and storage system, a prototype app software with graphic user interface on iOS device was built to control the progress of the data recording. All the sensed physiological signals were transmitted from the sensing devices to the iOS device through Bluetooth. Then, they were uploaded to the Dropbox cloud data server for the following data analysis.

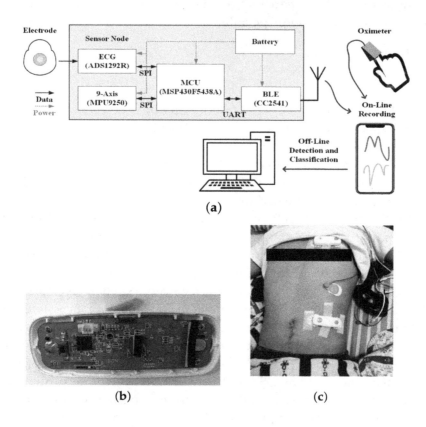

Figure 1. (a) Block diagram of the integrated sensing device and system; (b) photo of the sensing device; and (c) devices worn for sensing the ABD-TAA, THO-TAA and ECG signals.

2.3. Signal Preprocessing

Figure 2 displays the processing diagram of the proposed AHI evaluation system. Six channels of the ABD-TAA and THO-TAA signals were passed through six-order low-pass filters with a 0.8-Hz cut-off frequency and then converted into two respiratory motion signals, namely THO and ABD. Subsequently, the THO and ABD signals were segmented by a 10-s window and the SpO_2 signal was segmented by a 20-s window. Nine features in each segment were generated. These features were used to classify four types of sleep breathing events with an LSTM-RNN classifier. SpO_2 desaturation and sleep–wake detectors were used to improve the results of the LSTM-RNN classifier for the AHI evaluation. The algorithm is detailed step by step as follows.

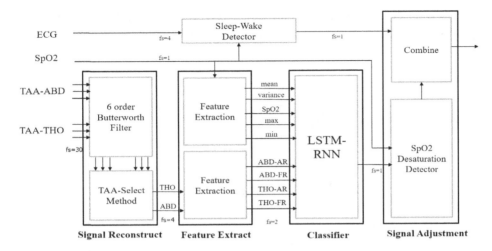

Figure 2. Processing diagram of the proposed AHI evaluation system.

Each TAA sensor sampled a three-axis acceleration vector at a time. Typically, principle component analysis (PCA) is used to combine the three-dimensional (3D) acceleration vector into 1D signal for the following analysis. Although PCA is suitable when the recording time is short, this approach is insufficient for overnight recording. The PCA could possibly distort the useful information of sleep breathing features because of the nonstationarity, particularly when the selected axis is switched frequently because of change in the sleep position. Thus, a TAA selection method was proposed to avoid this problem as shown in Figure 3. Three-dimensional TAA signals were first segmented by 30-s window with a 10-s time step. The number of periodic peaks was counted in a segment of an axis. Then, the axis with the most similar number of peaks to the human average respiration rate (6–9 peaks per 30 s) was selected as the output axis. After determining the selected axes of five successive segments, the most frequent axis in the previous five segments was selected as the output signal for the following analysis, as depicted in Figure 3a. If two axes had equal appearances, the axis with the larger magnitude was selected, as depicted in Figure 3b.

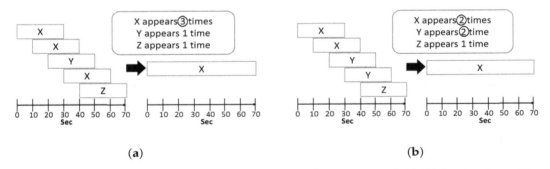

(a)   (b)

Figure 3. (**a**) TAA selection with the most appearances of one axis; and (**b**) TAA selection with equal appearances of two axes.

2.4. Feature Extraction

The preprocessed 1D THO and ABD signals were used to generate the features for sleep breathing event classification. The most obvious feature of the OSA event is the paradox between the THO and ABD signals. For the CSA event, the signal strengths of the THO and ABD signals are extremely small and exhibit small frequency deviation (e.g., the cardiogenic artifact). Because distinguishing HYP events in the ABD and THO signals is difficult, SpO_2 is incorporated to detect the HYP events.

2.4.1. Features of the THO and ABD signals

The THO and ABD signals are denoted as Y_{tho} and Y_{abd}, respectively. The THO and ABD signals were segmented using a 10-s window with a step of 0.5 s for feature extraction. According to the aforementioned physiological properties of the OSA, CSA and HYP events, the amplitude ratios (ARs) and the frequency ratios (FRs) [23] were considered as follows:

$$AR_{tho}(n) = \frac{Q_{95}(\tilde{A}_{tho}(t)\chi_{CW(n)})}{Q_{95}(\tilde{A}_{tho}(t)\chi_{PW(n)})}$$

$$AR_{abd}(n) = \frac{Q_{95}(\tilde{A}_{abd}(t)\chi_{CW(n)})}{Q_{95}(\tilde{A}_{abd}(t)\chi_{PW(n)})}.$$

(1)

$$FR_{tho}(n) = \log_{10}\left(\frac{\int_{0.8}^{1.5} |\mathcal{F}(Y_{tho}(t)\chi_{CW(n)})(\xi)|^2 d\xi}{\int_{0.1}^{0.8} |\mathcal{F}(Y_{tho}(t)\chi_{CW(n)})(\xi)|^2 d\xi}\right)$$

$$FR_{abd}(n) = \log_{10}\left(\frac{\int_{0.8}^{1.5} |\mathcal{F}(Y_{abd}(t)\chi_{CW(n)})(\xi)|^2 d\xi}{\int_{0.1}^{0.8} |\mathcal{F}(Y_{abd}(t)\chi_{CW(n)})(\xi)|^2 d\xi}\right)$$

(2)

where χ is the indicator function (1 or 0) for the windowing segmentation of input signals; Q_{95} represents the 95% quantile of the given function; $\tilde{A}_{tho}(t)$ and $\tilde{A}_{abd}(t)$ are the amplitudes of the THO and ABD signals, respectively, which were determined using the synchrosqueezing transform; and $\mathcal{F}$ represents the Fourier transform. CW represents the current window, that is, the nth CW is denoted as $CW(n) \subset \mathbb{R}$, where n is the index of segment. PW is the previous 60-s windowed signal before the current window. PW contains the baseline amplitude for AR. The nth PW associated with the nth CW is denoted as $PW(n) \subset \mathbb{R}$. Consequently, $AR_{tho}(n)$ and $AR_{abd}(n)$ represent the ARs and $FR_{tho}(n)$ and $FR_{abd}(n)$ represent the FRs of the THO and ABD signals, respectively, over the nth CW.

Synchrosqueezing transform (SST) is a novel nonlinear-type time–frequency analysis technique aiming to analyze complicated and nonstationary time series. It has been theoretically proved to enjoy several nice properties [24,25]. For our application, the main benefit of SST is an accurate estimation of the instantaneous frequency and the amplitude modulation of the respiratory signal. Moreover, the estimation does not depend on whether or not the oscillatory patter or wave-shape function is sinusoidal [26]. In addition, the SST is robust to various kinds of noise, including colored or even nonstationary random process [25].

The AR features were determined from the estimated amplitudes of the THO and ABD signals, which are denoted as $\tilde{A}_{tho}(t)$ and $\tilde{A}_{abd}(t)$, respectively, by using the synchrosqueezing transform. This step is critical because it suppresses the artifacts caused by the sudden change of body posture. The FR indicates the frequency distributions of the respiration and probably the cardiogenic artifact caused by heart beats. The integration range from 0.8 to 1.5 Hz in the numerator in (2) is the average range of heart beat rate. In our algorithm, the heart beat information was taken into account and the cardiogenic artifact indicates how silent the respiratory signal is. The detailed properties of the ARs and FRs of the THO and ABD signals can be obtained from [23].

2.4.2. Features of SpO$_2$ signal

SpO$_2$ is the percentage of oxyhemoglobin in hemoglobin. When sleep apnea and hypopnea events occur, SpO$_2$ decreases gradually until the subject breathes again. According to our data, the average delay time between an apnea (hypopnea) event and the 3% drop of SpO$_2$ was 19.3 ± 9.6 s. The average event duration is 20.2 ± 3.4. Figure 4a,b displays the distributions of the desaturation delay times of all events for the patients with AHI > 30 and AHI < 30, respectively. For patients with severe symptoms (AHI > 30), the desaturation distribution exhibits a high probability of error in which the previous respiratory event related to desaturation is labeled as the current event, that is, the desaturation drop of the previous respiratory event is almost adjacent to the current event. Therefore, features of SpO$_2$ were generated for every 20-s segment with a 20-s delay from the sampling point, as depicted in Figure 5. The minimum, maximum, mean and variance of the first derivative were used as the four features, and the original SpO$_2$ signal was also reserved as the baseline. To eliminate the variation of subjects, the SpO$_2$ signal was normalized by subtracting it by its median and dividing the obtained value by its standard deviation.

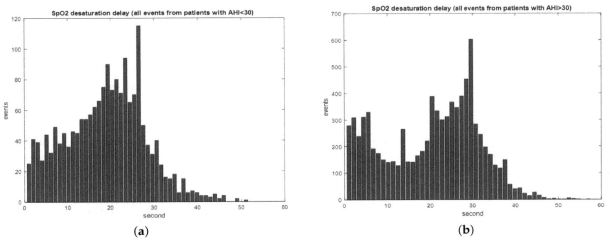

(a) (b)

Figure 4. (a) SpO$_2$ desaturation time of patients with AHI lower than 30; and (b) SpO$_2$ delay time of patients with AHI higher than 30.

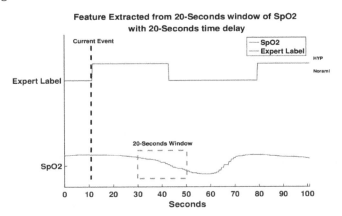

Figure 5. The decline of the SpO$_2$ signal occurs 20–40 s after abnormal events according to the physiological phenomenon.

2.5. Neutral Network Model, Event Classification and AHI Evaluation

2.5.1. Neural Network Model Classifier

The RNN based on the LSTM model, which was first presented by Hochreiter [27], was instrumental in solving many sequence problems with long-term dependency, such as language translation, speech recognition, image captioning and genomic information learning [28–31]. The features of the sleep breathing events based on THO/ABD and SpO$_2$ signals are time-varying and have long-term dependency. Therefore, an LSTM-RNN model was used to classify the sleep breathing events. The LSTM-RNN is an extension of the RNN and has more complex memory neurons than the RNN (Figure 6a). Unlike the original neuron with a simple loop in the RNN, every neuron in the RNN is replaced with an LSTM cell. An LSTM cell has three gates, namely the input, output and forget gates. These gates are scalars that are trained in every iteration to control the input, output and memory of every cell. Furthermore, the computation of output is reserved in the LSTM and combined with the new input. With the aforementioned design, the LSTM can thus deal with the long-term dependency problem, various desaturation times and many other subject variations for sleep breathing event classification.

Figure 6b illustrates the LSTM-RNN architecture, which has three layers, namely the input, LSTM-cell hidden and output layer. The input layer consists of nine neurons corresponding to nine extracted features from the THO/ABD and SpO$_2$ signals. The output layer contains four neurons representing four types of events, namely the OSA, CSA and HYP events and NOR breathing. The output of the network was normalized by using the softmax function. In total, 80 LSTM cells were utilized in the hidden layer according to the thumb of rule. The upper bound of the hidden neuron number was calculated by dividing the number of cases in the training dataset by the sum of the numbers of input and output layers in the network. The LSTM-RNN model was trained with 500 epochs of 500 batches of Adam gradient descents and a learning rate of 0.001. The activation function used in each layers was the rectified linear unit (ReLU) because of the benefit of sparsity and its capability of reducing the vanishing gradient. The loss function was used to compute the sum of cross entropy and L2 regularization with $\beta = 0.05$. Moreover, gradient clipping was added to the loss function to avoid the exploding gradient. Figure 7 illustrates the event detection results of 1-h segment for a patient. The PSG labeling results obtained from experts are displayed in the top panel of Figure 7. The middle panel displays the softmax output results of the LSTM-RNN classifier. In this panel, the four curves represent the probabilities of the four types of events. The decision rule of the LSTM-RNN classifier involves selecting the event with the highest probability in every time step, as depicted in the red line in the bottom panel. The LSTM-RNN classifier generates almost the same event states as PSG labeling does.

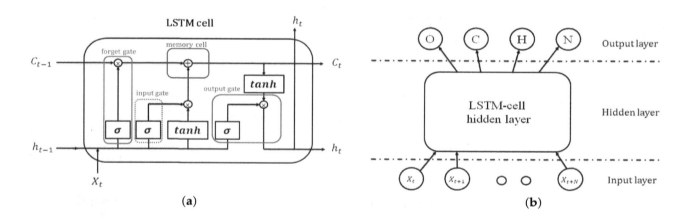

Figure 6. (a) X_t is the tth input feature, where $t = 1, 2, \ldots, N$. N is the total number of data points; C_t is the tth memory; h_t is the tth output; and σ and *tanh* represent the sigmoid and hyperbolic tangent function, respectively [27]. (b) LSTM-RNN architecture with the input layer, hidden layer and four-neuron output layer for classifying CSA, OSA, HYP and NOR states in every N seconds.

2.5.2. Oxygen Desaturation Detection

According to the 2014 guidelines from the American Academy of Sleep Medicine [3], a 3% drop of SpO$_2$ is considered as a potential sleep apnea and hypopnea event. Therefore, the proposed sleep breathing event classifier incorporates a SpO$_2$ desaturation detection scheme to capture every 3% drop in the SpO$_2$ signal (Figure 8). First, the difference of SpO$_2$ saturation signal was calculated and then convolved with a 20-s unity window to accumulate the difference. Afterwards, every desaturation with over 3% drop can be marked as an HYP event, which may not easily be detected using the LSTM-RNN classifier because limited CSA or OSA features can be extracted for the hypopnea event. Finally, the remarked signal was moved 20-s forward to compensate the delay of SpO$_2$ desaturation. Figure 9 illustrates the 1-h classification results of PSG labeling, the softmax outputs of the RNN and the outputs of the LSTM-RNN classifier with desaturation detection. By adding SpO$_2$ desaturation, the HYP softmax output exhibits higher probability than the NOR state. Therefore, the HYP events can be easily (see HYP softmax output) detected.

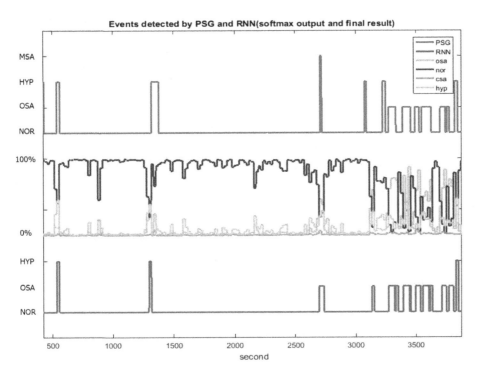

Figure 7. Event classification results of the PSG labeling, LSTM-RNN softmax outputs and final results of the LSTM-RNN classifier during 1-h sleep of a patient.

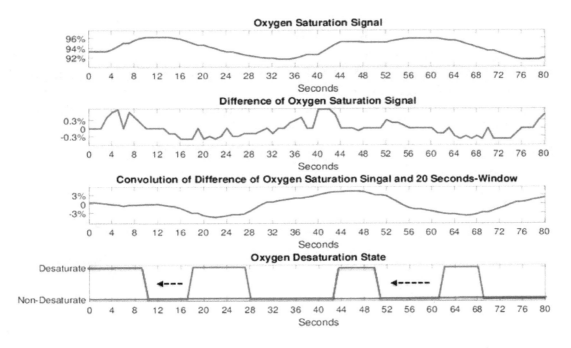

Figure 8. Processing steps for the oxygen desaturation detection.

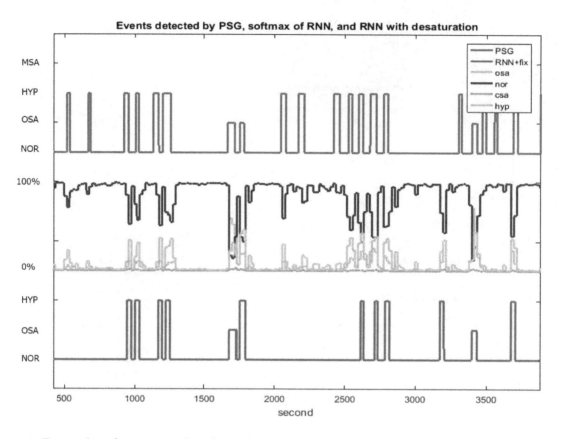

Figure 9. Event classification results of PSG labeling, the LSTM-RNN softmax outputs and the final results of the LSTM-RNN classifier with desaturation detection during 1-h sleep of a subject.

2.5.3. Sleep–Wake Classification

Because AHI is defined as the number of apnea and hypopnea events that occur during sleep, heart rate variability (HRV) was used in this study to detect the sleep and wake status during overnight sleep [32]. According to a previous study [33], a CNN was used to classify the sleep and wake status by using the instantaneous heart rate (IHR) signal converted from the ECG signal and SpO$_2$. Finally, the LSTM-RNN classification results and the sleep–wake state are combined to remove false positive events during the wake state. HRV is quantified by the intervals between successive heartbeats of ECG signals. HRV is estimated as the IHR per minute as follows:

$$\text{IHR}(r_i) = \frac{60}{r_i - r_{i-1}} \quad i = 2, \ldots, n, \tag{3}$$

where r_i denotes time instants in seconds when the ith R peak is detected. The unit of IHR is then beats per minute (bpm). Subsequently, the IHR signal along with the 20-s-delayed SpO$_2$ signal was segmented into 30-s epochs for the CNN network.

Figure 10a displays the CNN network used to classify the sleep and wake state. The input is first passed through five convolution layers and then two fully connected layers. Figure 10b illustrates each convolution layer. A single convolution layer has ten filters with a kernel size 8, and the stride is equal to 1 and 2. Each fully connected layer has 20 nodes, and every node is associated with a bias and ReLU activation function. Finally, a softmax function is applied before the output layer. Five minutes of the IHR and SpO$_2$ signals were used as inputs, which were normalized by subtracting the median value. The output was a 2D one-hot code for the sleep and wake states. L2 regularization was applied with $\beta = 0.3$. The CNN network was trained using the Adam gradient descent with a learning rate of 10^{-3}, a batch size of 100 and cross entropy as the loss function.

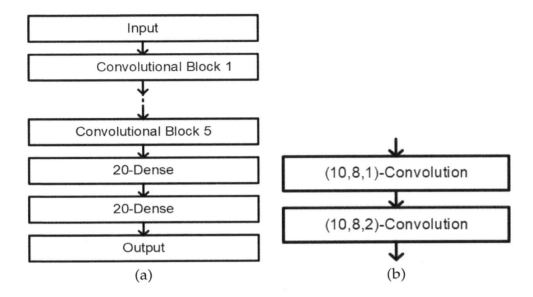

Figure 10. (**a**) Architecture of the one-dimensional CNN. The notation 20-Dense denotes that the fully connected layer possesses 20 nodes. For 5-min input signals, we used five convolution blocks [33]. (**b**) Architecture of a single convolution block. The notation (f, k, s)-convolution denotes that the convolutional layer has f filters with a kernel size k and stride s. The output of the block is half the size of the input [33]. A bias is added to the output of each filter, and the result is fed into a rectified linear unit (ReLU) activation function. A dropout with probability 0.5 is applied to the last layer and both fully-connected layers. The output of the network is normalized by the softmax function. An epoch is predicted to be wake if the output of the wake node is greater than or equal to that of the sleep node. We refer readers to Section 2.3 of [33] for more details.

3. Results

The clinic experiments were approved by the Institutional Review Board of the Chang Gung Memorial Hospital (CGMH: No. 201601576B0). Clinical patients at the sleep center in CGMH, Linkou, Taoyuan, Taiwan who were suspected of having sleep apnea were considered for this study. In total, 115 participants were examined in the clinical experiments. The demographic details of the participants are summarized in Table 1. The sleep experts identified the OSA, CSA, mixed sleep apnea (MSA) and HYP events from the overnight PSG signals of all patients. The remaining signals were NOR states. The MSA was regarded as the OSA in this study because of the similarity of physiological features. The training and testing databases had nearly the same distribution over various severity levels, as presented in Table 2.

Table 1. Demographic details of the 115 participants.

Severity	Gender	AHI (times/hr)	BMI (kg/m^2)	Age (year)	* TST (min)	** SE (%)	*** REM (%)	**** NREM (%)
Normal	all (9) male (6) female (3)	1.8 ± 1.6	23.2 ± 3.3	30.0 ± 8.2	312.9 ± 37.2	84.4 ± 9.9	15.4 ± 5.7	84.6 ± 5.7
Mild	all (17) male (13) female (4)	9.4 ± 2.4	25.6 ± 3.7	49.0 ± 11.3	313.4 ± 28.0	84.3 ± 7.3	17.8 ± 5.8	82.2 ± 5.8
Moderate	all (28) male (21) female (7)	21.7 ± 4.1	25.4 ± 2.7	48.5 ± 12.9	311.0 ± 40.7	83.9 ± 11.1	14.9 ± 5.6	85.1 ± 5.6
Severe	all (61) male (50) female (11)	61.1 ± 24.0	30.2 ± 6.0	50.3 ± 12.3	291.0 ± 52.6	79.4 ± 13.8	11.0 ± 6.2	89.0 ± 6.2

* TST, Total Sleep Time; ** SE, Sleep Efficiency; *** REM, Rapid Eye Movement Percentage; *** NREM, None Rapid Eye Movement Percentage.

Table 2. Distribution of the training and testing participants.

Level of Severity	Training Subjects	Testing Subjects	Total Subjects
Normal	6	3	9
Mild	9	8	17
Moderate	14	14	28
Severe	30	31	61
All levels	59	56	115

In our previous studies [23,34], SVM was used and followed by a state machine for screening OSAHS. The SVM model is divided into three types. First, the original SVM uses 50% of participants for training and 50% of participants for testing. Second, in the phenotype-based SVM [34], $K = 15$ nearest subjects of all data are selected according to gender, BMI and age with weights of 4, 2 and 1, respectively. Third, in the phenotype-based SVM with comorbidity information, the most similar 20 subjects are first selected and then the nearest 15 subjects are selected from these candidates using the K-nearest neighborhood method. For the LSTM-RNN model, the time step N was first evaluated for screening OSAHS. The detection performances of various Ns are presented in Table 3. When N was 20, the largest F_1 score was 0.72 ± 0.22 and the AHI difference was 8.1 ± 7.3. As the time step increased, the performance declined because the average duration of all events (apnea and hypopnea) was approximately 20 s (Figure 3).

Table 3. Sensitivity, precision, F_1 score and AHI difference of LSTM-RNN with different time steps (N).

Time Step (N)	Precision	Sensitivity	F_1 Score	AHI Difference
10 s	0.59 ± 0.25	0.88 ± 0.16	0.68 ± 0.24	9.7 ± 7.2
15 s	0.67 ± 0.23	0.74 ± 0.22	0.68 ± 0.21	8.8 ± 6.6
20 s	0.74 ± 0.22	0.73 ± 0.22	0.72 ± 0.22	8.1 ± 7.3
25 s	0.72 ± 0.22	0.75 ± 0.21	0.71 ± 0.21	8.7 ± 6.3
30 s	0.71 ± 0.21	0.77 ± 0.2	0.71 ± 0.2	8.6 ± 6.5

Precision = # of True Positive/(# of True Positive + # of False Positive); Sensitivity = # of True Positive/(# of True Positive + # of False Negative); F_1 Score = (2 × Precision · Sensitivity)/(Precision + Sensitivity).

LSTM-RNN with Oxygen Desaturation and Sleep–Wake Detection

Using the sleep–wake information of the overnight sleep, the classified sleep breathing events occurring when subjects were awake were eliminated. Thus, highly accurate sleeping hours for AHI evaluation could also be obtained in the experiment. Table 4 lists the sensitivity, precision, F_1 score and AHI difference for all subjects at various severity levels. We observed that sensitivity, precision and F_1 increased with the severity. The primary reason for this result was that the database size of the sleep breathing events for the severe group was considerably larger than that for the normal, mild and moderate groups. Compared with the generic SVM (F_1 score of 65% ± 26%) in Table 5, the proposed LSTM-RNN with oxygen desaturation and sleep–wake detection had a higher F_1 score (71% ± 22%) with respect to the PSG labeling of the sleep experts. The average AHI difference of the proposed LSTM-RNN model was 5.0 ± 4.5, which is smaller than that of the generic SVM model. Table 6 lists the confusion matrix of the classification of the proposed LSTM-RNN model with oxygen desaturation and sleep–wake detection for different severity levels. The severity classification achieved an accuracy of 89.3%.

Table 7 presents the confusion matrix of the classification of OSA, CSA and HYP events and NOR breathing. The overall event-by-event classification accuracy was 83.3%. The NOR breathing and OSA events could be well identified, whereas the identification of HYP events was difficult because of the lack of obvious information for HYP events. Some CSA events were classified as OSA events mainly because the OSA events had more than twice the CSA events in the database. However, the accuracy of distinguishing abnormal events was still 92.3%. This detection accuracy approximates the recommended intra-class correlation (95%) for the reliability of different scorers by [35]. This difference is very close to traditional subjective interpretation. Therefore, the proposed portable sensing system and OSAHS event identification algorithm can be reliable for the OSAHS screening in the home environment.

Table 4. Sensitivities, precisions, F_1 scores and AHI differences of LSTM-RNN with oxygen desaturation and sleep–wake detection for different severity groups.

LSTM-RNN Model	Sensitivity	Precision	F_1 Score	AHI Difference
Normal	0.62 ± 0.44	0.16 ± 0.15	0.23 ± 0.2	4.9 ± 4.4
Mild	0.62 ± 0.16	0.48 ± 0.14	0.54 ± 0.13	2.4 ± 1.7
Moderate	0.64 ± 0.2	0.77 ± 0.15	0.68 ± 0.16	5.8 ± 5.7
Severe	0.81 ± 0.13	0.86 ± 0.07	0.83 ± 0.09	5.7 ± 4.0
All levels	0.73 ± 0.2	0.74 ± 0.23	0.71 ± 0.22	5.0 ± 4.5

Table 5. Comparison of the LSTM-RNN and SVM models with oxygen desaturation.

Model + Oxygen Desaturation	Original SVM [23]	Phenotype SVM [34]	Phenotype SVM+ Comoribidity [34]	LSTM-RNN
Precision	0.77 ± 0.25	0.74 ± 0.27	0.74 ± 0.28	0.72 ± 0.22
Sensitivity	0.63 ± 0.27	0.64 ± 0.27	0.65 ± 0.27	0.81 ± 0.2
F1 score	0.65 ± 0.26	0.65 ± 0.26	0.65 ± 0.29	0.72 ± 0.22
AHI difference	10.6 ± 13.4	9.8 ± 10.0	9.0 ± 11.8	6.0 ± 5.2

Table 6. Confusion matrix of the LSTM-RNN model with oxygen desaturation and sleep–wake detection.

LSTM-RNN with Desaturation and Awake Detection		Expert Label Normal	Mild	Moderate	Severe
RNN Label	Normal	3	0	0	0
	Mild	0	8	3	0
	Moderate	0	0	11	3
	Severe	0	0	0	28
Accuracy		89.28%			

Table 7. Confusion matrix of the OSA, CSA and HYP events and NOR breathing for the LSTM-RNN model with oxygen desaturation and sleep–wake detection.

Four Events Types Classification in LSTM-RNN		Expert Label Normal	OSA	CSA	HYP
RNN Label	Normal	37,788	232	470	1824
	OSA	1391	7485	2132	1213
	CSA	21	35	1855	32
	HYP	556	1703	149	2138
Accuracy		83.34%			

4. Discussion

From the clinical perspective, through the proposed LSTM-RNN classifier with the TAA, ECG and SpO_2 signals, the respiratory events (apnea vs. hypopnea) and pattern (obstructive vs. central) can be effectively detected by the proposed system. Moreover, sleep–wake status be identified by using a CNN algorithm with instantaneous heart rate derived from ECG and SpO_2 signals. According to the heat rate and rhythm information in the ECG signal, our sensing devices and algorithm fully meet the requirements of AASM "SCOPER" (sleep, cardiovascular, oximetry, position, effort and respiratory) criteria for the home-base OSAHS detection. Compared with other Level 3 home-base equipments for sleep event screening using fewer sensors and channels for reducing sleep interference, the proposed sensing system and classification algorithm can provide better sleep quality and higher accuracy without sacrificing any useful information. The proposed system and algorithm can also support an effective early diagnosis and early treatment possibility for a clinically vital disease with high prevalence and low diagnostic and treatment rates.

From the hardware perspective, as suggested by a preliminary result provided in [33], the sleep–wake classification can be conducted accurately through PPG. This indicates that the ECG signal can be replaced by the PPG signal. Because only the partial information SpO_2 of the PPG signal was considered, one channel can be reduced in the next-generation sensing device.

From the algorithmic perspective, the following aspects should be considered to further improve the algorithm. The signal quality was considered in this study. The robustness properties of the feature extraction algorithm was simply focused on avoiding the impact of the inevitable noise and artifact. In addition to using the existing signal quality index (SQI) for the ECG or PPG signal, a suitable SQI should be developed for the ABD-TAA and THO-TAA signals. By incorporating these indices into the algorithm, the algorithm performance should be improved. This possibility will be explored in future study.

Limitation

This discussion is not complete without mentioning its limitation. First, the data were collected in a hospital environment designed for type I sleep screening. Additional data should be collected at the home-base environment to further confirm the applicability of the proposed model and algorithm. Another limitation is the database size. According to the encouraging positive results provided by the phenotype-based SVM, we expect to achieve a superior result if the database size increases. Specifically, with a larger database, we can have more cases with similar phenotype to build up an accurate model for each new-arriving patient.

5. Conclusions

In this study, a series of classification and detection algorithms was developed for screening sleep apnea patients by using a pulse oximeter and a wireless sensing system with TAA and ECG sensors. The features were extracted from the THO/ABD and SpO_2 signals and then used for training the LSTM-RNN classifier. The proposed system incorporates an SpO_2 desaturation detector and an ECG-based sleep–wake detector to improve the overall classification performance of the LSTM-RNN classifier. The severity group classification based on the AHI evaluation results of the proposed algorithm achieved an accuracy of 89.3%, and the sleep breathing event classification achieved an accuracy of 92.3%. Thus, we believe that the proposed screening system and classification algorithms can establish a solid foundation for the clinical screening of OSAHS.

This study has some potential future works. The proposed LSTM-based neural network has been proven to be effective in identifying several sleep apnea event types in this work. Since the proposed portable sensing system was designed for a homecare screening system, the LSTM-based neural network can be customized for individual person by using distributed learning techniques, which can be achieved by adopting phenotype information such as gender, weight, age and other personal physical information so as to enhance the personalized and high-accuracy sleep disorder screening system. Moreover, the proposed sensing system and APP software on a smartphone can record overnight data. To realize home-based screening or monitoring, the off-line data analysis (detection and event classification algorithms) on the PC can be further replaced by cloud-based analysis. That is, the user can upload the data by smartphone to a cloud server, and the data are then analyzed on the cloud server. Accordingly, the results can be easily viewed by the remote users such as doctors or caregivers.

Author Contributions: Conceptualization, Y.-L.L. and Y.-H.H.; methodology, Y.-H.H., P.-C.H., H.-P.M. and H.-T.W.; software, H.-C.C.; validation, H.-C.C., H.-T.W. and Y.-H.H.; formal analysis, H.-C.C.; investigation, H.-T.W.; data curation, Y.-L.L., P.-C.H. and H.-P.M.; writing—original draft preparation, Y.-H.H. and H.-C.C.;

writing—review and editing, Y.-L.L. and H.-T.W.; supervision, Y.-H.H.; and funding acquisition, Y.-L.L. and Y.-H.H. All authors have read and agreed to the published version of the manuscript.

References

1. Peppard, P.E.; Young, T.; Barnet, J.H.; Palta, M.; Hagen, E.W.; Hla, K.M. Increased prevalence of sleep-disordered breathing in adults. *Am. J. Epidemiol.* **2013**, *177*, 1006–1014. [CrossRef] [PubMed]

2. Kapur, V.K.; Auckley, D.H.; Chowdhuri, S.; Kuhlmann, D.C.; Mehra, R.; Ramar, K.; Harrod, C.G. Clinical Practice Guideline for Diagnostic Testing for Adult Obstructive Sleep Apnea: An American Academy of Sleep Medicine Clinical Practice Guideline. *J. Clin. Sleep Med.* **2017**, *15*, 479–504. [CrossRef] [PubMed]

3. Berry, R.B. The AASM Manual for the Scoring of Sleep and Associated Events. Available online: http://aasm.org/clinical-resources/scoring-manual/ (accessed on 25 October 2020)

4. Pevernagie, D.A.; Gnidovec–Strazisar, B.; Grote, L.; Heinzer, R.; McNicholas, W.T.; Penzel, T.; Randerath, W.; Schiza, S.; Verbraecken, J.; Arnardottir, E. S. On the rise and fall of the apnea–hypopnea index: A historical review and critical appraisal. *J. Sleep Res.* **2020**. [CrossRef] [PubMed]

5. Corral-Peñafiel, J.; Pepin, J.-L.; Barbe, F. Ambulatory monitoring in the diagnosis and management of obstructive sleep apnoea syndrome. *Eur. Respir. Rev.* **2013**, *22*, 312-324. [CrossRef]

6. Collop, N.A.; Anderson, W.M.; Boehlecke, B.; Claman, D.; Goldberg, R.; Gottlieb, D.J.; Hudgel, D.; Sateia, M.; Schwab, R. Clinical guidelines for the use of unattended portable monitors in the diagnosis of obstructive sleep apnea in adult patients. *J. Clin. Sleep Med.* **2007**, *3*, 737–747.

7. Li, K.; Pan, W.; Li, Y.; Jiang, Q.; Liu, G. A method to detect sleep apnea based on deep neural network and hidden Markov model using single-lead ECG signal. *Neurocomputing* **2018**, *294*, 94–101. [CrossRef]

8. Jung, D.W.; Hwang, S.H.; Yoon, H.N.; Lee, Y.J.G; Jeong, D.U.; Park, K.S. Nocturnal Awakening and Sleep Efficiency Estimation Using Unobtrusively Measured Ballistocardiogram. *IEEE Trans. Biomed. Eng.* **2014**, *61*, 131–1138. [CrossRef] [PubMed]

9. Almazaydeh, L.; Faezipour, M.; Elleithy, K. A neural network system for detection of obstructive sleep apnea through SpO_2 signal features. *Int. J. Adv. Comput. Sci. Appl.* **2012**, *3*, 7–11. [CrossRef]

10. Avci, C.; Akba, A. Sleep apnea classification based on respiration signals by using ensemble methods. *Bio-Med. Mater. Eng.* **2015**, *26*, S1703–S1710. [CrossRef]

11. Jane, R.; Fiz, J.A.; Solà-Soler; Mesquita, J.; Morera, J. Snoring Analysis for the Screening of Sleep Apnea Hypopnea Syndrome with a Single-Channel Device Developed using Polysomnographic and Snoring Databases. In Proceeding of 33rd Annual International Conference of the IEEE Engineering in Medicine an Biology Society (EMBC), Boston, MA, USA, 30 August–3 September 2011; pp. 8331–8333.

12. Eiseman, N.A.; Westover, M.B.; Mietus, J.E.; Thomas, R.J.; Bianchi, M.T. Classification algorithms for predicting sleepiness and sleep apnea severity. *J. Sleep Res.* **2012**, *21*, 101–112. [CrossRef]

13. De Chazal, P.; Sadr, N. Sleep apnoea classification using heart rate variability, ECG derived respiration and cardiopulmonary coupling parameters. In Proceeding of 38th Annual International Conference of the IEEE Engineering in Medicine and Biology Society (EMBC), Orlando, FL, USA, 16–20 August 2016; pp. 3203–3206.

14. Rodrigues, P.P.; Santos, D.F.; Leite, L. Obstructive sleep apnoea diagnosis: The Bayesian network model revisited. In Proceeding of 28th International Symposium on Computer-Based Medical Systems, Sao Carlos, Brazil, 22–25 June 2015; pp. 115–120

15. Dey, D; Chaudhuri, S.; Munshi, S. Obstructive sleep apnoea detection using convolutional neural network based deep learning framework. *Biomed. Eng. Lett.* **2018**, *8*, 95–100. [CrossRef] [PubMed]

16. Quiceno-Manrique, A.; Alonso-Hernandez, J.; Travieso-Gonzalez, C.; Ferrer-Ballester, M.; Castellanos-Dominguez, G. Detection of obstructive sleep apnea in ECG recordings using time-frequency distributions and dynamic features. In Proceeding of 31st IEEE Annual International Conference of the IEEE Engineering in Medicine and Biology Society (EMBS), Minneapolis, MN, USA, 3–6 September 2009; pp. 5559–5562.

17. Mendez, M.; Ruini, D.; Villantieri, O.; Matteucci, M.; Penzel, T.; Bianchi, A. Detection of sleep apnea from surface ECG based on features extracted by an autoregressive model. In Proceeding of 29th IEEE International Conference on Engineering in Medicine and Biology Society (EMBS), Lyon, France, 22–26 August 2007; pp. 6105–6108.

18. Novak, D.; Mucha, K.; Al-Ani, T. Long short-term memory for apnea detection based on heart rate variability. In Proceeding of 30th IEEE Annual International Conference of the IEEE Engineering in Medicine and Biology Society (EMBS), Vancouver, BC, Canada, 20–25 August 2008; pp. 5234–5237.

19. Ng, A.; Chung, J.; Gohel, M.; Yu, W.; Fan, K.; Wong, T. Evaluation of the performance of using mean absolute amplitude analysis of thoracic and abdominal signals for immediate indication of sleep apnoea events. *J. Clin. Nursing* **2008**, *17*, 2360–2366. [CrossRef] [PubMed]

20. Garde, A.; Dekhordi, P.; Ansermino, J. M.; Dumont, G. A. Identifying individual sleep apnea/hypoapnea epochs using smartphone-based pulse oximetry. In Proceeding of 38th IEEE Annual International Conference of the IEEE Engineering in Medicine and Biology Society (EMBS), Orlando, FL, USA, 16–20 August 2016; pp. 3195–3198.

21. Mendonca, F.; Mostafa, S.S.; Ravelo-Garcia, A.G.; Morgado-Dias, F.; Penzel, T. A Review of Obstructive Sleep Apnea Detection Approaches. *IEEE J. Biomed. Health Inf.* **2019**, *23*, 825–837. [CrossRef] [PubMed]

22. Collop, N.A.; Tracy, S.L.; Kapur, V.; Mehra, R.; Kuhlmann, D.; Fleishman, S.A.; Ojile, J.M. Obstructive sleep apnea devices for out-of-center (OOC) testing: Technology evaluation. *J. Clin. Sleep Med.* **2011** *7*, 531–548. [CrossRef]

23. Lin, Y.Y.; Wu, H.T.; Hsu, C.A.; Huang, P.C.; Huang, Y.H.; Lo, Y.L. Sleep apnea detection based on thoracic and abdominal movement signals of wearable piezo-electric bands. *IEEE J. Biomed. Health Inf.* **2017**, *21*, 1533–1545. [CrossRef]

24. Daubechies, I.; Lu, J.; Wu, H.-T. Synchrosqueezed Wavelet Transforms: An empirical mode decomposition-like tool. *Appl. Comput. Harmon. Anal.* **2011**, *30*, 243–261. [CrossRef]

25. Chen, Y.-C.; Cheng, M.-Y.; Wu, H.-T. Nonparametric and adaptive modeling of dynamic seasonality and trend with heteroscedastic and dependent errors. *J. R. Stat. S.* **2014**, *76*, 651–782. [CrossRef]

26. Wu, H.-T. Instantaneous frequency and wave shape function (I). *Appl. Comput. Harmon. Anal.* **2013**, *35*, 181–199. [CrossRef]

27. Hochreiter, S.; Schmidhuber, J. Long short-term memory. *Neural Comput.* **1997**, *9*, 1735–1780. [CrossRef]

28. Auli, M.; Galley, M.; Quirk, C.; Zweig, G. Joint language and translation modeling with recurrent neural networks. In Proceedings of Conference on Empirical Methods in Natural Language Processing, Seattle, WA, USA, 18–21 October 2013; pp.1044–1054.

29. Sutskever, I.; Vinyals, O.; Le, Q.V. Sequence to sequence learning with neural networks. In Proceeding of Advances in Neural Information Processing Systems (NIPS), Montreal, QC, Canada, 8–13 December 2014; pp. 3104–3112.

30. Vinyals, O.; Toshev, A.; Bengio, S.; Erhan, D. Show and tell: A neural image caption generator. In Proceedings of the IEEE Conference on Computer Version and Pattern recognition, Boston, MA, USA, 7–12 June 2015; pp. 3156–3164.

31. Lipton, Z.C.; Kale, D.C.; Elkan, C.; Wetzel, R. Learning to Diagnose with LSTM Recurrent Neural Networks. Available online: https://arxiv.org/abs/1511.03677 (accessed on 25 October 2020)

32. Snyder, F.; Hobson, J.A.; Morrison, D.F.; Goldfrank, F. Changes in respiration, heart rate, and systolic blood pressure in human sleep. *Eur. J. Appl. Physiol.* **1964**, *19*, 417–422. [CrossRef]

33. Malik, J.; Lo, Y.L.; Wu, H.T. Sleep-wake classification via quantifying heart rate variability by convolutional neural network. *Physiol. Meas.* **2018**, *39*, 085004. [CrossRef] [PubMed]

34. Wu, H.T.; Wu, J.C.; Huang, P. C.; Lin, T.Y.; Wang, T.; Huang, Y.H.; Lo, Y.L. Phenotype-based and self-learning inter-individual sleep apnea screening with a level IV-like monitoring system. *Front. Physiol.* **2018**, *9*, 723. [CrossRef]

35. Whitney, C.W.; Gottlieb, D.J.; Redline, S.; Norman, R.G.; Dodge, R.R.; Shahar, E.; Surovec, S.; Nieto, F.J. Reliability of scoring respiratory disturbance indices and sleep staging. *Sleep* **1998**, *21*, 749–757. [CrossRef]

2

Electroactive Hydrogels Made with Polyvinyl Alcohol/Cellulose Nanocrystals

Tippabattini Jayaramudu [1,2], Hyun-U Ko [1], Hyun Chan Kim [1], Jung Woong Kim [1], Ruth M. Muthoka [1] and Jaehwan Kim [1,*]

[1] Center for Nanocellulose Future Composites, Department of Mechanical Engineering, Inha University, 100 Inha-Ro, Nam-Gu, Incheon 22212, Korea; mr.jayaramudu@gmail.com (T.J.); lostmago@naver.com (H.-U.K.); Kim_HyunChan@naver.com (H.C.K.); jw6294@naver.com (J.W.K.); mwongelinruth@gmail.com (R.M.M.)
[2] Laboratory of Material Sciences, Instituto de Quimica de Recursos Naturales, Universidad de Talca, Talca 747, Chile
* Correspondence: jaehwan@inha.ac.kr

Abstract: This paper reports a nontoxic, soft and electroactive hydrogel made with polyvinyl alcohol (PVA) and cellulose nanocrystal (CNC). The CNC incorporating PVA-CNC hydrogels were prepared using a freeze–thaw technique with different CNC concentrations. Fourier transform infrared spectroscopy, thermogravimetric analysis, X-ray diffraction and scanning electron microscopy results proved the good miscibility of CNCs with PVA. The optical transparency, water uptake capacity and mechanical properties of the prepared hydrogels were investigated in this study. The CNC incorporating PVA-CNC hydrogels showed improved displacement output in the presence of an electric field and the displacement increased with an increase in the CNC concentration. The possible actuation mechanism was an electrostatic effect and the displacement improvement of the hydrogel associated with its enhanced dielectric properties and softness. Since the prepared PVA-CNC hydrogel is nontoxic and electroactive, it can be used for biomimetic soft robots, actively reconfigurable lenses and active drug-release applications.

Keywords: electroactive hydrogel; polyvinyl alcohol; cellulose nanocrystals; freeze–thaw method; actuation

1. Introduction

Hydrogels are hydrophilic three-dimensional network structures that are cross-linked physically or chemically and which maintain their structural integrity during formation [1]. They can hold large amounts of water molecules/biological solutions, which turn them into soft and viscoelastic materials. The soft, flexible, elastic and wet features of the hydrogels promote them as potential candidates for various biomedical and pharmaceutical applications including diapers, contact lenses, membranes, tissue engineering, drug delivery systems and biosensors [2–5]. Stimuli–response hydrogels change their structure (especially volume and shape) due to such conditions as pH, ionic strength, temperature and electric field [6,7]. Several studies revealed that acrylic acid and its polymers, as well as other hydrogels based on polymeric materials, are electric or pH responsive. However, acrylic acid is known to be toxic in nature [8]. This toxicity problem can be overcome by blending or reinforcing natural polymers into synthetic polymers. Accordingly, natural polymer-based hydrogels can show stimuli-responsive behavior, resulting in their high number of potential applications including biomimetic soft robots, haptic actuators, artificial muscles, active tunable lenses and active drug release. Thus far, many natural polymers have been used to develop hydrogels such as chitosan, cellulose, whey protein and carboxymethyl cellulose [9–13]. Among them, cellulose has merits in terms of renewability, biocompatibility, abundance, low price, superior mechanical properties and easy chemical modification.

Cellulose consists of crystal and amorphous parts connected in a row. Cellulose nanocrystal (CNC), a rod-like shaped nanocrystal, can be isolated from cellulose resources including wood pulp, tunicates, bacterial cellulose, cotton, ramie, hemp as well as other agricultural residues by treating them with acid hydrolysis [14–16]. CNC has a high degree of crystallinity, mechanical properties and a specific surface area [17,18]. The typical width of CNCs is in the range of 5–50 nm, but their length and width depend on the source and the process conditions. CNC produced by sulfuric acid hydrolysis is electrostatically stable and easily dispersed in polar aqueous suspensions due to the sulfate ester groups on their surfaces [19–22]. Based on their attractive characteristics, CNCs have been used as reinforcing agents for a wide range of applications in packaging films, nanocomposites, microchips, tissue engineering, actuators and sensors [23–27].

In hydrogels, reinforcement technology is playing a key role [21,26–29]. Cellulose can easily interact with various polar and water-soluble polymer materials. Thus, blending of CNC with hydrogels can reinforce the hydrogels in terms of mechanical properties and electromechanical properties. Especially the integration of CNC in hydrogels can increase their dielectric constant so as to improve its electroactive properties. With this background, this study aims to improve the transparency and electroactive properties of hydrogels by incorporating CNC into polyvinyl alcohol (PVA) to develop nontoxic electroactive hydrogels. PVA hydrogel was reported as an electroactive material [30] and showed higher transparency when the hydrogels were prepared using the solvent mixture of dimethyl sulfoxide (DMSO) and water (80:20 wt.%) [31]. PVA and CNC are known to be nontoxic. The basic physical properties of the prepared hydrogels including the swelling behavior, transparency and surface morphology were investigated using the water uptake capacity test, UV-vis spectroscopy and scanning electron microscopy (SEM). To study the CNC interaction and its structural and thermal characteristics, the prepared hydrogels were tested using Fourier transform infrared (FTIR) spectroscopy, X-ray diffraction (XRD) and thermogravimetric analysis (TGA). The mechanical properties of the prepared hydrogels were characterized using a universal testing machine. Furthermore, the actuation properties of the prepared hydrogels were tested by applying actuation voltage.

2. Materials and Methods

2.1. Materials

Cellulose cotton pulp (MVE, DPw-4580) of 98% purity was obtained from Buckeye Technology Inc. Poly (vinyl alcohol) (Mw = 85,000~124,000 g/mole, 99% hydrolyzed), sulfuric acid (H_2SO_4) and sodium hydroxide were purchased from Sigma-Aldrich Korea, Gyeonggi-do, South Korea. Dimethyl sulfoxide (DMSO) was purchased from Dae Jung chemicals & Metals Co. Ltd. (Gyeonggi-do, South Korea) Deionized (DI) water was used throughout the experiments.

2.2. Preparation of CNC

In this study, CNC was prepared using acid hydrolysis treatment. The preparation of CNC was described in Reference [19,20]; following is a brief explanation. The cotton pulp (20.0 g), a source of cellulose, was dispersed in H_2SO_4 (175 mL of 30% (v/v) aqueous) under mechanical stirring with 200 rpm and 6 h at 60 °C. An alkaline (NaOH, 1 M) pre-treatment was carried out on the cotton pulp to remove the non-cellulosic components and to prior obtain the high yield of CNC. The acid hydrolysis resulted in a suspension, and it was diluted (Ph = 7) by adding excessive deionized (DI) water, followed by centrifugation (11,000 rpm and 10 min). After this, the CNC suspension was homogenized and dialyzed overnight. A certain amount of homogenized CNC was dispersed in 20 mL of solvent mixture of DMSO and DI water (80:20 wt.%) by sonication for 1 h. Finally, 1% of CNC suspension was obtained and stored at room temperature until use.

2.3. Preparation of PVA-CNC Hydrogels

For the preparation of the PVA-CNC hydrogels, 9 wt.% PVA solution and 1 wt.% CNC suspension were used. The transparent PVA solution was prepared by dissolving 9 g of PVA in a 91 g solvent mixture of DMSO and DI water (80:20 wt.%) by continuous stirring at 80 °C for 8 h under a nitrogen atmosphere. To the PVA solution, different amounts of 1 wt.% CNC suspension were added, while the weight of the PVA-CNC mixtures was kept constant at 20 g. After adding the CNC suspension, the PVA-CNC mixtures were sonicated for 20 min and then subjected to magnetic stirring for another 2 h (200 rpm) at 80 °C to obtain a homogeneous mixture. Finally, PVA-CNC hydrogels were obtained via a freeze–thaw process. The PVA-CNC mixtures were poured into a petri dish and subjected to three freeze–thaw cycles consisting of a 12 h freezing step at −20 °C, followed by a 6 h thawing step at room temperature. After finishing the three freeze and thaw steps, PVA-CNC hydrogels were formed. The prepared hydrogels were immersed in 100 mL of DI water in order to remove solvents and water-soluble/unreacted materials [32,33]. The DI water was changed every 8 h up to 3 days. The thickness of the prepared hydrogels was 4 ± 0.05 mm. The prepared PVA-CNC hydrogels were kept in DI water until use. The sample codes of the PVA-CNC hydrogels were designated as PVA-CNCx according to the amount of CNC suspension used in the hydrogels. Table 1 provides the feed composition ratio of PVA to CNC.

Table 1. Feed composition ratio of PVA-CNC hydrogels.

Hydrogels	Weight of 9 wt.% PVA (g)	Weight of 1% wt. CNCs (g)
PVA	20	0
PVA-CNC1	17	3
PVA-CNC2	15	5
PVA-CNC3	13	7

3. Characterization

3.1. Physical Properties

A water uptake capacity test of the prepared PVA-CNC hydrogels was carried out. The hydrogels were dried in an oven for 24 h at 60 °C until their weight reached saturation. The weight of the dried hydrogels were noted and immersed in a 100 mL beaker containing 50 mL distilled water at room temperature to equilibrate for up to 48 h. Then the samples were taken out and blotted with wiper paper to remove water on their surface and again reweighed using an analytical balance (GH-200, A&D weighing, Tokyo, Japan). The water uptake ratio, W.U., can be represented using the following equation:

$$W.U._{(g/g)} = (W_{wet} - W_{dry})/W_{dry}, \tag{1}$$

where W_{wet} and W_{dry} denote the weight of the equilibrated hydrogel at 48 h and initial weight of the dried hydrogel, respectively.

The optical transparency of the prepared PVA-CNC hydrogels was measured using a UV-visible spectrophotometer (HP8452A, Agilent, Santa Clara, CA, USA). For the measurement, the hydrogels were cut into the desired shape and the spectra range of 200–800 nm wavelengths were recorded.

A Scanning electron microscope (SEM, S-4000, Hitachi, Tokyo, Japan) was used to observe morphologies of the prepared hydrogels. To prepare specimens, the prepared hydrogels were freeze-dried and coated with platinum. The images were taken using the SEM, at 15 kV accelerating voltage.

3.2. FTIR, XRD and TGA

FTIR spectroscopy was used to study the transmission of light and the interaction of CNCs of the prepared PVA-CNC hydrogels. For the FTIR analysis, the samples were completely dried in a vacuum oven at 60 °C for 6 h. The FTIR spectra were recorded on a FTIR spectrometer (Bruker Optics, Billerica, MA, USA) with the range of 400–4000 cm^{-1} using the KBr disk pellet method and averaging 16 scans.

XRD patterns of the prepared CNC, PVA, and PVA-CNC hydrogels were recorded using an X-ray diffractometer (DMAX 2500, Rigaku, Japan), with Cu Kα radiation source (λ = 0.1542 nm) at 40 kV and 300 mA. The scan speed was 2° per min and the spectra of 2θ (Bragg angle) ranged from 2.5 to 60°. The thermal stability of the prepared CNC, PVA and PVA-CNC hydrogels was studied using a TGA (STA 409 PC, NETZSCH , Selb, Germanay) at a constant heating rate of 10 °C/min in the range of 30–600 °C under a constant nitrogen flow (20 mL/min).

3.3. Mechanical Testing

The compression test of the PVA-CNC hydrogels was conducted at a fully-hydrated stage and was followed by the ASTM D-882-97 test method using a universal test machine (Won Shaft Jeong Gong, Gyeonggi-do, South Korea) under the ambient condition with compression rate of 0.0005 mm/s. The size of the specimens was 20 × 20 × 5 mm^3. The specimen was kept between two parallel plates and the upper plate pressed the specimen until it reached the maximum value.

3.4. Actuation Test

The actuation test was carried out using a laser displacement sensor (Keyance LK-G85, Tokyo, Japan), a high voltage amplifier (Model 10/10, Trek, Lockport, NY, USA) and a function generator (33220A, Agilent, Santa Clara, CA, USA). Figure 1 shows the schematic setup of the actuation test. Before conducting the actuation test, the hydrogel specimens (10 × 10 × 4 mm^3) were equilibrated in DI water for 24 h and kept between two electrodes (polyimide tape attached to indium tin oxide coated glass (ITO glass)). A high voltage was applied on the electrodes via the function generator and the high voltage amplifier. The displacement of the hydrogel specimen was measured using the laser displacement sensor along with a data acquisition system (Pulse, B&K, Nærum, Denmark) connected to personal laptop. The actuation test was conducted at a constant environmental condition (25 °C, 95% RH) using an environmental chamber.

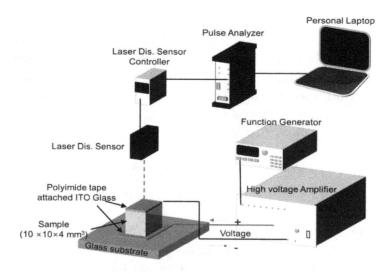

Figure 1. Schematic setup of the actuation test.

4. Results and Discussion

4.1. Physical Properties

The water uptake ratios of the pure PVA and PVA-CNC hydrogels were calculated using Equation (1). Figure 2A shows the results for the pure PVA and the hydrogels. As the CNC concentration increased, the water uptake ratio consistently increased from 220% to 250%. This might be due to the fact that the hydrogen bonds between the CNC and PVA chains decreased the residual hydrogen bonds in the PVA chains, which resulted in increased water uptake [34].

The optical transparency of the prepared hydrogels was measured using the UV-vis spectroscopy at 300 to 700 nm. Figure 2B shows the optical transparency of the pure PVA and PVA-CNC hydrogels. The optical transparency taken at 500 nm of pure PVA was 92.4% and it decreased to 91.0, 77.7 and 75.9%, as the CNC concentration in the PVA-CNC hydrogels increased. Increasing the CNC concentration reduced the transparency due to CNC aggregation, which enhanced the turbidity of PVA hydrogel so as to decrease its transparency [20].

The SEM images of PVA-CNC3 hydrogel were taken to observe the morphology of the hydrogel. Figure 3A,B shows the surface morphologies of the pure PVA and PVA-CNC3 hydrogel, respectively. The pure PVA showed a smooth surface morphology, meanwhile the CNC-incorporated PVA-CNC3 hydrogel exhibited a uniform but rough surface. The CNCs were shown to be well-dispersed in the hydrogel. The cross-sectional SEM image of the PVA-CNC3 hydrogel (Figure 3C) showed that the rod-shaped CNCs were dispersed in the cross-sectional image of the hydrogel. This uniform dispersion might be associated with the interaction between the PVA and the CNC.

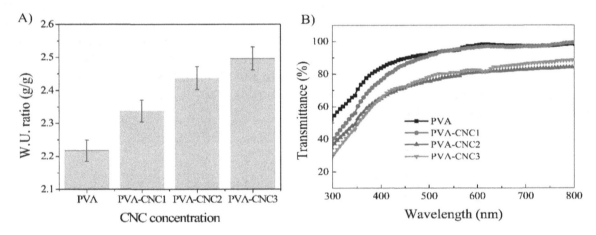

Figure 2. (**A**) Water uptake capacity of pure PVA and PVA-CNC hydrogels and (**B**) Optical transparency of the pure PVA and PVA-CNC hydrogels.

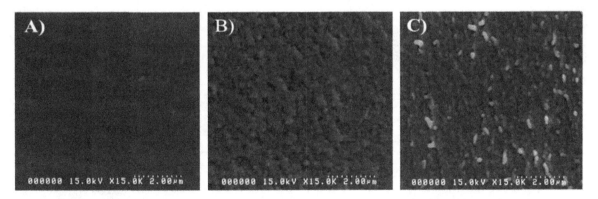

Figure 3. SEM images: (**A**) the pure PVA, (**B**) surface of PVA-CNC3 hydrogel and (**C**) cross-section of PVA-CNC3 hydrogel.

4.2. FTIR, XRD and TGA

To study the transmission of light and the interactions of CNC in the prepared PVA-CNC hydrogels, FTIR spectroscopy analysis was performed. Figure 4 shows the FTIR spectra of the prepared CNC, PVA, and PVA-CNC3 hydrogel. The O-H stretching vibration of the pure PVA is shown at 3422 cm^{-1}. The characteristic peaks at 1070 cm^{-1} and 2901 cm^{-1} are related to stretching vibrations of the C-O and C-H. The peak at 1628 cm^{-1} is related to an acetyl group (C=O), which is induced from the preparation of PVA. A bending vibration related to CH$_2$ groups is observed in the region of 1430–1446 cm^{-1} [10]. The FTIR spectra of the prepared CNC indicates the characteristic peaks assigned to cellulose I structures: Peaks are shown at 3374 cm^{-1} (O-H region), 2900 cm^{-1} (C-H stretching vibration), 1430 cm^{-1} (CH$_2$ symmetric bending) and 1320 cm^{-1} (CH$_2$ wagging at C-6). Peaks at 1065 cm^{-1}, 1124 cm^{-1} and 1160 cm^{-1} demonstrate the presence of sulfate ester bonds, which are induced by the sulfuric acid hydrolysis for CNC preparation [35]. In the case of the PVA-CNC3 hydrogel, the O-H stretching vibration peak shifted to 3402 cm^{-1} due to the overlap of intermolecular hydrogen bonded O-H peaks from PVA-PVA and CNC-CNC. There is a new peak at 3201 cm^{-1} on the FTIR spectrum of PVA-CNC3. This peak might correspond to intermolecular hydrogen bonded between PVA and CNC. The result shows that CNC and PVA are well-interacted. This gives rise to the increase in the water uptake capacity of PVA-CNC hydrogels.

Figure 5A represents XRD patterns that give crystalline information for the pure PVA, CNC and PVA-CNC3 hydrogel. PVA is known to be semi-crystalline in nature and the pure PVA shows the main strong diffraction intensity characteristic peak at 2θ = 19.5° [36] and the CNC sample exhibits four well-defined diffraction peaks at 2θ = 14.6, 16.2, 22.5, and 34.4°, which correspond to a typical cellulose I structure [22]. Note that the PVA-CNC3 hydrogel exhibits a similar diffraction peak at 2θ = 19.6°, with decreased intensity, and a shoulder peak at 2θ = 22.4°, with increased intensity, which suggests the physical interaction of PVA and CNC. This observation indicates that the incorporation of CNCs in PVA does not affect the crystalline structure of the PVA matrix. This means that the CNCs are well-dispersed in the PVA matrix so as to form the PVA-CNC hydrogel [37]. This fact was also confirmed for the FTIR spectra shown in Figure 4.

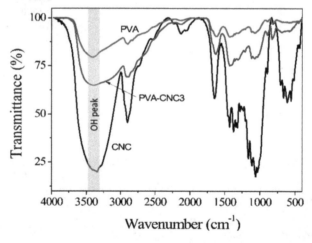

Figure 4. FTIR spectra of CNC, PVA, and PVA-CNC3 hydrogel.

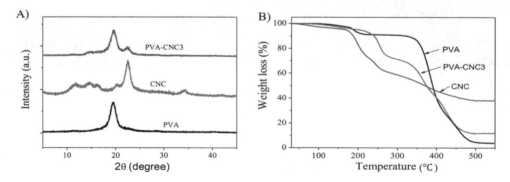

Figure 5. (**A**) X-ray diffraction patterns of CNC, PVA, and PVA-CNC3 hydrogel, (**B**) TGA curves of the pure PVA, CNC and PVA-CNC3 hydrogel.

TGA measures the weight changes as a function of temperature. As the temperature increases, the weight of the sample decreases, indicating the continuous decomposition of the sample. Figure 5B shows the TGA curves of the pure PVA, CNC and PVA-CNC3 hydrogel. Below 150 °C, a minor weight loss occurred in all samples near 89 °C, which is associated with the evaporation of the absorbed water molecules. The pure PVA hydrogel showed mainly two weight-loss steps. The first weight loss started from 179 °C and finished at 216 °C (the weight loss was 8.9%), and was mainly associated with the dehydration of the hydroxyl groups by applying heat. The second weight loss started at 345 °C and degraded rapidly up to 500 °C (the weight loss was 95.4%), which was due to the degradation of the main chain. The PVA-CNC3 hydrogel showed two weight loss steps. The weight loss started from 212 °C and continually decreased up to 500 °C and a maximum 88.4% of weight loss was observed. Note that the PVA-CNC3 hydrogel showed higher thermal stability than the pure PVA, which might be due to the formation of the intermolecular bond between the CNC and the PVA. A similar observation has been reported previously [38,39]. In addition, the TGA spectrum of the CNC sample showed that the starting degradation temperature (160 °C) was lower than that of the pure PVA and the PVA-CNC3 hydrogel because CNC has many hydroxyl groups on its surface [40].

4.3. Mechanical Testing

The mechanical properties of the pure PVA and PVA-CNC hydrogels were studied using the universal testing machine. The test specimens were fully hydrated in distilled water. Figure 6A shows the compressional stress–strain curves of the pure PVA and PVA-CNC hydrogels with various CNC concentrations. Figure 6B shows the compressive modulus values of the hydrogels with different CNC concentrations. The modulus decreased with the increasing CNC concentration. The compressive modulus decrease of the PVA-CNC hydrogels can be surmised from the water uptake results. The mechanical property was inversely proportional to the water uptake capacity in the hydrogels: Increasing the water uptake capacity decreased the compressive modulus, due to the softening of the hydrogel structures. The CNC concentration plays an important role in the successful dispersion and formation of strong interfaces within the PVA polymer matrix. When the CNC concentration is above a critical value, the compressive strength of the hydrogels could be significantly decreased due to poor dispersion of the CNC as well as limited interfacial interaction between the CNC and PVA [41]. The compressive modulus of the pure PVA hydrogel was 82 kPa, and as the CNC concentration increased, it gradually decreased to 7 kPa for the PVA-CNC3 hydrogel.

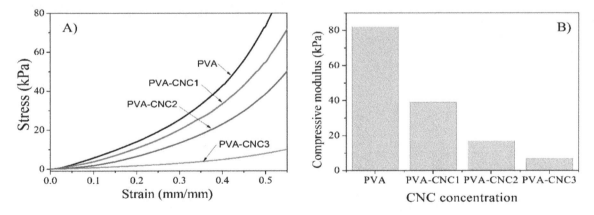

Figure 6. (**A**) Compressive stress–strain curves of PVA, PVA-CNC composite hydrogels and (**B**) compressive modulus.

Figure 7 shows the formation of PVA-CNC hydrogels. The hydroxyl groups of the PVA as well as on the surface of the CNC can interact with each other to form hydrogen bonds. However, as a large amount of CNC is dispersed in the hydrogel, for example PVA-CNC3, it seems that CNC aggregation occurs due to the hydrophilic nature of CNC, resulting in the evenly rough surface of the hydrogel.

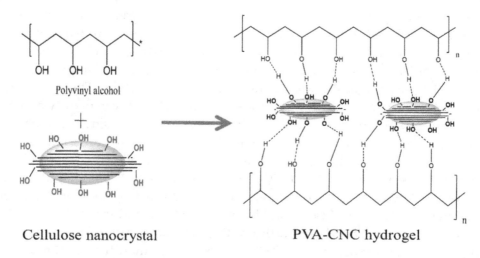

Figure 7. Formation of the PVA-CNC hydrogel.

4.4. Actuation Test

A soft actuator deforms in the presence of an external electric field. In this study, the deformation was defined as displacement and investigated in terms of the applied electric field and frequency. The actuation test of the prepared hydrogels was carried out in an aqueous swollen state in the DI water of the PVA-CNC hydrogels. Figure 8 shows the displacement of the hydrogels in terms of CNC concentration with the applied voltage and the frequency. Figure 8A shows the displacement of the hydrogels with a voltage change at 0.1 Hz. The displacement increased with increased voltage as well as increased CNC concentration. The maximum displacement of 14.4 μm was shown from the PVA-CNC3 hydrogel at 1.6 kV. This displacement corresponded to 3600 ppm strain and the applied voltage does corresponded to 0.4 V/μm electric field strength. This actuation performance is better than the cellulose hydrogel case (1800 ppm at 0.25 V/μm) [10]. Figure 8B displays the frequency-dependent displacement of the hydrogels under a constant voltage of 1.6 kV. The displacement output decreased with an increasing frequency. The CNC concentration played a significant role in the electroactive behavior of the PVA-CNC hydrogels, and the higher CNC concentration exhibited larger displacement than the pure PVA case. The PVA-CNC3 hydrogel showed higher displacement than the other hydrogels. This result is associated with the interfacial polarization between CNCs and the PVA polymer matrix [42]. It is a known fact that dispersed CNCs in a polymer matrix increases its dielectric properties, which is beneficial to improving its electroactive behavior.

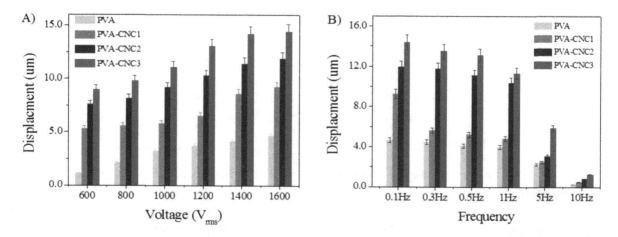

Figure 8. Actuation results for the pure PVA and PVA-CNC hydrogels: (**A**) actuation voltage variation at 0.1 Hz and (**B**) actuation frequency at 1.0 kV.

Generally, an electroactive response occurs through a combination of piezoelectricity, electrostriction, flexoelectricity, electrostatic effect (Coulombic force), electrophoretic effect, electrochemical effect (ion migration) and electroosmotic interaction [5]. In the PVA/DMSO hydrogel, electrostrictive interaction was claimed as the mechanism causing its electroactive response since the displacement was proportional to the square of the electrical actuation voltage [30]. In some electroactive materials, it is hard to clarify the mechanism because although the same materials are used, different morphologies or physical/chemical properties could result in different mechanisms of electroactive behavior.

The prepared PVA-CNC hydrogel is not an ionic hydrogel. Although a sulfate ester bond peak was observed from the FTIR, this peak was caused by the sulfuric acid hydrolysis for the CNC preparation. During the CNC preparation, sulfuric acid was applied to isolate CNC from the pulp and some of the sulfuric ions remained on the surface of the CNCs. However, the remnant sulfuric ions were not significant because CNCs were dialyzed and washed with DI water several times. Thus, we believe that the prepared hydrogel was a nonionic hydrogel and the ion migration effect was not significant in the prepared hydrogel.

8

When the displacement and voltage curves are considered, as shown in Figure A, the displacements increased linearly or quadratically with the actuation voltage, as well as CNC concentration. This may give piezoelectricity in the hydrogel. However, it is very hard to possess dipole domains in the hydrogel. Thus, the prepared hydrogel was far from a piezoelectric material. On the other hand, as increasing the CNC concentration causes the compressive modulus to decrease, which is beneficial in terms of increasing the electrostatic effect associated with the Coulombic force. Under Coulombic force, a large strain can be produced when the electroactive material is soft. This is a well-known fact for dielectric elastomer electroactive polymers. In summary, since the PVA-CNC hydrogel is a soft, nonionic hydrogel, and it has high dielectric properties, the electrostatic effect may be its dominant actuation mechanism.

5. Conclusions

In this research, nontoxic, soft and electroactive PVA-CNC hydrogels were prepared using the freeze–thaw process with different CNC concentrations, and their characteristics were analyzed. The water uptake capacity of the hydrogels increased and the compressive modulus decreased as the CNC concentration increased. The optical transparency of the prepared hydrogels was inversely proportional to the CNC concentration. The thermogravimetric analysis and scanning electron microscopy results showed good miscibility of CNC with PVA. The CNC incorporated PVA-CNC hydrogels showed an improved displacement output in the presence of the electric field and with the increasing CNC concentration. The maximum 3600 ppm strain was produced under 0.4 V/μm electric field strength from the PVA-CNC3 hydrogel. The displacement improvement of the PVA-CNC hydrogels is associated with their enhanced dielectric properties and reduced compressive modulus. Since the PVA-CNC hydrogel is nonionic, soft, and it possible has strong dielectric properties, the electrostatic effect may be its dominant actuation mechanism. Since the prepared PVA-CNC hydrogel is nontoxic and electroactive, it may be a promising material for biomimetic soft robots, actively reconfigurable lenses and active drug-release.

Author Contributions: Conceptualization, T.J. and J.K.; Methodology, T.J. and H.K.; Validation, J.K.; Formal Analysis, T.J. and H.K.; Investigation, T.J., H.C.K and J.W.K; Resources, H.C.K.; Data Curation, T.J.; Writing-Original Draft Preparation, T.J.; Writing-Review & Editing, R.M. and J.K.; Visualization, T.J. and H.K.; Supervision, J.K.; Project Administration, J.W.K.; Funding Acquisition, J.K.

References

1. Du, X.; Zhou, J.; Shi, J.; Xu, B. Supramolecular hydrogelators and hydrogels: From soft matter to molecular biomaterials. *Chem. Rev.* **2015**, *115*, 13165–13307. [CrossRef] [PubMed]

2. Zolfagharian, A.; Kouzani, A.Z.; Khoo, S.Y.; Moghadam, A.A.A.; Gibson, I.; Kaynak, A. Evolution of 3D printed soft actuators. *Sens. Actuator A Phys.* **2016**, *250*, 258–272. [CrossRef]

3. Kwon, I.C.; Bae, Y.H.; Kim, S.W. Characteristics of charged networks under an electric stimulus. *J. Polym. Sci. Part B Polym. Phys.* **1994**, *32*, 1085–1092. [CrossRef]

4. Sun, S.; Wong, Y.W.; Yao, K.; Mak, A.F. A study on mechano-electro-chemical behavior of chitosan/poly (propylene glycol) composite fibers. *J. Appl. Polym. Sci.* **2000**, *76*, 542–551. [CrossRef]

5. Koetting, M.C.; Peters, J.T.; Steinchen, S.D.; Peppas, N.A. Stimulus-responsive hydrogels: Theory, modern advances, and applications. *Mater. Sci. Eng. R* **2015**, *93*, 1–49. [CrossRef] [PubMed]

6. Kim, S.J.; Lee, K.J.; Kim, S.I.; Lee, Y.M.; Chung, T.D.; Lee, S.H. Electrochemical behavior of an interpenetrating polymer network hydrogel composed of poly (propylene glycol) and poly (acrylic acid). *J. Appl. Polym. Sci.* **2003**, *89*, 2301–2305. [CrossRef]

7. Wandera, D.; Wickramasinghe, S.R.; Husson, S.M. Stimuli-responsive membranes. *J. Membr. Sci.* **2010**, *357*, 6–35. [CrossRef]

8. Jayaramudu, T.; Li, Y.; Ko, H.U.; Shishir, I.R.; Kim, J. Poly (acrylic acid)-Poly (vinyl alcohol) hydrogels for reconfigurable lens actuators. *Int. J. Precis. Eng. Manuf. Green Technol.* **2016**, *3*, 375–379. [CrossRef]

9. Yuan, N.; Xu, L.; Zhang, L.; Ye, H.; Zhao, J.; Liu, Z.; Rong, J. Superior hybrid hydrogels of polyacrylamide enhanced by bacterial cellulose nanofiber clusters. *Mater. Sci. Eng. C Mater. Biol. Appl.* **2016**, *67*, 221–230. [CrossRef] [PubMed]

10. Jayaramudu, T.; Ko, H.U.; Zhai, L.; Li, Y.; Kim, J. Preparation and characterization of hydrogels from polyvinyl alcohol and cellulose and their electroactive behavior. *Soft Matter* **2017**, *15*, 64–72. [CrossRef]

11. Kamal, M.R.; Khoshkava, V. Effect of cellulose nanocrystals (CNC) on rheological and mechanical properties and crystallization behavior of PLA/CNC nanocomposites. *Carbohydr. Polym.* **2015**, *123*, 105–114. [CrossRef] [PubMed]

12. Khoshkava, V.; Kamal, M.R. Effect of cellulose nanocrystals (CNC) particle morphology on dispersion and rheological and mechanical properties of polypropylene/CNC nanocomposites. *ACS Appl. Mater. Interfaces* **2014**, *6*, 8146–8157. [CrossRef] [PubMed]

13. Jayaramudu, T.; Raghavendra, G.M.; Varaprasad, K.; Sadiku, R.; Raju, K.M. Development of novel biodegradable Au nanocomposite hydrogels based on wheat: For inactivation of bacteria. *Carbohydr. Polym.* **2013**, *92*, 2193–2200. [CrossRef] [PubMed]

14. Kim, J.H.; Shim, B.S.; Kim, H.S.; Lee, Y.J.; Min, S.K.; Jang, D.; Kim, J. Review of nanocellulose for sustainable future materials. *Int. J. Precis. Eng. Manuf. Green Technol.* **2015**, *2*, 197–213. [CrossRef]

15. Azizi Samir, M.A.S.; Alloin, F.; Dufresne, A. Review of recent research into cellulosic whiskers, their properties and their application in nanocomposite field. *Biomacromolecules* **2005**, *6*, 612–626. [CrossRef] [PubMed]

16. Mueller, S.; Weder, C.; Foster, E.J. Isolation of cellulose nanocrystals from pseudostems of banana plants. *RSC Adv.* **2014**, *4*, 907–915. [CrossRef]

17. Gao, F. *Advances in Polymer Nanocomposites: Types and Applications*; Woodhead Publishing: Cambridge, UK, 2012; pp. 131–155, ISBN 978-1-84569-940-6.

18. George, J.; Sabapathi, S.N. Cellulose nanocrystals: Synthesis, functional properties, and applications. *Nanotechnol. Sci. Appl.* **2015**, *8*, 45–54. [CrossRef] [PubMed]

19. Gao, X.; Sadasivuni, K.K.; Kim, H.C.; Min, S.K.; Kim, J. Designing pH-responsive and dielectric hydrogels from cellulose nanocrystals. *J. Chem. Sci.* **2015**, *127*, 1119–1125. [CrossRef]

20. Sadasivuni, K.K.; Ponnamma, D.; Ko, H.U.; Zhai, L.; Kim, H.C.; Kim, J. Electroactive and optically adaptive bionanocomposite for reconfigurable microlens. *J. Phys. Chem. B* **2016**, *120*, 4699–4705. [CrossRef] [PubMed]

21. Domingues, R.M.; Silva, M.; Gershovich, P.; Betta, S.; Babo, P.; Caridade, S.G.; Gomes, M.E. Development of injectable hyaluronic acid/cellulose nanocrystals bionanocomposite hydrogels for tissue engineering applications. *Bioconjug. Chem.* **2015**, *26*, 1571–1581. [CrossRef] [PubMed]

22. Kumar, A.; Negi, Y.S.; Choudhary, V.; Bhardwaj, N.K. Characterization of cellulose nanocrystals produced by acid-hydrolysis from sugarcane bagasse as agro-waste. *J. Mater. Phys. Chem.* **2014**, *2*, 1–8. [CrossRef]

23. Favier, V.; Chanzy, H.; Cavaille, J.Y. Polymer nanocomposites reinforced by cellulose whiskers. *Macromolecules* **1995**, *28*, 6365–6367. [CrossRef]

24. Capadona, J.R.; Van Den Berg, O.; Capadona, L.A.; Schroeter, M.; Rowan, S.J.; Tyler, D.J.; Weder, C. A versatile approach for the processing of polymer nanocomposites with self-assembled nanofibre templates. *Nat. Nanotechnol.* **2007**, *2*, 765–769. [CrossRef] [PubMed]

25. Einchhorn, S.J.; Dufresne, A.; Aranguren, M.M.; Capadona, J.R.; Rowan, S.J.; Weder, C.; Veigel, S. Review: Current international research into cellulose nanofibres and composites. *J. Mater. Sci.* **2010**, *45*, 1–33. [CrossRef]

26. McKee, J.R.; Hietala, S.; Seitsonen, J.; Laine, J.; Kontturi, E.; Ikkala, O. Thermoresponsive nanocellulose hydrogels with tunable mechanical properties. *ACS Macro Lett.* **2014**, *3*, 266–270. [CrossRef]

27. Yang, J.; Zhang, X.M.; Xu, F. Design of cellulose nanocrystals template-assisted composite hydrogels: Insights from static to dynamic alignment. *Macromolecules* **2015**, *48*, 1231–1239. [CrossRef]

28. Ooi, S.Y.; Ahmad, I.; Amin, M.C.I.M. Cellulose nanocrystals extracted from rice husks as a reinforcing material in gelatin hydrogels for use in controlled drug delivery systems. *Ind. Crops Prod.* **2016**, *93*, 227–234. [CrossRef]

29. De France, K.J.; Chan, K.J.; Cranston, E.D.; Hoare, T. Enhanced mechanical properties in cellulose nanocrystal–poly (oligoethylene glycol methacrylate) injectable nanocomposite hydrogels through control of physical and chemical cross-linking. *Biomacromolecules* **2016**, *17*, 649–660. [CrossRef] [PubMed]

30. Liang, S.; Xu, J.; Weng, L.; Zhang, L.; Guo, X.; Zhang, X. Biologically Inspired Path-Controlled Linear Locomotion of Polymer Gel in Air. *J. Phys. Chem. B* **2007**, *111*, 941–945. [CrossRef] [PubMed]

31. Hou, Y.; Chen, C.; Liu, K.; Tu, Y.; Zhang, L.; Li, L. Preparation of PVA hydrogel with high-transparence and investigations of its transparent mechanism. *RSC Adv.* **2015**, *5*, 24023–24030. [CrossRef]

32. Jayaramudu, T.; Raghavendra, G.M.; Varaprasad, K.; Sadiku, R.; Ramam, K.; Raju, K.M. Iota-Carrageenan-based biodegradable Ag^0 nanocomposite hydrogels for the inactivation of bacteria. *Carbohydr. Polym.* **2013**, *95*, 188–194. [CrossRef] [PubMed]

33. Jayaramudu, T.; Raghavendra, G.M.; Varaprasad, K.; Raju, K.M.; Sadiku, E.R.; Kim, J. 5-Fluorouracil encapsulated magnetic nanohydrogels for drug-delivery applications. *J. Appl. Polym. Sci.* **2016**, *133*, 43921. [CrossRef]

34. Kudo, S.; Otsuka, E.; Suzuki, A. Swelling Behavior of Chemically Crosslinked PVA Gels in Mixed Solvents. *J. Polym. Sci. Part B Polym. Phys.* **2010**, *48*, 1978–1986. [CrossRef]

35. Xu, X.; Shen, Y.; Wang, W.; Sun, C.; Li, C.; Xiong, Y.; Tu, J. Preparation and in vitro characterization of thermosensitive and mucoadhesive hydrogels for nasal delivery of phenylephrine hydrochloride. *Eur. J. Pharm. Biopharm.* **2014**, *88*, 998–1004. [CrossRef] [PubMed]

36. Bajpai, A.K.; Gupta, R. Synthesis and characterization of magnetite (Fe$_3$O$_4$)—Polyvinyl alcohol-based nanocomposites and study of superparamagnetism. *Polym. Compos.* **2010**, *31*, 245–255. [CrossRef]

37. Kakroodi, A.R.; Cheng, S.; Sain, M.; Asiri, A. Mechanical, thermal, and morphological properties of nanocomposites based on polyvinyl alcohol and cellulose nanofiber from Aloe vera rind. *J. Nanomater.* **2014**, *2014*, 903498. [CrossRef]

38. Abitbol, T.; Johnstone, T.; Quinn, T.M.; Gray, D.G. Reinforcement with cellulose nanocrystals of poly (vinyl alcohol) hydrogels prepared by cyclic freezing and thawing. *Soft Matter* **2011**, *7*, 2373–2379. [CrossRef]

39. Kaneko, D.; Shimoda, T.; Kaneko, T. Preparation methods of alginate micro-hydrogel particles and evaluation of their electrophoresis behavior for possible electronic paper ink application. *Polym. J.* **2010**, *42*, 829–833. [CrossRef]

40. Han, J.; Lei, T.; Wu, Q. High-water-content mouldable polyvinyl alcohol-borax hydrogels reinforced by well-dispersed cellulose nanoparticles: Dynamic rheological properties and hydrogel formation mechanism. *Carbohydr. Polym.* **2014**, *102*, 306–316. [CrossRef] [PubMed]

41. Tanpichai, S.; Oksman, K. Cross-linked nanocomposite hydrogels based on cellulose nanocrystals and PVA: Mechanical properties and creep recovery. *Compos. Part A Appl. Sci. Manuf.* **2016**, *88*, 226–233. [CrossRef]

42. Ko, H.U.; Kim, H.C.; Kim, J.W.; Zhai, L.; Jayaramudu, T.; Kim, J. Fabrication and characterization of cellulose nanocrystal based transparent electroactive polyurethane. *Smart Mater. Struct.* **2017**, *26*, 085012. [CrossRef]

3

Non-Contact Monitoring of Breathing Pattern and Respiratory Rate via RGB Signal Measurement

Carlo Massaroni [1,*], Daniela Lo Presti [1], Domenico Formica [2], Sergio Silvestri [1] and Emiliano Schena [1]

[1] Unit of Measurements and Biomedical Instrumentation, Department of Engineering, Università Campus Bio-Medico di Roma, 00128 Rome, Italy; d.lopresti@unicampus.it (D.L.P.); s.silvestri@unicampus.it (S.S.); e.schena@unicampus.it (E.S.)

[2] Unit of Neurophysiology and Neuroengineering of Human-Technology Interaction, Department of Engineering, Università Campus Bio-Medico di Roma, 00128 Rome, Italy; d.formica@unicampus.it

[*] Correspondence: c.massaroni@unicampus.it

Abstract: Among all the vital signs, respiratory rate remains the least measured in several scenarios, mainly due to the intrusiveness of the sensors usually adopted. For this reason, all contactless monitoring systems are gaining increasing attention in this field. In this paper, we present a measuring system for contactless measurement of the respiratory pattern and the extraction of breath-by-breath respiratory rate. The system consists of a laptop's built-in RGB camera and an algorithm for post-processing of acquired video data. From the recording of the chest movements of a subject, the analysis of the pixel intensity changes yields a waveform indicating respiratory pattern. The proposed system has been tested on 12 volunteers, both males and females seated in front of the webcam, wearing both slim-fit and loose-fit t-shirts. The pressure-drop signal recorded at the level of nostrils with a head-mounted wearable device was used as reference respiratory pattern. The two methods have been compared in terms of mean of absolute error, standard error, and percentage error. Additionally, a Bland–Altman plot was used to investigate the bias between methods. Results show the ability of the system to record accurate values of respiratory rate, with both slim-fit and loose-fit clothing. The measuring system shows better performance on females. Bland–Altman analysis showed a bias of -0.01 breaths·min^{-1}, with respiratory rate values between 10 and 43 breaths·min^{-1}. Promising performance has been found in the preliminary tests simulating tachypnea.

Keywords: measuring system; measurements; contactless; respiratory rate; breathing pattern

1. Introduction

Accurate measurement of vital signs and physiological parameters, such as body temperature, pulse rate, blood pressure, and respiratory rate, plays a pivotal role in the healthcare sector and management of patients. Among these, the respiratory rate (f_R) is still considered the neglected vital sign in both the clinical practice and sports activity monitoring [1,2]. Temporal changes in the respiratory rate may indicate relevant variations of the physiological status of the subject, even better than other vital signs (e.g., pulse rate) [2] and it is found to be more discriminatory between stable and unstable patients than pulse rate [1].

In a clinical setting, the respiratory rate is an early indicator of physiological deterioration [3] and a predictor of potentially dangerous adverse events [1]. Indeed, respiratory rate is an important predictor of cardiac arrest and of unplanned intensive care unit admission [1], as well as an independent prognostic marker for risk assessment after acute myocardial infarction [4]. Besides, it is fundamental in the early detection and diagnosis of dangerous conditions such as sleep apnea [5], sudden infant death syndrome, chronic obstructive pulmonary disease, and respiratory depression in post-surgical patients [6]. In intensive care units, the respiratory waveform and f_R are typically recorded. In mechanically ventilated patients, such data can be obtained directly by the mechanical ventilator traces [7] or retrieved by pulse oximetry sensors [8]. However, f_R is typically collected at regular interval by operators (i.e., every 8–10 h) in the clinical setting outside this ward, while is often neglected in home monitored people and patient [1].

Conventional methods for measuring respiratory parameters require sensing elements in contact with the patient [9]. These methods are mainly based on the analysis of several parameters sampled from the inspiratory and/or expiratory flow. Differently, approaches based on the measurement of respiratory-related chest and abdominal movements have been also adopted [10]. Sensors may be directly attached on the torso [11] or integrated into clothing fibers. Several sensors have been used as resistive sensors, capacitive sensors, inductive sensors. Such monitoring systems must be worn and powered [11]. Additionally, they may cause undesirable skin irritation and discomfort, especially when long-term monitoring is required or during sleep. Substantial evidence indicates all these contact-based measurement techniques may influence the underlying physiological parameters being measured [12].

Contactless monitoring systems may overcome these issues related to placing sensors on patients and influence the measurand [13]. Mainly, solutions based on the analysis of depth changes of the torso using time-of-flight sensors [14] during breathing, low-power ultra wideband impulse radio radar [15,16], and laser Doppler vibrometers [17–19] have been designed and tested. Principal limitations of such solutions are related to the high cost of the instrumentation, need for specialized operators, and, in some cases, a low signal-to-noise ratio. Contactless monitoring systems based on the use of optical sensors are gaining preeminence in the field of respiratory monitoring mainly because of recent progress in video technology. Commercial and industrial cameras may be exciting solutions as they provide low-cost and easy-to-use non-contact approaches for measuring and monitoring physiological signals [4]. Some attempts have been made to record respiratory parameters from breathing-related movements of thoraco-abdominal area, face area, area at the edge of the shoulder, pit of the neck [20–25]. Then, different approaches have been also used to post-process the video to extract the respiratory-related signal mainly based on image subtraction [26], optical flow analysis [27], Eulerian Video Magnification [24] and Independent Component Analysis (ICA) applied to pixel intensity changes [28]. By the review of the literature, there is a lack of results about accuracy of such methods in the monitoring of eupneic respiratory pattern and f_R monitoring, since the majority of the cited studies present proof of concepts and preliminary tests, but accuracy evaluation is not performed. When available, typically a frequency-domain analysis is carried out to extract the frequency content of the respiratory-related video signal and to measure the average respiratory rate. Since analysis with these techniques requires the recording of the torso movement, clothing can influence the data quality and validity of the methods. However, no studies have focused on such potential influences on respiratory pattern and f_R measurement. Only a preliminary study of our research group tried to investigate this influencing factor in [29].

In this paper, we present a measuring system capable of non-contact monitoring of respiratory pattern by using RGB video signal acquired from a single built-in high-definition webcam. The aim of this study is three-fold: (i) the development of the measuring system and the related algorithm for the extraction of breath-by-breath f_R values; (ii) the evaluation of the error between the breath-by-breath f_R values retrieved by using the proposed measuring system and those recorded with a reference instrument; and (iii) the analysis of influence of clothing (i.e., slim-fit and loose-fit) and sex on the performance of the proposed method.

2. Measuring System

The proposed measuring system is composed of a hardware module (i.e., a built-in webcam) for video recording and an algorithm for (i) preprocessing of the video to obtain a respiratory signal, and (ii) event detection, segmentation and extraction of breath-by-breath f_R values. The working principle of the method used to extract respiratory information from a video is explained in the following section.

2.1. Light Intensity Changes Caused by Respiration

Each video can be considered a series of f frames (i.e., polychromatic images), where f is the number of the frames collected. Each frame is an image composed of three images in the red (R), green (G) and blue (B) channels. Each image in the R, G and B channels is a matrix composed of pixels. The size of the matrix (of dimensions x along the x-axis , and y along the y-axis) depends on the resolution of the camera used for the data collection. Each pixel assumes a value representing the color light intensity: the value 0 means black, whereas the maximum value is the white. The numerical values of each pixel depend on the number of bytes used to represent a given R, G, B channel. When considering commercial 8-bit/channel cameras (24-bit for RGB colors), the maximum value is 2^8 (i.e., 255 colors including zero).

When an object is recorded by a video, the pixel of each frame of the video assume an intensity level caused by the light reflected from the object over a two-dimensional grid of pixels. In the RGB color model separate intensity signals corresponding to each channel—$V_R(x,y,f), V_G(x,y,f), V_B(x,y,f)$—can be recorded at each frame f. The measured intensity of any reflected light (V) can be decomposed into two components: (i) intensity of illumination (I), and (ii) reflectance of the surface (R):

$$V(x,y,f) = I(x,y,f) \cdot R(x,y,f). \tag{1}$$

The respiratory activity causes the periodic movement of the chest wall. During inspiration, the ribcage widens: it results in an upward movement of the thorax; during expiration, the opposite occurs. By considering the chest wall covered by clothing as the surface framed by the camera, and the intensity of illumination almost constant, the changes of intensity of reflected light between two consecutive frames can be considered caused by the movement of the chest surface. Breathing-related chest movements are transmitted to the clothing (e.g., t-shirts, sweaters), so the subsequent changes of V can be used to collect respiratory patterns and events indirectly. Loose- or slim-fit clothing differently adhere to the skin. In the case of slim-fit clothing, we can hypothesize the complete transfer of chest wall movement to the side of the t-shirt framed by the camera, whereas only a partial transfer in the case of loose-fit clothing.

2.2. Hardware for Video Data Recording

The proposed system needs to collect a video of a person seated in front of the camera (Figure 1). The hardware module consists of a built-in CCD RGB webcam (iSight camera) integrated into a MacBook Pro laptop (by Apple Inc., California, USA). This camera is used to collect video with a resolution of 1280·720 pixel. Video images are recorded at 24-bit RGB with three channels, 8 bits per channel. A bespoke interface was developed in MATLAB (MathWorks, Massachusetts, USA) to record the video and pre-process the data (i.e., images) collected with the camera. The video is collected for 120 s at a frame rate of 30 Hz, which is enough to register the breathing movements.

2.3. Algorithm for the Preprocessing of the Video

The preprocessing of the recorded video is performed off-line via a bespoke algorithm developed in MATLAB, which is an upgraded version of the algorithm presented in our previous papers [29,30]. Several steps must be followed as shown in Figure 1.

Basically, after the video is loaded, the user (i.e., the one who is designated to analyze the data) is asked to select one pixel (with coordinates x_P, y_P) at the level of the jugular notch (i.e., the anatomical point near the suprasternal notch) in the first frame of the video. This anatomical marker has been chosen because it is easily identifiable (see Figure 1).

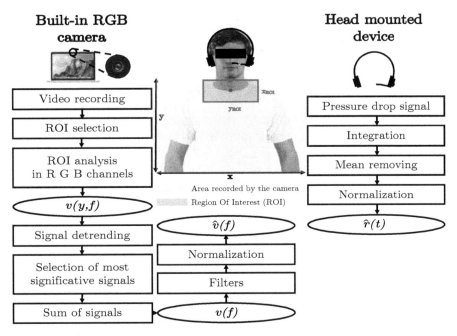

Figure 1. Flowchart presenting all the steps carried out to extract the respiratory pattern from video recorded with the built-in camera (on the left) and from the pressure-drop signal collected at the level of nostrils with the reference device (on the right). Region Of Interest (ROI) is the red rectangle; the area recorded by the camera is highlighted with the blue rectangle, the black point is the pixel (with coordinates x_P, y_P) at the level of the jugular notch.

Automatically a rectangular region of interest (in short ROI) is delineated, with dimensions $x_{ROI} \times y_{ROI}$:

$$x_{ROI} = [x_P - \tfrac{1}{100} \cdot 15 \cdot x, x_P + \tfrac{1}{100} \cdot 15 \cdot x],$$

$$y_{ROI} = [y_P - \tfrac{1}{100} \cdot 15 \cdot y, y_P + \tfrac{1}{100} \cdot 15 \cdot y], \tag{2}$$

where x and y are the x-axis and y-axis frame dimensions (related to camera resolution), respectively.

The selected ROI is then split into three same-size images corresponding to the red, green, and blue channels. At each frame f, the intensity components of each channel $I(x, y, c, f)$ are obtained, where c is the color channel (i.e., red (R), green (G), and blue (B)). Then, the intensity components are averaged for each line y of the ROI according to Equation (3):

$$v(y, f) = \frac{1}{x_{ROI}} \cdot \sum_{x=1}^{x_{ROI}} \left(\sum_{c=R,G,B} I(x, y, c, f) \right), \tag{3}$$

where $y \in y_{ROI}$.

From each $v(y, f)$, the mean of the signal is removed from the signal itself (i.e., the signal is detrended). The standard deviation of each $v(y, f)$ signal is then calculated. The 5% of the $v(y, f)$ with the higher standard deviations are selected. The 5% value was selected with an empirical approach using data from previous experiments carried out on volunteers aimed at calibrating the algorithm. The 5% of the $v(y, f)$ are used to calculate the mean value considering the selected lines at each frame. The $v(f)$ signal is obtained with this procedure. At that point, filters were applied to the $v(f)$ signal. For filtering the signal and to emphasize the respiratory content, adequate cut-off frequencies and bandwidth need to be defined. A bandpass configuration was chosen, by fixing the low cut-off frequency around 0.05 Hz, to avoid the slow signal variations unrelated to respiratory movements and a high cut-off frequency around 2 Hz. In this way, the changes generated by the respiratory movements recorded to the webcam sensor can be adequately isolated and relayed to the subsequent elaboration stages. A third order Butterworth digital filter was employed. Finally, the $v(f)$ signal is normalized to obtain $\hat{v}(f)$ as reported in the following Equation (4):

$$\hat{v}(f) = \frac{v(f) - \mu(v(f))}{\sigma(v(f))} \qquad (4)$$

where $\mu(v(f))$ and $\sigma(v(f))$ are the mean and standard deviation of signal $v(f)$, respectively.

The signal $\hat{v}(f)$ is used for extracting respiratory temporal information (i.e., period duration—T_R and respiratory rate—f_R) since $\hat{v}(f)$ would be proportional to the changes in the intensity component, and thus to the underlying respiratory signal of interest (Figure 2). A window of 60 s is shown in Figure 2B. In this figure the apnea phase of about 5 s used for synchronizing reference signal and video-derived signal in the experimental trials is not shown (see Section 3.1).

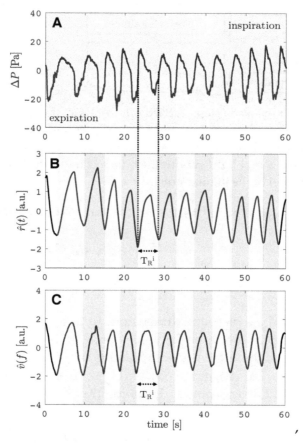

Figure 2. (A) ΔP signal recorded by the reference instrument at the level of the nostrils. In grey, the signal collected during the inspiration (positive pressure), while in green, the signal recorded during the expiration (negative pressure). (B) Reference respiratory pattern signal ($\hat{r}(t)$) obtained from data processing of ΔP signal. (C) Respiratory pattern signal obtained from the proposed measuring system ($\hat{v}(f)$). Figure in (B) and (C) show similar patterns: during the inspiratory phase the signal increases, while during the expiratory phase they decrease. The duration of one breath ($T_R(i)$) is shown on both the $\hat{r}(t)$ and $\hat{v}(f)$ signals.

3. Tests and Experimental Trials

3.1. Participants and Tests

In this study, we enrolled 12 participants (6 males and 6 females) with a mean age 24 ± 4 years old, mean height of 165 ± 15 cm, mean body mass of 60 ± 10 kg). All the participants provided informed consent. We have created a data set for evaluation of the proposed system. We aim to cover normal breathing (i.e., respiratory frequency in the range 8–25 breaths·min^{-1}), abnormal breathing (i.e., tachypnea) and apnea stages.

Each participant was invited to sit on a chair in front of the web camera at a distance of about 1.2 m. The user adjusted the screen of the laptop in order to record the trunk area (as shown in Figure 1). All the experiments were carried out indoor (in a laboratory room) and with a stable amount of light delivered by neon lights and three windows as sources of illumination. The participants' shoulders were turned towards the furnishings of the room. The windows were lateral to the scene recorded by the camera. Other people were in the room during the data collection but not allowed to pass near the shooting area.

Participants were asked to keep still and seated, and to breathe spontaneously by facing the webcam. Each volunteer was called to breathe quietly for around 5 s, simulate an apnea of duration <10 s, and then to breathe quietly at self-paced f_R for all the duration of the trial (120 s). Each volunteer carried out two trials with the same experimental design: in the first trial, the participant wore a loose-fit t-shirt; in the second trials, a slim-fit t-shirt. Two volunteers were also invited to simulate abnormal breathing (i.e., tachypnea) that is characterized by high f_R values (>35 bpm).

At the same time, respiratory pattern was recorded with a reference instrument described in the following Section 3.2.

3.2. Reference Instrument and Signal

For registering reference pattern, a head-mounted wearable device was used. We already used this system in a similar scenario [31]. This device is based on the recording of the pressure-drop (ΔP) that occurs during the expiratory/inspiratory phases of respiration at the level of nostrils. The device consists of a cannula attached to the jaw with tape: one piece of tape at the end of the nostrils in order to collect part of the nasal flow while the other tap is connected to a static tap of a differential digital pressure sensor (i.e., Sensirion—model SDP610, pressure range up to ±125 Pa). The pressure data were recorded with a dedicated printed circuit board described in [31], at 100 Hz of sample rate. Data were sent to a remote laptop via a wireless connection and archived.

Negative pressure was collected during the expiratory phase and positive pressure during the inspiratory phase, as can be seen in Figure 2A. Then, a temporal standard cumulative trapezoidal numerical integration of the ΔP signal was carried out to obtain a smooth respiratory signal for further analysis ($r(t)$) and to emphasize the maximum and minimum peaks. Afterward, such integrated $r(t)$ has been filtered using a bandpass Butterworth filter in the frequency range 0.05–2 Hz and normalized as in Equation (4) and $\hat{r}(t)$ has been obtained. This $\hat{r}(t)$ is the reference respiratory pattern signal, then used to extract breath-by-breath f_R reference values (i.e., $f_R(i)$).

As shown in Figure 2B, one breath is the portion of the signal between the starting point of the inspiration and the end of the following expiration. During the inspiratory phase, the ΔP signal pass from 0 to positive values (grey area in Figure 2A), and $r(t)$ is an increasing signal. During the expiratory phase, the opposite situation: ΔP signal passes from 0 to negative values (green area in Figure 2A), and $\hat{r}(t)$ is a decreasing signal.

3.3. Respiratory Rate Calculation

The breathing rate can be extracted from both the reference signal $\hat{r}(t)$ and $\hat{v}(f)$ either in the frequency or time domains [21,32]. The analysis in the time domain requires the identification of specific points on the signal. Mainly, two different approaches may be used: (i) based on the identification of the maximum and minimum points; or (ii) the zero-crossing point individuation on the signals. In this work, we used a zero-crossing-based algorithm. We used the same algorithm for the event detection on both the reference signal $\hat{r}(t)$ and $\hat{v}(f)$. The algorithm provides the detection of the zero-crossing points on the signal based on signum function. It allows determining the onset of each respiratory cycle, characterized by a positive going zero-crossing value. The signum function of a real number x is defined as in the following Equation (5):

$$sgn(x) : \begin{cases} -1 & \text{if } x_i < 0, \\ 0 & \text{if } x_i = 0, \\ 1 & \text{if } x_i > 0, \end{cases} \tag{5}$$

where x_i is the value x of the signal for frame index i corresponding to the onset of a respiratory cycle. Then, the algorithm provides the location of local minimum points on the signal and their indices between respiratory cycle onsets determined in the first step.

The duration of each i-th breath—$T_R(i)$—is then calculated as the time elapsed between two consecutive minima points (expressed in s). Consequently, the i-th breath-by-breath breathing rate $f_R(i)$, expressed in breaths per minute (bpm), is calculated as in Equation (6):

$$f_R(i) = \frac{60}{T_R(i)}. \tag{6}$$

3.4. Data Analysis

We recorded the breath-by-breath respiratory rate with our system and the reference instrument and evaluated the discrepancies coming from their comparison. Signals obtained from the measuring system have been compared to the reference signals. Firstly the $\hat{r}(t)$ and $\hat{v}(f)$ were synchronized to be directly compared. We used the apnea stage to detect a common event on both signals. All the analysis were carried out on both the $\hat{r}(t)$ and $\hat{v}(f)$ that occur after the first end expiratory point after the apnea stage. The breath-by-breath f_R values have been compared between instruments by extracting such values with the time-domain analysis from $\hat{r}(t)$ (i.e., $f_R(i)$) and $\hat{v}(f)$ (i.e., $\hat{f}_R(i)$).

To compare the values gathered by the reference instrument and computed by the video-based method, we use the mean absolute error (MAE) as in Equation (7):

$$MAE = \frac{1}{n} \cdot \sum_{i=1}^{n} |\hat{f}_R(i) - f_R(i)|, \tag{7}$$

where n is the number of breaths recognized by the algorithm for each subject in the trial.

Then, the standard error of the mean (SE) is calculated as in Equation (8):

$$SE = \frac{SD}{\sqrt{n}}, \tag{8}$$

where SD is the standard deviation of the absolute difference between estimations and reference data $\hat{f}_R(i) - f_R(i)$. Standard error was used to provide a simple estimation of uncertainty.

Lastly, the percentage difference between instruments was calculated as in Equation (9), per each volunteer:

$$\%E = \frac{1}{n} \cdot \sum_{n} \frac{\hat{f}_R(i) - f_R(i)}{f_R(i)} \cdot 100. \tag{9}$$

Additionally, we used the Bland–Altman analysis to investigate the agreement between the proposed method and the reference, in the whole range of f_R measurement. With this graphical method we investigated if the differences between the two techniques against the averages of the two techniques presented a tendency at the different f_R collected during the trials. The Bland–Altman analysis was used to obtain the mean of the Differences (MOD) and the limits of Agreements (LOAs) values [33] that are typically reported in other studies and extremely useful when comparing our results with the relevant scientific literature [2].

To fulfill the scope of this paper we carried out three separate analyses using these metrics for comparisons. Firstly, we used the data collected with slim-fit and loose-fit clothing to investigate the influence of clothing on the performance of the proposed method, using both male and female data.

Then, we separately use the data collected from male and from female to investigate the influence of sex on performance. Lastly, the overall performance of the proposed measuring system has been tested considering all the breath-by-breath f_R (n = 411). Preliminary tests have been also done using data collected from two volunteers during tachypnea.

4. Experimental Results

The detection of apnea stages used for synchronizing the signals on $\hat{r}(t)$ and $\hat{v}(f)$ was always possible. Therefore, no trials were excluded from the analysis. During the apnea, the signal collected by the reference instrument is a constant and null ΔP; constant signals were also found in $\hat{v}(f)$.

Table 1 summaries the number of breaths, average $\hat{f}_R$ and f_R values, MAE, SE and %E for each subject, at the two t-shirt fittings. MAE value was always lower than 0.78 bpm, while standard error was <0.24 bpm in all the volunteers. %E values were both negative and positive: the maximum value was 0.62%. The performance of the proposed method in the measurement of breath-by-breath respiratory frequencies can be appreciated in Figure 3.

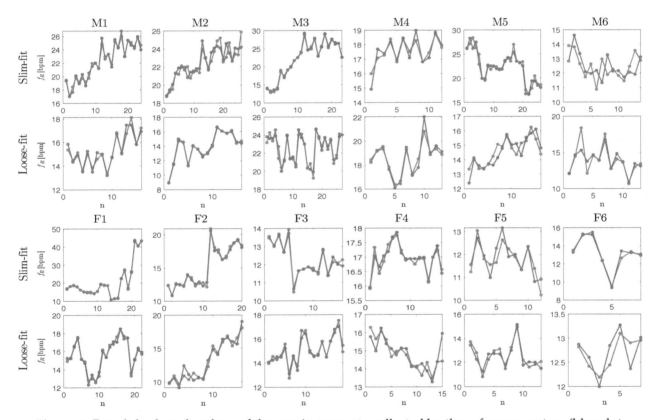

Figure 3. Breath-by-breath values of the respiratory rate collected by the reference system (blue dots and lines) and by the proposed measuring system (orange dots and lines). Data from male (i.e., M1, M2, M3, M4, M5, M6) and female (F1, F2, F3, F4, F5, F6) volunteers wearing slim-fit and loose-fit clothing are reported. Details about MAE, SE and %E values per each volunteer with slim-fit and loose-fit clothing are reported in Table 1.

4.1. Influence of Clothing Type

The influence of clothing was investigated by analyzing the difference (i.e., $\hat{f}_R(i) - f_R(i)$) distribution considering all the data obtained from male and female together. Since the sample size and bin width of the histograms are different between slim-fit (n = 211) and loose-fit (n = 203) data, it is difficult to compare them. So, we normalize the histograms so that all the bar heights add to 1, and we use a uniform bin width (0.1 bpm). With the slim-fit clothing, the 28% of the differences between the two instruments were in the range ±0.1 bpm (94% of data in the range ±1 bpm), while with the loose-fit clothing only 19% of data (94% of data in the range ±1 bpm). For details refers to Figure 4A. The Bland–Altman showed a bias of -0.02 ± 1.07 bpm and 0.01 ± 0.98 bpm in the case of loose-fit and slim-fit clothing, respectively. From the Bland–Altman plot, neither proportional error nor magnitude of measurements dependence were found.

Table 1. Breath-by-breath analysis: average $\hat{f}_R$, average f_R, mae, se and %e values per each volunteer at the different t-shirt fitting. MAE: Mean Absolute Error ; SE: Standard Error of the mean.

Vol.	T-Shirt Fitting	# Breaths	$\hat{f}_R$ [bpm]	f_R [bpm]	MAE [bpm]	SE [bpm]	%E [%]
M1	slim	24	22.29	22.28	0.76	0.18	−0.52
	loose	16	15.33	15.31	0.27	0.05	0.18
M2	slim	17	13.90	13.86	0.58	0.09	0.46
	loose	26	22.48	22.39	0.14	0.02	0.28
M3	slim	23	22.21	22.18	0.27	0.04	0.14
	loose	27	22.55	22.55	0.35	0.0	0.04
M4	slim	12	17.53	17.55	0.32	0.09	0.19
	loose	13	18.57	18.52	0.33	0.09	−0.16
M5	slim	26	22.32	22.46	0.65	0.13	−0.52
	loose	16	14.51	14.60	0.43	0.08	−0.62
M6	slim	14	12.49	12.51	0.78	0.14	0.21
	loose	13	13.82	13.92	0.60	0.24	−0.10
F1	slim	23	20.62	20.67	0.24	0.04	−0.13
	loose	22	15.61	15.57	0.23	0.03	0.26
F2	slim	20	15.08	15.07	0.27	0.04	0.14
	loose	16	13.14	13.07	0.60	0.10	0.55
F3	slim	16	12.27	12.30	0.11	0.02	−0.15
	loose	19	15.08	15.06	0.25	0.04	0.18
F4	slim	17	16.96	16.95	0.11	0.02	0.07
	loose	15	14.85	14.78	0.37	0.10	0.53
F5	slim	12	11.83	11.78	0.35	0.07	0.50
	loose	13	12.50	12.55	0.36	0.04	−0.32
F6	slim	8	13.16	13.14	0.23	0.08	0.17
	loose	7	12.71	12.69	0.23	0.07	0.16
Overall	-	414	-	-	0.39	0.02	0.07

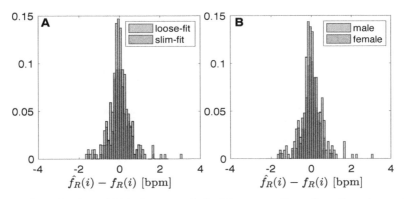

Figure 4. Difference distribution: (**A**) influence of clothing type (i.e., slim-fit vs loose-fit); (**B**) influence of sex (i.e., male vs female).

4.2. Influence of Sex

The influence of sex on the performance of the measuring system was investigated by analyzing the difference $(\hat{f}_R(i) - f_R(i))$ distribution considering all the data obtained from data collection carried out with slim-fit and loose-fit clothing. Normalized histograms with uniform bin widths (0.1 bpm) were used since the difference sample size between male data ($n = 226$) and female data ($n = 188$). In the male group, 21% of data show difference between instrument in the range ±0.1 bpm (90% of data in the range ±1 bpm), while in the female group was 27% of the data (98% of data in the range ±1 bpm). Figure 4B shows the two distributions. The Bland–Altman analysis revealed a bias of 0.01 ± 1.22 bpm (see Figure 5C) and -0.01 ± 0.73 bpm (see Figure 5D) for male and female volunteers, respectively. All the f_R values recorded by the male volunteers are between 10 and 30 bpm (mean 19.14 bpm, SD 4.55 bpm). In female volunteers, five f_R values over 25 bpm can be observed in Figure 5D, while 96% of the data are in the range of 10–20 bpm (mean 14.99 bpm, SD 4.47). Bland–Altman analysis shows the absence of proportional error and magnitude of measurements dependence.

4.3. Overall Performance

All the $f_R(i)$ extracted from $\hat{r}(t)$ and $\hat{v}(f)$ per each subject with slim-fit and loose-fit clothing are presented in Figure 3. Data extracted from signal collected with the proposed measuring system follow the data extracted from reference signal in each subject, both a low f_R and high f_R. Similar variations in f_R estimates can be clearly observed in that figure.

Figure 5A shows the difference distribution of all the 414 breaths collected: the 24% of the differences are in the interval of ±0.1 bpm, and only 6% of data shows differences higher than ±1 bpm. Bland–Altman analysis (Figure 5B) demonstrates a bias with a MOD close to 0 (i.e., -0.01 bpm) and LOAs of 1.02 bpm. Bland–Altman analysis allows us to assess the absence of proportional error and magnitude of measurements dependence.

4.4. Preliminary Results during Tachypnea

The proposed measuring system has also been preliminarily tested on two subjects during tachypnea. Figure 6 reports two examples of 30 s data collection on two volunteers. By applying the algorithm for the f_R calculation, we found a MAE of 1.05 bpm, a SE 0.13 bpm and a %E of -0.24% for the first volunteer; second volunteer data show a MAE of 0.48 bpm, SE of 0.08 bpm and %E of 0.04%. Due to the small sample size, Bland–Altman was not used to summarize bias between methods.

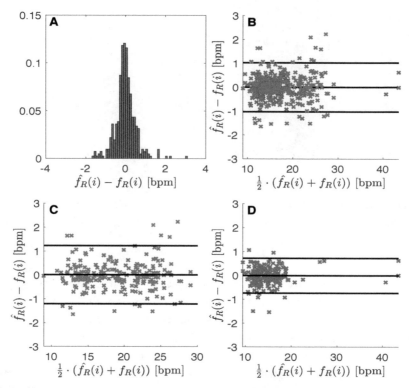

Figure 5. (**A**) Difference distribution between proposed method and reference respiratory rate values; (**B**) Bland–Altman plot obtained considering all the data recorded by male and female volunteers: black line is the MOD, red lines are the LOAs (i.e., ±1.96 times the standard deviation); (**C,B**) Bland–Altman plot obtained considering data recorded by male volunteers; (**D**) Bland–Altman plot obtained considering data recorded by female volunteers.

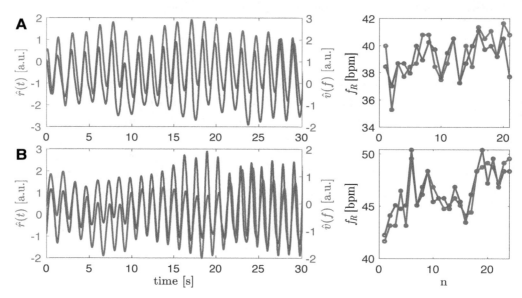

Figure 6. Two patterns collected from two volunteers simulating tachypnea. In blue, the reference signal $\hat{r}(t)$, in orange the $\hat{v}(f)$ signal. In the first volunteer (**graphs A**), the average $\hat{f}_R$ is 39.14 bpm while the average f_R is 39.34 bpm. In the second volunteer (**graphs B**), the average $\hat{f}_R$ is 46.44 bpm while the average f_R is 46.28 bpm.

5. Discussion

In this paper, a single built-in camera system is proposed for the extraction of the respiratory pattern and the estimation of breath-by-breath f_R. The built-in camera of a commercial laptop allows the non-intrusive, ecological, and low-cost recording of chest wall movement. The algorithm for the processing of images allows (i) the chest wall video recording at sufficient frame rate (i.e., 30 Hz), (ii) the selection of a pixel for further semi-automatic selection of a ROI for the measurement of the pixel intensity change, in order to extract video-based respiratory pattern $\hat{v}(f)$, and (iii) the post-processing of the $\hat{v}(f)$ signal to estimate breath-by-breath f_R values. The proposed system has been tested on healthy participants. Tests were carried out on male and female participants wearing both slim-fit and loose-fit t-shirts to simulate real respiratory monitoring conditions (e.g., a subject at home, patient in a medical room, etc.). In the literature, rarely authors take into account the influence of sex and clothing when camera-based methods are used. Additionally, in this paper, we used an unobtrusive head-mounted wearable as reference instrument to not compromise the area recorded by the camera.

Signals obtained with the proposed method allow clear identification of the apnea stages, breathing pattern at quiet pace and during tachypnea in all the trials. Considering the breath-by-breath $f_R(i)$ values, we obtained comparable MAE and SE values in the two groups (slim-fit vs. loose-fit). From the analysis of the bias revealed by the Bland–Altman plots, we found slightly better results with volunteers wearing slim-fit clothing (LOAs of ±0.98 bpm against ±1.07 bpm with loose-fit clothing). These results confirm those obtained in [29]. Considering the sex, results demonstrated good performance with both males and females with slightly lower bias in females (-0.01 ± 0.73 bpm) than in males (0.01 ± 1.22 bpm). By considering all 414 breaths, the Bland–Altman analysis demonstrates a bias of -0.01 ± 1.02 bpm of the proposed method when compared to the f_R values gathered by the reference instrument. The method proposed in [20] achieves bias of -0.32 ± 1.61 bpm when tested in similar setting and participants. Then, the bias we found is comparable with the one reported in [34] (i.e., -0.02 ± 0.83 bpm) where the pseudo-Wigner–Villetime frequency analysis was used (with a f_R resolution of 0.7324 bpm). The performances we obtained are better than those obtained in [35] where the average f_R were considered (bias of 0.37 ± 1.04 bpm), and advanced signal and video processing techniques, including developing video magnification, complete ensemble empirical mode decomposition with adaptive noise, and canonical correlation analysis were used in the post-processing phase. When compared to depth sensors used on participant in supine position [16], our method demonstrates comparable results with simplicity and cost ($\sim0.01 \pm 0.96$ bpm in [16]). Despite the absence of contact with the subject, the proposed method shows overall performance similar to those obtained with wearable device for f_R monitoring requiring direct contact with the torso (e.g., garment with optical fibers showed bias of -0.02 ± 2.04 bpm in [36], during quiet breathing). In contrast to other research studies, we did not use a background behind the user to test the system in conditions resembling real application scenarios. Further tests might be focused on extracting respiratory volumes by using a more structured environment during video collection as in [37].

One of the main limitations of this study is the limited number of subjects included in the analysis. For this reason, we did not perform any statistical analysis because population size does not allow any statistically significative conclusions. Additionally, we tested the proposed method at one distance between camera and subject (i.e., 1.2 m).

Further effort will be mainly devoted to addressing these points. Tests will be carried out to investigate the performance of the system in different scenarios at different subject–camera relative distances, and on many subjects. Furthermore, performance of the method will be tested in a wide range of atypical respiratory pattern (i.e., tachypnea, deep breaths, Cheyne-Stokes) and in extracting additional respiratory parameters (e.g., duration of expiratory and inspiratory parameters, inter-breathing variations). We are already testing the validity of additional techniques based on pixel flow analysis to remove unrelated breathing movements. Additionally, we are working on feature selection approaches to use the proposed method for respiratory monitoring when small movements of the user happen. We hope to use the proposed measuring system for respiratory monitoring even with undesired subject' motion, also by implementing a fully automatic process to detect ROI from video frames. These steps will allow automatic and long-term data collection.

Author Contributions: Conceptualization, C.M. and E.S.; Data curation, C.M.; Formal analysis, C.M.; Funding acquisition, C.M.; Investigation, C.M., D.L.P. and D.F.; Methodology, C.M., D.L.P., D.F., S.S. and E.S.; Project administration, C.M.; Resources, C.M. and E.S.; Software, C.M.; Supervision, C.M., D.F., S.S. and E.S.; Validation, C.M.; Visualization, C.M., D.L.P., D.F., S.S. and E.S.; Writing—original draft, C.M.; Writing—review & editing, D.L.P., D.F., S.S. and E.S.

References

1. Cretikos, M.A.; Bellomo, R.; Hillman, K.; Chen, J.; Finfer, S.; Flabouris, A. Respiratory rate: The neglected vital sign. *Med. J. Aust.* **2008**, *188*, 657–659. [PubMed]

2. Nicolò, A.; Massaroni, C.; Passfield, L. Respiratory frequency during exercise: The neglected physiological measure. *Front. Physiol.* **2017**. [CrossRef] [PubMed]

3. Smith, I.; Mackay, J.; Fahrid, N.; Krucheck, D. Respiratory rate measurement: A comparison of methods. *Br. J. Healthc. Assist.* **2011**, *5*, 18–23. [CrossRef]

4. Barthel, P.; Wensel, R.; Bauer, A.; Müller, A.; Wolf, P.; Ulm, K.; Huster, K.M.; Francis, D.P.; Malik, M.; Schmidt, G. Respiratory rate predicts outcome after acute myocardial infarction: A prospective cohort study. *Eur. Heart J.* **2012**, *34*, 1644–1650. [CrossRef] [PubMed]

5. Younes, M. Role of respiratory control mechanisms in the pathogenesis of obstructive sleep disorders. *J. Appl. Physiol.* **2008**, *105*, 1389–1405. [CrossRef] [PubMed]

6. Rantonen, T.; Jalonen, J.; Grönlund, J.; Antila, K.; Southall, D.; Välimäki, I. Increased amplitude modulation of continuous respiration precedes sudden infant death syndrome: Detection by spectral estimation of respirogram. *Early Hum. Dev.* **1998**, *53*, 53–63. [CrossRef]

7. Schena, E.; Massaroni, C.; Saccomandi, P.; Cecchini, S. Flow measurement in mechanical ventilation: A review. *Med. Eng. Phys.* **2015**, *37*, 257–264. [CrossRef]

8. Brochard, L.; Martin, G.S.; Blanch, L.; Pelosi, P.; Belda, F.J.; Jubran, A.; Gattinoni, L.; Mancebo, J.; Ranieri, V.M.; Richard, J.C.M.; et al. Clinical review: Respiratory monitoring in the ICU-a consensus of 16. *Crit. Care* **2012**, *16*, 219. [CrossRef]

9. Massaroni, C.; Nicolò, A.; Lo Presti, D.; Sacchetti, M.; Silvestri, S.; Schena, E. Contact-based methods for measuring respiratory rate. *Sensors* **2019**, *19*, 908. [CrossRef]

10. Massaroni, C.; Di Tocco, J.; Presti, D.L.; Longo, U.G.; Miccinilli, S.; Sterzi, S.; Formica, D.; Saccomandi, P.; Schena, E. Smart textile based on piezoresistive sensing elements for respiratory monitoring. *IEEE Sens. J.* **2019**. [CrossRef]

11. Dionisi, A.; Marioli, D.; Sardini, E.; Serpelloni, M. Autonomous wearable system for vital signs measurement with energy-harvesting module. *IEEE Trans. Instrum. Meas.* **2016**, *65*, 1423–1434. [CrossRef]

12. Gilbert, R.; Auchincloss, J., Jr.; Brodsky, J.; Boden, W.A. Changes in tidal volume, frequency, and ventilation induced by their measurement. *J. Appl. Physiol.* **1972**, *33*, 252–254. [CrossRef] [PubMed]

13. Al-Naji, A.; Gibson, K.; Lee, S.H.; Chahl, J. Monitoring of cardiorespiratory signal: Principles of remote measurements and review of methods. *IEEE Access* **2017**, *5*, 15776–15790. [CrossRef]

14. Deng, F.; Dong, J.; Wang, X.; Fang, Y.; Liu, Y.; Yu, Z.; Liu, J.; Chen, F. Design and Implementation of a Noncontact Sleep Monitoring System Using Infrared Cameras and Motion Sensor. *IEEE Trans. Instrum. Meas.* **2018**, *67*, 1555–1563. [CrossRef]

15. Lai, J.C.Y.; Xu, Y.; Gunawan, E.; Chua, E.C.; Maskooki, A.; Guan, Y.L.; Low, K.; Soh, C.B.; Poh, C. Wireless Sensing of Human Respiratory Parameters by Low-Power Ultrawideband Impulse Radio Radar. *IEEE Trans. Instrum. Meas.* **2011**, *60*, 928–938. [CrossRef]

16. Bernacchia, N.; Scalise, L.; Casacanditella, L.; Ercoli, I.; Marchionni, P.; Tomasini, E.P. Non contact measurement of heart and respiration rates based on Kinect™. In Proceedings of the 2014 IEEE International Symposium on Medical Measurements and Applications (MeMeA), Lisbon, Portugal, 11–12 June 2014, pp. 1–5.

17. Marchionni, P.; Scalise, L.; Ercoli, I.; Tomasini, E. An optical measurement method for the simultaneous assessment of respiration and heart rates in preterm infants. *Rev. Sci. Instrum.* **2013**, *84*, 121705. [CrossRef] [PubMed]

18. Scalise, L.; Ercoli, I.; Marchionni, P.; Tomasini, E.P. Measurement of respiration rate in preterm infants by laser Doppler vibrometry. In Proceedings of the 2011 IEEE International Workshop on Medical Measurements and Applications Proceedings (MeMeA), Bari, Italy, 30–31 May 2011; pp. 657–661.

19. Sirevaag, E.J.; Casaccia, S.; Richter, E.A.; O'Sullivan, J.A.; Scalise, L.; Rohrbaugh, J.W. Cardiorespiratory interactions: Noncontact assessment using laser Doppler vibrometry. *Psychophysiology* **2016**, *53*, 847–867. [CrossRef] [PubMed]

20. Lin, K.Y.; Chen, D.Y.; Tsai, W.J. Image-Based Motion-Tolerant Remote Respiratory Rate Evaluation. *IEEE Sens. J.* **2016**. [CrossRef]

21. Massaroni, C.; Lopes, D.S.; Lo Presti, D.; Schena, E.; Silvestri, S. Contactless Monitoring of Breathing Patterns and Respiratory Rate at the Pit of the Neck: A Single Camera Approach. *J. Sens.* **2018**, *2018*, 4567213. [CrossRef]

22. Bartula, M.; Tigges, T.; Muehlsteff, J. Camera-based system for contactless monitoring of respiration. In Proceedings of the 2013 35th Annual International Conference of the IEEE Engineering in Medicine and Biology Society (EMBC), Osaka, Japan, 3–7 July 2013; pp. 2672–2675.

23. Koolen, N.; Decroupet, O.; Dereymaeker, A.; Jansen, K.; Vervisch, J.; Matic, V.; Vanrumste, B.; Naulaers, G.; Van Huffel, S.; De Vos, M. Automated Respiration Detection from Neonatal Video Data. In Proceedings of the International Conference on Pattern Recognition Applications and Methods ICPRAM, Lisbon, Portugal, 10–12 January 2015; pp. 164–169.

24. Antognoli, L.; Marchionni, P.; Nobile, S.; Carnielli, V.; Scalise, L. Assessment of cardio-respiratory rates by non-invasive measurement methods in hospitalized preterm neonates. In Proceedings of the 2018 IEEE International Symposium on Medical Measurements and Applications (MeMeA), Rome, Italy, 11–13 June 2018; pp. 1–5.

25. Bernacchia, N.; Marchionni, P.; Ercoli, I.; Scalise, L. Non-contact measurement of the heart rate by a image sensor. In *Sensors*; Springer: Berlin, Germany, 2015; pp. 371–375.

26. Bai, Y.W.; Li, W.T.; Chen, Y.W. Design and implementation of an embedded monitor system for detection of a patient's breath by double Webcams in the dark. In Proceedings of the 12th IEEE International Conference on e-Health Networking Applications and Services (Healthcom), Lyon, France, 1–3 July 2010; pp. 93–98.

27. Janssen, R.; Wang, W.; Moço, A.; De Haan, G. Video-based respiration monitoring with automatic region of interest detection. *Physiol. Meas.* **2015**. [CrossRef]

28. Poh, M.Z.; McDuff, D.J.; Picard, R.W. Advancements in noncontact, multiparameter physiological measurements using a webcam. *IEEE Trans. Biomed. Eng.* **2011**, *58*, 7–11. [CrossRef] [PubMed]

29. Massaroni, C.; Schena, E.; Silvestri, S.; Taffoni, F.; Merone, M. Measurement system based on RBG camera signal for contactless breathing pattern and respiratory rate monitoring. In Proceedings of the 2018 IEEE International Symposium on Medical Measurements and Applications (MeMeA), Rome, Italy, 11–13 June 2018; pp. 1–6.

30. Massaroni, C.; Nicolò, A.; Girardi, M.; La Camera, A.; Schena, E.; Sacchetti, M.; Silvestri, S.; Taffoni, F. Validation of a wearable device and an algorithm for respiratory monitoring during exercise. *IEEE Sens. J.* **2019**. [CrossRef]

31. Taffoni, F.; Rivera, D.; La Camera, A.; Nicolò, A.; Velasco, J.R.; Massaroni, C. A Wearable System for Real-Time Continuous Monitoring of Physical Activity. *J. Healthc. Eng.* **2018**, *2018*, 1878354. [CrossRef]

32. Welch, P. The use of fast Fourier transform for the estimation of power spectra: A method based on time averaging over short, modified periodograms. *IEEE Trans. Audio Electroacoust.* **1967**, *15*, 70–73. [CrossRef]

33. Altman, D.G.; Bland, J.M. Measurement in medicine: The analysis of method comparison studies. *Statistician* **1983**, *32*, 307–317. [CrossRef]

34. Reyes, B.A.; Reljin, N.; Kong, Y.; Nam, Y.; Chon, K.H. Tidal Volume and Instantaneous Respiration Rate Estimation using a Volumetric Surrogate Signal Acquired via a Smartphone Camera. *IEEE J. Biomed. Health Inform.* **2017**, *21*, 764–777. [CrossRef] [PubMed]

35. Al-Naji, A.; Chahl, J. Simultaneous tracking of cardiorespiratory signals for multiple persons using a machine vision system with noise artifact removal. *IEEE J. Translat. Eng. Health Med.* **2017**, *5*, 1–10. [CrossRef] [PubMed]

36. Massaroni, C.; Venanzi, C.; Silvatti, A.P.; Lo Presti, D.; Saccomandi, P.; Formica, D.; Giurazza, F.; Caponero, M.A.; Schena, E. Smart textile for respiratory monitoring and thoraco-abdominal motion pattern evaluation. *J. Biophotonics* **2018**, *11*, e201700263. [CrossRef] [PubMed]

4

A Soft Polydimethylsiloxane Liquid Metal Interdigitated Capacitor Sensor and its Integration in a Flexible Hybrid System for On-Body Respiratory Sensing

Yida Li [1,*,†], Suryakanta Nayak [1,†], Yuxuan Luo [1], Yijie Liu [1],
Hari Krishna Salila Vijayalal Mohan [1], Jieming Pan [1], Zhuangjian Liu [2], Chun Huat Heng [1]
and Aaron Voon-Yew Thean [1,*]

[1]   Department of Electrical and Computer Engineering, National University of Singapore, 4 Engineering
      Drive 3, Singapore 117583, Singapore; suryakanta.nayak@nus.edu.sg (S.N.); elelyux@nus.edu.sg (Y.L.);
      liuyijie1987@outlook.com (Y.L.); harikrishnasv@nus.edu.sg (H.K.S.V.M.); e0361620@u.nus.edu (J.P.);
      elehch@nus.edu.sg (C.H.H.)
[2]   Institute of High Performance Computing, A*STAR Research Entities, 1 Fusionopolis Way, #16-16 Connexis,
      Singapore 138632, Singapore; liuzj@ihpc.a-star.edu.sg
*   Correspondence: elelyida@nus.edu.sg (Y.L.); aaron.thean@nus.edu.sg (A.V.-Y.T.)
†   Equal contributions.

Abstract: We report on the dual mechanical and proximity sensing effect of soft-matter interdigitated (IDE) capacitor sensors, together with its modelling using finite element (FE) simulation to elucidate the sensing mechanism. The IDE capacitor is based on liquid-phase GaInSn alloy (Galinstan) embedded in a polydimethylsiloxane (PDMS) microfludics channel. The use of liquid-metal as a material for soft sensors allows theoretically infinite deformation without breaking electrical connections. The capacitance sensing is a result of E-field line disturbances from electrode deformation (mechanical effect), as well as floating electrodes in the form of human skin (proximity effect). Using the proximity effect, we show that spatial detection as large as 28 cm can be achieved. As a demonstration of a hybrid electronic system, we show that by integrating the IDE capacitors with a capacitance sensing chip, respiration rate due to a human's chest motion can be captured, showing potential in its implementation for wearable health-monitoring.

Keywords: stretchable; polydimethylsiloxane; liquid-metal; capacitor

---

1. Introduction

Soft electronics that enable conformal contacts on irregular surfaces is an emerging area with increasing importance. The development of this technology is expected to enhance human–machine interfaces to cover areas such as medical and e-health applications, robotics, and communications [1–12]. Flexible and stretchable electronics are vigorously studied for the choice of materials and integration strategies [5–7,9,10,13]. However, flexible electronics is only suitable for a non-conformal substrate that is static or does not undergo significant strain in the x-y axes during operation [7,13]. Stretchable electronics, on the other hand, offers more degrees of freedom that can theoretically tolerate mechanical strain in all three axes. This leads to increasing interest in the field of wearable devices for health-monitoring. In such applications, soft sensors with a Young's modulus that matches that of skin are particularly attractive. This allows for prolonged human body attachment for continuous health monitoring [5,9,13,14]. Hence, besides the functionality of the sensor, there is a need to address the mechanical robustness and the system integration strategies with high performance integrated circuits (IC) [5,7,9,13,15–18]. This calls for novel materials and approaches, such as the use of liquid metal or stretchable conducting materials, in place of conventional metal materials that are rigid [19–21]. Several studies have reported soft-matter capacitors comprising of a microfludics channel of liquid-metal (Galinstan) and described the theoretical model of capacitance change effect under mechanical deformation [22,23]. While there are reports of sensors with similar structures being used for bio-sensing and proximity sensing, the implementation of such sensors in real systems is still lacking [24,25].

In this work, we report on the experimental characterization together with a finite element (FE) simulation model of soft interdigitated (IDE) capacitors sensors. The IDE capacitor was fabricated from serpentine microfluidics channels of GaInSn liquid alloy (Galinstan) embedded in a polydimethylsiloxane (PDMS) matrix. The soft IDE capacitor, besides responding to perpendicular strains in the x-y axes, also responded to proximity sensing of a human finger that has not been reported before. In addition, previous reports have not described the IDE capacitor using FE simulation with proper boundary conditions. We will address these in this paper. Experimentally, the opposite capacitance change in the x and y directions allows for detection of direction specific strain with a resolution of 0.02 pF/(% engineering strain) as verified by our FE simulation model. Proximity sensing is achieved via the modifications of the capacitor's fringing E-field by the surrounding dielectric medium [26]. We show that spatial detection as large as 28 cm can be achieved by varying a human's finger distance to the IDE capacitor. The described FE simulation model provides a design guideline for future implementation of such a class of sensors. Finally, as a demonstration of a hybrid electronic system, we show that when the IDE capacitor sensor attached to a human chest is integrated with a functional capacitance sensing chip, it can be used for on-body respiratory sensing by utilizing the proximity effect, thus demonstrating its potential as a soft sensor suitable for use in wearables for health monitoring.

2. Fabrication Process of Soft PDMS-Liquid Metal IDE Capacitor

The stretchable capacitor was composed of two layers of PDMS (Dow Corning Sylgard 184). The first layer consisted of a microfluidics channel in the form of an IDE design, fabricated using a soft lithography approach [9]. Special design care in providing for the inlet and outlet points were necessary to ensure the Galinstan filled the microfludics channel properly without trapped air. The master mold was made using a permanent resist (SU-8 3050, Microchem, Westborough, MA, USA), where the PDMS pre-polymer was casted over the pre-fabricated design to a thickness of ~500 μm and removed after curing by peeling. The second layer consisted of a plain piece of PDMS molded to the same thickness of ~500 μm. For the formation of the closed microfluidics channel, the two PDMS layers were surface treated using a light remote O_2 plasma treatment before contacting with each other. A post-baking step (90 °C, 2 h) ensured a permanent bond of the two layers of PDMS. Finally, the microfluidics channel was completely filled with Galinstan using a needle and syringe approach. The Galinstan was injected from the inlet point while air was extracted from the outlet point simultaneously to allow the complete fill of the microfluidics channel. The height of the Galinstan electrodes was dependent on the master mold, and was 100 μm in this case [9,27,28]. Figure 1a,b shows the fabrication process flow of the soft IDE capacitor, and a photo image of the fabricated IDE soft capacitors with various sizes, respectively.

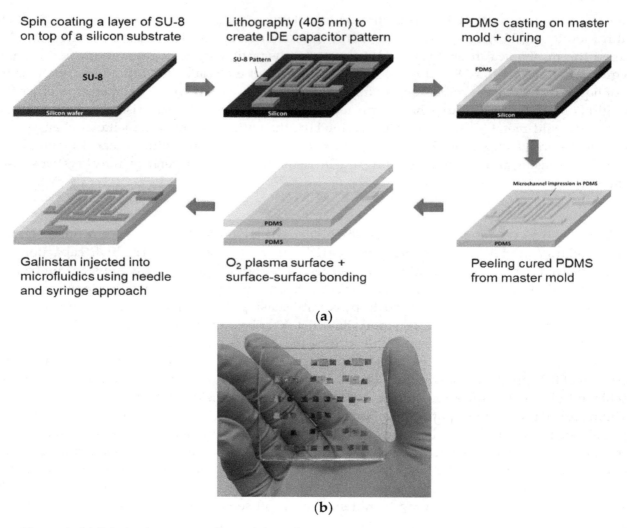

Spin coating a layer of SU-8 on top of a silicon substrate

Lithography (405 nm) to create IDE capacitor pattern

PDMS casting on master mold + curing

Galinstan injected into microfluidics using needle and syringe approach

O₂ plasma surface + surface-surface bonding

Peeling cured PDMS from master mold

(a)

(b)

Figure 1. (**a**) Fabrication process flow of the soft IDE capacitor, and (**b**) photo image of the fabricated IDE soft capacitors of various sizes. The height of the liquid metal electrode was 100 μm.

While encapsulated in the elastomer matrix, the PDMS provided good barrier resistance to moisture as reported earlier, which otherwise would cause the oxidation of the Galinstan [9,28]. We immersed the soft IDE capacitor in water for a period of 10 min and no visible and electrical change to the capacitor were observed. Hence, this allows for its use without degradation in practical environment. For electrical contact to the IDE capacitor, short sections of tungsten (W) wires (Goodfellow, 125 μm, Huntingdon, UK) perforated the PDMS into the Galinstan reservoir and was resealed with PDMS to avoid leakage.

3. Electrical Characterization and Modelling of a Static IDE Capacitor

The capacitance of all the fabricated IDE capacitors were first measured and calibrated using a benchtop LCR meter (Keysight E4980A, Santa Rosa, CA, USA) at 1 kHz. In this set of measurements, parasitic capacitance from the connecting wires to the LCR meter caused an offset to the intrinsic capacitance by a fixed positive value. From the linear fit of the data points, the parasitic capacitance was extracted as the y-intercept when the electrode length was zero. Correcting for the parasitic capacitance, the actual capacitance of the IDE capacitors ranged from 1.05 pF to 2.40 pF. Figure 2 shows the as-measured capacitance across a total electrode length from 15 mm to 44 mm, together with the corrected capacitance values and modeled values based on empirical equations. The corrected capacitances agree very well with the capacitor model. It should be noted that the main discrepancy between actual values and measured values comes from the wires' parasitic capacitances of ~0.68 pF. In subsequent measurements, the wires' parasitic capacitances were removed from the measured values.

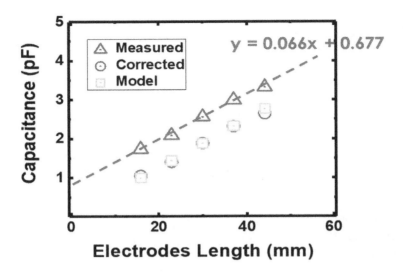

Figure 2. As-measured capacitance across a total electrode length from 15 mm to 44 mm, together with the corrected capacitance values and modeled values based on empirical equations indicated in the legends.

In our IDE capacitor design, the electrodes were of non-negligible thickness, and that was advantageous to enhance its capacitance and sensitivity. As such, a single coplanar capacitor model was not sufficient. Instead, we used a combination of co-planar capacitor and bi-planar capacitor model connected in parallel, as shown by the schematic in Figure 3.

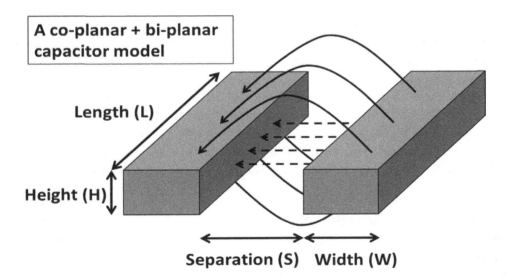

Figure 3. Schematic showing the electric field lines connecting two electrodes of the IDE capacitor. Due to the non-negligible thickness of the electrode, the two contributions of the electric field lines are the direct field lines, and the fringing field lines connected in parallel.

In this model, the electric field lines consist of those that flows directly between the sides of the two electrodes, as well as the fringing field lines that flow from the top and bottom of the electrodes. Further, the effective capacitance of such a structure is described using Equations (1) and (2) for the coplanar model, and Equation (3) for the parallel plate model.

$$C = \frac{\epsilon_r l \ln\left(-\frac{2}{\sqrt[4]{1-\frac{s^2}{(s+2w)^2}}-1}\left(\sqrt[4]{1-\frac{s^2}{(s+2w)^2}}-1\right)\right)}{377\pi V_o}, \quad for\ 0 < \frac{s}{s+2w} \le \frac{1}{\sqrt{2}} \qquad (1)$$

$$C = \frac{\epsilon_r l}{377\pi V_o \ln\left(-\frac{2}{\sqrt{\frac{s}{s+2w}}-1}\left(\sqrt{\frac{s}{s+2w}}-1\right)\right)}, \quad for\ \frac{1}{\sqrt{2}} < \frac{s}{s+2w} \le 1 \qquad (2)$$

$$C = \epsilon_r \frac{A}{d} \qquad (3)$$

where ε is the dielectric constant of the PDMS matrix, A is the area of the electrode given by channel length × height of the microfluidics channel, and d is the spacing (100 µm) between the electrodes. The above model for a static IDE capacitor was found to be in excellent agreement with experimental values, plotted out together with the measured capacitance in Figure 2, validating the accuracy of the model.

Fassler and co-workers have attempted to study the relationship between the deformation of IDE capacitors and the effect on its capacitance using empirical equations [23]. In their model, they assume that the electrode thickness plays a negligible role in the capacitance, and use only a single co-planar model. However, the thickness of the electrode does contribute to the effective capacitance and should be accounted for as described in Equation (3). In addition, the study is only limited to mechanical strains in the x-y axes. Although model has been reported to predict the change in such a capacitor due to the deformation of the system, it is done by setting assumptions, and does not allow for dynamic boundaries conditions. In addition, the model does not take into account the modifications of electric field lines due to an external change in dielectric material, which we termed as the proximity effect in this work. This effect is similar to reported works on electric-field sensing but has not been discussed thus far for IDE capacitors [26]. Hence, in this work, we further the study by modelling both the IDE capacitor's deformation and proximity effect using FE simulation. This allows for dynamic boundary conditions to be set. By coupling the simulated results together with experimental measurements, we elucidated the mechanism of capacitance sensing. The FE simulation was performed using Abaqus and the setup is described in Appendix A of this paper. Separately, for the following functional tests described in the following sections, a larger IDE capacitor was fabricated in order to achieve a higher sensitivity and easier handling. The new IDE capacitor was fabricated using the same process flow described earlier and the base capacitance was ≈9.6 pF after the parasitic capacitance correction.

3.1. Functional Test—Strain Effect

The mechanical deformation of the IDE capacitor led to a change in its geometry and a resultant change in capacitance. As the IDE capacitor was strained in the x-axis (space between electrodes pulled apart), the adjacent electrodes increased in distance from each other, causing a reduction in the capacitance. On the other hand, when the IDE capacitor was strained in the y-axis (electrodes elongating), the effect of the electrode elongating and a decrease in distance between adjacent electrodes resulted in an increase of the capacitance. In the FE simulation, we applied the same boundary condition at both ends of the PDMS during the stretching action. Figure 4a shows the FE simulation model where we applied a fixed constraint on one side and a stretched displacement condition on the other side, while Figure 4b,c shows the experimental measurements, FE simulated values of the capacitance change w.r.t to the two different strain directions up to 50%, and a comparison to the model described by Fassler et al. [23]. Good agreement between experimental and simulated values was obtained, validating the accuracy of the FE model. On the other hand, though showing a similar trend, there existed some error between the measured values as compared to earlier proposed model, thus showing the advantage of FE simulation in such a study [23]. Finally, the IDE capacitor demonstrated a resolution up to 0.02 pF/(% engineering strain).

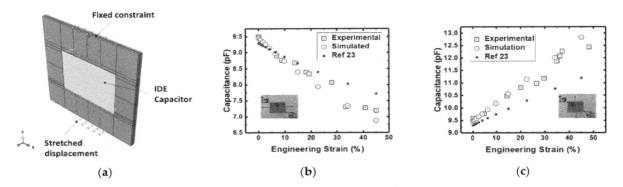

Figure 4. (**a**) FE simulation model where a fixed constraint was applied to one side and a stretched displacement condition was applied to the other side. Stretching in both x- and y-axes was simulated. (**b**) Relationship between capacitance and the x-axis strain. and (**c**) relationship between capacitance and y-axis strain comparison between experimental, FE simulated, and the earlier model proposed [23].

3.2. Proximity Effect

In this section, we describe the proximity sensing effect of the IDE capacitor through the disturbance of the E-field lines with objects placed at different distances from it. Figure 5a shows the testing setup photo images where the IDE capacitor was connected to a precision impedance analyzer (Agilent 4294A, Santa Clara, CA, USA) for capacitance measurement. The corresponding capacitance was measured as a human finger was moved between different distances from the surface of the IDE capacitor, as shown in Figure 5a. The proximity sensing mechanism is described as follows. Capacitive sensors use capacitive transducers to detect the proximity of a body, and are broadly classified in three modes: transmit mode, shunt mode, and loading mode [26]. Our setup behaved as a transmit mode where one side of the electrodes acted as a transmitter, and the other side as a receiver. Figure 5b shows an illustration of the different capacitance paths of the system as a human finger approached. The original capacitor electric field was now coupled to the receiver side through the human finger, creating two parasitic capacitances (C_1 and C_2) in series. Thus, the effective capacitance of the system increased based on the capacitance summation rule in a parallel configuration between the intrinsic capacitance C_0 and the parasitic capacitances C_1 and C_2. C_0, C_1, and C_2 were, in turn, dependent on the distance of the human finger from the capacitor due to the strength of the electric-field coupling. The further away the finger was from the capacitor, the weaker the coupling and the smaller the effective capacitance. In our experiment, a reduction of capacitance was seen as the finger moved towards the capacitor, while capacitance increased when the finger moved away from the capacitor. The proximity effect could be felt by the sensor from a distance as far as 28 cm. Compared with the dielectric property of air, human tissue is considered to be a conductive material. From the perspective of electrostatics, the boundary of human tissue was assumed to be a floating electrode, where the total electrical charge at the surface was equal to zero. The entire FE simulation model had a volumetric size of 10 cm × 5 cm × 3 cm, and the IDE capacitor, air, and the human finger model is shown in Figure 5c.

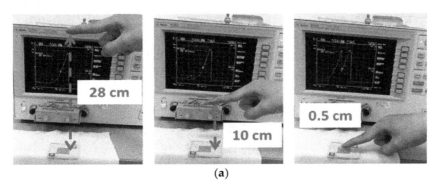

(**a**)

Figure 5. *Cont.*

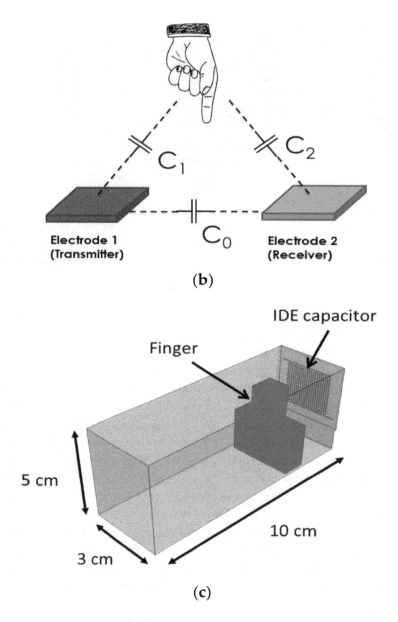

(b)

(c)

Figure 5. (**a**) Photo images showing the testing setup where a human finger is positioned at different positions above the IDE capacitor. (**b**) Illustration of the different capacitance paths as a human finger approaches the capacitor. C_0 is the intrinsic capacitance and $C_1 C_2$ are the parasitic capacitances. (**c**) FE model in the numerical simulation (finger and IDE capacitor indicated) with a size of 10 cm × 5 cm × 3 cm.

Figure 6a,b shows the capacitance versus distance of a human finger placed above the IDE capacitor up to 28 cm (both experimental and simulated indicated in legend), and time based capacitance measurements as the finger hovers above the IDE capacitor at a height of ~1–3 cm, respectively. In this simulation, a simple numerical finger model was constructed (Appendix A). The main factors resulting in the discrepancy between the experimental and simulated values were due to the leaky fringe electrical field and the finger model difference. In addition, the simulated distance was limited at 10 cm due to calculation complexity beyond that. Nonetheless, the trend of the capacitance change agreed very well in both experimental and simulation, and the most sensitive region lay within 1 cm from the IDE capacitor. The disturbance in the field line resulted from the float electrical potential. When the distance between the finger model and sensor was within 1 cm, the leaky fringe electrical field around the finger became large, resulting in a significant capacitance change.

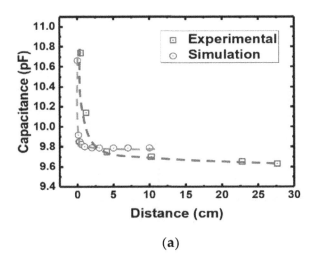

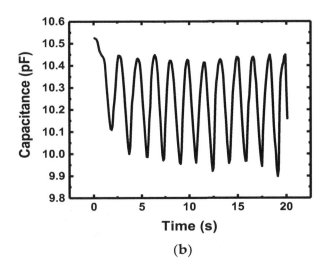

(a)   (b)

Figure 6. (**a**) Measured capacitance w.r.t. various distances a human finger was placed from the IDE capacitor, and (**b**) transient capacitance plot when a human finger hovered above the IDE capacitor in a cyclic manner at a height of ~1–3 cm above.

4. Demonstration of an IDE Capacitor Based Flexible Hybrid Respiratory System

Complementary Metal Oxide Semiconductor (CMOS) chips and printed circuit boards (PCBs) integrated with soft components allow them to be interfaced comfortably with the human body. The co-design of composite materials and electronic circuits/system in a monolithic form of a flexible hybrid electronic system provides the guideline for on-body wearables. In this section, we demonstrate a prototype hybrid flexible respiratory system by integrating the IDE capacitor to a rigid capacitance sensing circuit using external wires [29]. In subsequent measurements, the capacitance data measured by the chip is transmitted wirelessly via Wi-Fi protocol through a Raspberry Pi to a computer for readout. In the current setup, the IDE capacitor was connected to the external chip using tungsten wires. More reliable interconnects suitable for flexible system integration will be further investigated [30].

The human body respiratory detection was achieved by utilizing the proximity sensing effect of the IDE capacitor, where the sensor was attached to the human chest. The expansion and contraction of the chest caused change in the effective dielectric constant of the surrounding medium and disturbed the electrical field lines. This allowed for the respiratory motion to be picked up in a straightforward manner. Hence, the sensor was placed at a location where chest motion was obvious in this demonstration. Figure 7a shows the photo image of the integrated system attached to a human chest, while Figure 7b shows the logged capacitance values by the circuitry over 50 s. During the respiratory rate tracking, the sensor and electronics were fully covered up by clothing. Notwithstanding the slight motion of the clothing during breathing, we did not observe any distortion to the acquired waveform. Although noise was present in the collected capacitance data, the undulating trace indicated the respiratory motion was clearly visible over a range of ~0.2 pF. We demonstrate two different respiratory rates of 20/min and 60/min as shown in Figure 7b. In both cases, the sensor responded adequately, and the captured rates matched with manual counting. The implementation shown here is straightforward but effective, thus paving the way for such sensor to be implemented in a wearable medical device.

System Overview

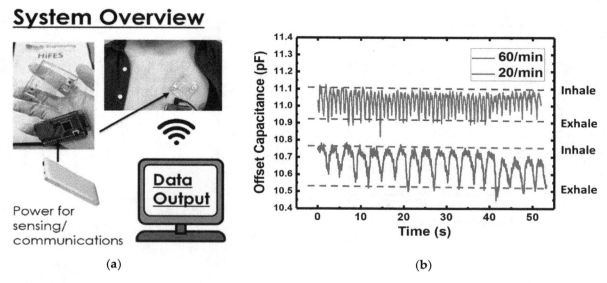

(a)   (b)

Figure 7. (**a**) System overview of the respiratory tracker with a photo image of the patch attached to a human chest, and (**b**) time dependence capacitance values measured by the capacitance chip as the human subject was breathing over 50 s. Two different respiratory rates were demonstrated as indicated in the legend.

5. Conclusions

In summary, we describe in detail the fabrication and electrical characterization of a soft PDMS-Galinstan based IDE capacitor. An FE simulation model was developed that allowed for dynamic boundary conditions to be applied, matching with experiments. With the Galinstan electrode completely encapsulated in the soft PDMS matrix, the IDE capacitor was mechanically robust to physical deformation as well as moisture. In addition to strain sensing in both the x and y axes, we show the proximity effect of such a class of soft sensors by modifying the surrounding dielectric medium. The disturbance of the electrical field lines by surrounding objects resulted in a change in effective dielectric constant, and consequently, a change in the capacitance. This effect allowed for spatial detection, and we showed experimentally that a sensing distance up to 28 cm can be achieved. The FE simulation elucidated the capacitance change mechanism and provide a guideline for more different applications. Finally, we demonstrate for the first time the use of an IDE capacitor based flexible hybrid electronics respiratory system utilizing the proximity effect. An accurate human breathing pattern was successfully tracked, paving the way for its use as a part of continuous health monitoring applications.

Author Contributions: Conceptualization, Y.L. (Yida Li), Y.L. (Yuxuan Luo), S.N., C.H.H., and A.V.-Y.T.; Methodology, Y.L. (Yida Li), Y.L. (Yuxuan Luo), and S.N.; Software, Y.L. (Yijie Liu) and Z.L.; Validation, Y.L. (Yida Li), Y.L. (Yuxuan Luo), and S.N.; Formal Analysis, Y.L. (Yida Li); Investigation, Y.L. (Yida Li), Y.L. (Yuxuan Luo), and S.N.; Resources, Z.L., C.H.H., and A.V.-Y.T.; Data Curation, Y.L. (Yida Li), Y.L. (Yuxuan Luo), and S.N.; Writing—Original Draft Preparation, Y.L. (Yida Li); Writing—Review and Editing, All; Supervision, C.H.H. and A.V.-Y.T.; Funding Acquisition, C.H.H. and A.V.-Y.T.

Appendix A

The finite element (FE) model was built up and simulated using commercial software Abaqus for non-linear FE analysis. We constructed two FE models to simulate the effect on the capacitance of the sensor due to deformation and proximity. In the FE model, the PDMS substrate was modelled using a C3D8RH element. PDMS was modelled using a hyperelastic material model (Mooney–Rivlin model in Abaqus) and was incompressible. The material parameters used were equivalent to the initial Young's modulus = 1 MPa and Poisson's ration = 0.49, obtained experimentally. Since the channels were completely filled with a nearly incompressible fluid, the surface-based fluid cavity capability was used, and the pressure applied by the fluid on the surface of channel was determined using the cavity volume.

To obtain the capacitance of the deformed sensor, the steady-state linear electrical–mechanical analysis (piezoelectric elements in Abaqus) was performed on the deformed solid mesh, where the piezoelectric constants were set to zero and the dielectric constant parameter was 2.62. In order to obtain the capacitance, an electrical potential ΔU was applied on the interfaces between the elastomeric matrix and liquid metal at the left and right channels. The charge Q in the channel was calculated using numerical simulation and the capacitance was then obtained as:

$$C = \frac{Q}{\Delta U}$$

In the proximity sensing simulation, the human finger was modelled as a simple model with dimensions as shown in Figure A1. In this model, the human finger was regarded as a near perfect conductor compared with the PDMS and air. To determine the capacitance of the position sensor, the human was set to a floating electrical potential, where the net surface electrical charge was zero. The resulting capacitance as a result of the finger distance to the sensor was extracted using the same methodology as the deformation model described in the previous paragraph.

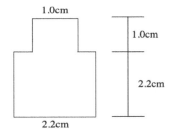

Figure A1. Shape and dimensions of the finger model. In this model, the thickness used was 1 cm.

References

1. So, J.-H.; Thelen, J.; Qusba, A.; Hayes, G.J.; Lazzi, G.; Dickey, M.D. Reversibly deformable and mechanically tunable fluidic antennas. *Adv. Funct. Mater.* **2009**, *19*, 3632–3637. [CrossRef]
2. Kim, J.; Banks, A.; Xie, Z.; Heo, S.Y.; Gutruf, P.; Lee, J.W.; Xu, S.; Jang, K.-I.; Liu, F.; Brown, G.; et al. Miniaturized flexible electronic systems with wireless power and near-field communication capabilities. *Adv. Funct. Mater.* **2015**, *25*, 4761–4767. [CrossRef]
3. Roberts, P.; Damian, D.D.; Shan, W.; Lu, T.; Majidi, C. Soft-matter capacitive sensor for measuring shear and pressure deformation. In Proceedings of the 2013 IEEE International Conference on Robotics and Automation, Karlsruhe, Germany, 6–10 May 2013; pp. 3529–3534.
4. Miyamoto, A.; Lee, S.; Cooray, N.F.; Lee, S.; Mori, M.; Matsuhisa, N.; Jin, H.; Yoda, L.; Yokota, T.; Itoh, A.; et al. Inflammation-free, gas-permeable, lightweight, stretchable on-skin electronics with nanomeshes. *Nat. Nanotechnol.* **2017**, *12*, 907–913. [CrossRef] [PubMed]
5. Xu, S.; Zhang, Y.; Jia, L.; Mathewson, K.E.; Jang, K.-I.; Kim, J.; Fu, H.; Huang, X.; Chava, P.; Wang, R.; et al. Soft microfluidic assemblies of sensors, circuits, and radios for the skin. *Science* **2014**, *344*, 70–74. [CrossRef]
6. Rogers, J.; Malliaras, G.; Someya, T. Biomedical devices go wild. *Science Advances* **2018**, *4*, eaav1889. [CrossRef] [PubMed]
7. Khan, Y.; Garg, M.; Gui, Q.; Schadt, M.; Gaikwad, A.; Han, D.; Yamamoto, N.A.D.; Hart, P.; Welte, R.; Wilson, W.; et al. Flexible hybrid electronics: Direct interfacing of soft and hard electronics for wearable health monitoring. *Adv. Funct. Mater.* **2016**, *26*, 8764–8775. [CrossRef]

8. Sheng, L.; Teo, S.; Liu, J. Liquid-metal-painted stretchable capacitor sensors for wearable healthcare electronics. *J. Med Boil. Eng.* **2016**, *36*, 265–272. [CrossRef]

9. Li, Y.; Luo, Y.; Nayak, S.; Liu, Z.; Chichvarina, O.; Zamburg, E.; Zhang, X.; Liu, Y.; Heng, C.H.; Thean, A.V.-Y. A stretchable-hybrid low-power monolithic ecg patch with microfluidic liquid-metal interconnects and stretchable carbon-black nanocomposite electrodes for wearable heart monitoring. *Adv. Electron. Mater.* **2019**, *5*, 1800463. [CrossRef]

10. Shay, T.; Velev, O.D.; Dickey, M.D. Soft electrodes combining hydrogel and liquid metal. *Soft Matter* **2018**, *14*, 3296–3303. [CrossRef] [PubMed]

11. Jin, H.; Matsuhisa, N.; Lee, S.; Abbas, M.; Yokota, T.; Someya, T. Enhancing the performance of stretchable conductors for e-textiles by controlled ink permeation. *Adv. Mater.* **2017**, *29*, 1605848. [CrossRef]

12. Cooper, C.B.; Arutselvan, K.; Liu, Y.; Armstrong, D.; Lin, Y.; Khan, M.R.; Genzer, J.; Dickey, M.D. Stretchable capacitive sensors of torsion, strain, and touch using double helix liquid metal fibers. *Adv. Funct. Mater.* **2017**, *27*, 1605630. [CrossRef]

13. Gao, W.; Emaminejad, S.; Nyein, H.Y.Y.; Challa, S.; Chen, K.; Peck, A.; Fahad, H.M.; Ota, H.; Shiraki, H.; Kiriya, D.; et al. Fully integrated wearable sensor arrays for multiplexed in situ perspiration analysis. *Nature* **2016**, *529*, 509–514. [CrossRef]

14. Liu, Y.; Pharr, M.; Salvatore, G.A. Lab-on-skin: A review of flexible and stretchable electronics for wearable health monitoring. *ACS Nano* **2017**, *11*, 9614–9635. [CrossRef] [PubMed]

15. Herbert, R.; Kim, J.-H.; Kim, Y.S.; Lee, H.M.; Yeo, W.-H. Soft material-enabled, flexible hybrid electronics for medicine, healthcare, and human-machine interfaces. *Materials* **2018**, *11*, 187. [CrossRef] [PubMed]

16. Schwartz, D.E.; Rivnay, J.; Whiting, G.L.; Mei, P.; Zhang, Y.; Krusor, B.; Kor, S.; Daniel, G.; Ready, S.E.; Veres, J.; et al. Flexible hybrid electronic circuits and systems. *IEEE J. Emerg. Sel. Top. Circuits Syst.* **2017**, *7*, 27–37. [CrossRef]

17. Sears, N.C.; Berrigan, J.D.; Buskohl, P.R.; Harne, R.L. Dynamic response of flexible hybrid electronic material systems. *Compos. Struct.* **2019**, *208*, 377–384. [CrossRef]

18. Tong, G.; Jia, Z.; Chang, J. Flexible hybrid electronics: Review and challenges. In Proceedings of the 2018 IEEE International Symposium on Circuits and Systems (ISCAS), Florence, Italy, 27–30 May 2018; pp. 1–5.

19. Abu-Khalaf, J.M.; Al-Ghussain, L.; Al-Halhouli, A.a. Fabrication of stretchable circuits on polydimethylsiloxane (pdms) pre-stretched substrates by inkjet printing silver nanoparticles. *Materials* **2018**, *11*, 2377. [CrossRef] [PubMed]

20. Rogers, J.A.; Someya, T.; Huang, Y. Materials and mechanics for stretchable electronics. *Science* **2010**, *327*, 1603–1607. [CrossRef] [PubMed]

21. Matsuhisa, N.; Inoue, D.; Zalar, P.; Jin, H.; Matsuba, Y.; Itoh, A.; Yokota, T.; Hashizume, D.; Someya, T. Printable elastic conductors by in situ formation of silver nanoparticles from silver flakes. *Nat. Mater.* **2017**, *16*, 834–840. [CrossRef] [PubMed]

22. Lazarus, N.; Meyer, C.D.; Bedair, S.S.; Nochetto, H.; Kierzewski, I.M. Multilayer liquid metal stretchable inductors. *Smart Mater. Struct.* **2014**, *23*, 085036. [CrossRef]

23. Fassler, A.; Majidi, C. Soft-matter capacitors and inductors for hyperelastic strain sensing and stretchable electronics. *Smart Mater. Struct.* **2013**, *22*, 055023. [CrossRef]

24. Staginus, J.; Aerts, I.M.; Chang, Z.-y.; Meijer, G.C.M.; de Smet, L.C.P.M.; Sudhölter, E.J.R. Capacitive response of pdms-coated ide platforms directly exposed to aqueous solutions containing volatile organic compounds. *Sensors Actuators B: Chem.* **2013**, *184*, 130–142. [CrossRef]

25. Ma, M.; Wang, Y.; Liu, F.; Zhang, F.; Liu, Z.; Li, Y. Passive wireless LC proximity sensor based on LTCC technology. *Sensors* **2019**, *19*, 1110. [CrossRef]

26. Smith, J.; White, T.; Dodge, C.; Paradiso, J.; Gershenfeld, N.; Allport, D. Electric field sensing for graphical interfaces. *IEEE Comput. Graph. Appl.* **1998**, *18*, 54–60. [CrossRef]

27. Dickey, M.D. Stretchable and soft electronics using liquid metals. *Adv. Mater.* **2017**, *29*, 1606425. [CrossRef]

28. Zhang, B.; Dong, Q.; Korman, C.E.; Li, Z.; Zaghloul, M.E. Flexible packaging of solid-state integrated circuit chips with elastomeric microfluidics. *Sci. Rep.* **2013**, *3*, 1098. [CrossRef]

29. Luo, Y.; Heng, C. An 8.2 μw 0.14 mm^2 16-channel cdma-like period modulation capacitance-to-digital converter with reduced data throughput. In Proceedings of the 2018 IEEE Symposium on VLSI Circuits, Honolulu, HI, USA, 18–22 June 2018; pp. 165–166.

5

Materials and Devices for Biodegradable and Soft Biomedical Electronics

Rongfeng Li †, **Liu Wang** † **and Lan Yin** *

School of Materials Science and Engineering, The Key Laboratory of Advanced Materials of Ministry of Education, State Key Laboratory of New Ceramics and Fine Processing, Tsinghua University, Beijing 100084, China; luckylrf@163.com (R.L.); liuwang@mail.tsinghua.edu.cn (L.W.)
* Correspondence: lanyin@tsinghua.edu.cn
† These authors contributed equally to this work.

Abstract: Biodegradable and soft biomedical electronics that eliminate secondary surgery and ensure intimate contact with soft biological tissues of the human body are of growing interest, due to their emerging applications in high-quality healthcare monitoring and effective disease treatments. Recent systematic studies have significantly expanded the biodegradable electronic materials database, and various novel transient systems have been proposed. Biodegradable materials with soft properties and integration schemes of flexible or/and stretchable platforms will further advance electronic systems that match the properties of biological systems, providing an important step along the path towards clinical trials. This review focuses on recent progress and achievements in biodegradable and soft electronics for biomedical applications. The available biodegradable materials in their soft formats, the associated novel fabrication schemes, the device layouts, and the functionality of a variety of fully bioresorbable and soft devices, are reviewed. Finally, the key challenges and possible future directions of biodegradable and soft electronics are provided.

Keywords: biodegradable electronics; transient electronics; soft biomedical electronics; biodegradable materials

1. Introduction

With the growth of the global economy, and the development of science and technology, a massive assortment of electronics has been widely used in human society, which plays an important role in industrial processes, telecommunication, entertainment, healthcare, etc. [1–5]. Soft electronics that ensure conformal contact with nonplanar surfaces, such as soft biological tissues, are expected to play crucial roles in healthcare. The characteristic of these electronics is that they can significantly expand the capabilities of conventional rigid electronics in sensing, monitoring, diagnosing, and potentially intervening functions. The intimate contact between the soft device and the nonplanar object allows for high-quality data to be collected. Additionally, in the area of medical devices, soft electronics have similar mechanical properties to biological tissues and, thus, they cause minimal irritation to the human body.

On the other hand, biodegradable electronics possess unique characteristics and attract numerous research interests. The devices can dissolve, resorb, or physically disappear into physiological or environmental solutions, partially or completely, at controlled rates after the expecting working period [6–14]. Although long-lasting operation is one hallmark of traditional electronics, devices with biodegradability can potentially offer great benefits for temporary biomedical implants, green environmental electronics, and secured hardware. Biodegradable electronics can serve as temporary diagnostic and therapeutic platforms for important biological processes, e.g., wound healing and tissue regeneration, and they can be safely resorbed by the body after usage, eliminating a second surgery for device retrieval, and therefore avoiding associated infection risks and hospital costs [15]. Biodegradable electronics also provides an alternative way to alleviate issues that are associated with electronic waste (e-waste) [16], and they enable potential usage for security hardware, preventing unauthorized access of personal or security information [17,18].

Serving as medical implants, biodegradable electronics eliminate the potential retention of device materials, while soft electronics ensure conformal wrapping with the human body, as they are soft, curvilinear, and evolving [19]. Recent research on advanced materials [14], fabrication approaches [20], and design layouts [21] yield biodegradable and soft electronics that enable intimate integration into the body, with unique capabilities for diagnostic and therapeutic functions, which would otherwise be impossible when using conventional wafer-based electronics that are built upon non-degradable and rigid printed circuit boards. These emerging technologies provide critical tools that could have great potential to improve human health and enhance the understanding of biological systems.

This review specifically focuses on recent progress and achievements in electronics that combine both soft and biodegradable characteristics, targeting biomedical applications, while reviews on general transient electronics can be found elsewhere in references [6,13]. The available biodegradable materials in the soft formats, and their associated fabrication schemes are first reviewed, followed by the introduction of device layouts and the functionality of a variety of fully bioresorbable and soft devices, including solutions for power supply. Perspectives and the outlook of biodegradable soft electronics for clinical medicine are also provided at the end of the article.

2. Materials

A wide range of biodegradable materials have been explored to build biodegradable electronics. Traditional biodegradable materials are mostly based on polymers and magnesium alloys, and they serve mainly as structural components, e.g., cardiovascular stents and 3D scaffolds. As electronic properties are essential for constructing electronics, dissolvable inorganic materials with excellent operational characteristics are therefore also of great interest.

In addition to biodegradability, soft characteristics are another critical property to be considered for biomedical applications, in order to achieve minimal irritation to the body, and to obtain intimate contact with biological tissues. Soft materials should be able to survive mechanical deformations, and simultaneously, their functional properties should remain unaffected. The term "soft" can refer to flexible, foldable, stretchable, and twistable, and here, flexible materials are the focus.

The basic building blocks for electronic components are semiconductors, dielectrics, and conductors, and studies have developed strategies to ensure flexibility. The key method is to configure biodegradable inorganic semiconductors, dielectrics, and metals into thin film and open mesh formats, and to integrate them onto soft biodegradable polymeric or metal foil substrates. Through these techniques, biodegradable and flexible electronics that can adapt well to the soft nature of the human body.

In the following sections, inorganic biodegradable functional materials, substrate materials, and encapsulation materials, and organic functional materials will be reviewed respectively, in terms of their respective dissolution rates, mechanical properties, and biocompatibilities. Dissolution data from the literature of major inorganic materials are summarized in tables for better comparison. In all, dissolution rates of a wide range of biodegradable materials have been investigated in detail in simulated bio-fluids, such as phosphate-buffered saline (PBS), Hanks' solutions, artificial cerebrospinal fluid (ACSF), etc. A few studies have investigated the effects of proteins on the dissolution rates of Si. Strategies have been proposed to obtain soft biodegradable materials that combine both inorganic and organic components. Although detailed studies are needed to further reveal the pertinent biological influences, biodegradable materials of interest exhibit good biocompatibility through their evaluation in cell studies and animal trials.

2.1. Inorganic Functional Materials

Functional materials are key components for electronics, and they consist of semiconductors, conductive materials, and dielectric materials. Inorganic dissolvable thin-film materials that have been explored, include monocrystalline silicon (mono-Si), polycrystalline silicon (poly-Si), amorphous silicon (a-Si), germanium (Ge), silicon germanium alloy (SiGe), indium–gallium–zinc oxide (a-IGZO), and zinc oxide (ZnO) [22–27] for semiconductors; magnesium (Mg), molybdenum (Mo), tungsten (W), iron (Fe), and zinc (Zn) for conductive materials [23,27–29]; and magnesium oxide (MgO), silicon dioxide (SiO_2), and silicon nitride (SiN_x) for dielectric materials [14,20,30]. The acceptable levels of these elements can be informed from nutritional supplements. The recommended dietary allowance and tolerable upper intake levels of functional materials are summarized in Table 1. As is shown, Mg, Mo, Fe, and Zn are all necessary elements for the human body. It should be noticed that the mean intakes of Si in adult men and women are 40 and 19 mg day^{-1} respectively, and limited toxicity research on Si suggests that there is no risk of inducing adverse effects for the general population, based on the common intake level [31].The mean total Ge exposure for people is 4 μg day^{-1}, which can be absorbed from the intestinal tract and excreted largely through the kidneys [32–34]. In addition, W is usually found in rice, with concentrations of 7–283 μg kg^{-1} [35]. However, because of a lack of adequate and sufficient data for Si, Ge, and W, it is necessary to establish a recommended dietary allowance (RDA) and tolerable upper intake levels (UL).

Table 1. The recommended dietary allowance (RDA) and tolerable upper intake levels (UL) of biodegradable elements [31,36].

Life Stage	Category	Element			
		Mg (mg/day)	Mo (μg/day)	Fe (mg/day)	Zn (mg/day)
Infants 0–12 months	RDA	30–75	2–3	0.27–11	2–3
	UL	–	–	40	4–5
Children 1–8 years	RDA	80–130	17–22	7–10	3–5
	UL	65–110	300–600	40	7–12
Males ≥9 years	RDA	240–420	34–45	8–11	8–11
	UL	350	1100–2000	40–45	23–40
Females ≥9 years	RDA	240–320	34–45	8–15	8–9
	UL	350	1100–2000	40–45	23–40
Pregnancy 14–50 years	RDA	350–400	50	27	11–12
	UL	350	1700–2000	45	34–40
Lactation 14–50 years	RDA	310–360	50	9–10	12–13
	UL	350	1700–2000	45	34–40

Functional materials in the thin film format are adopted to assure flexibility, as well as reasonable degradation time frames. Studies have revealed that nanomembrane materials have high degrees of bendability, as the flexural rigidity and energy release rates scale down with thickness, enabling an intimate contact with non-planar and curvilinear surface [37]. Nanomembranes can be obtained by peeling the top membrane materials from commercially available wafers (e.g., silicon on insulator, SOI), which will be discussed later. Low-temperature deposition such as radiofrequency plasma-enhanced chemical vapor deposition (RF-PECVD) [38], electron cyclotron resonance (ECR) [39], and hot-wire chemical vapor deposition (HW-CVD) [40] can be used to fabricate high-quality functional thin films directly onto soft substrates. Additionally, solution-printing techniques have also been proposed as a low-cost alternative methods [41]. Another robust strategy for achieving soft materials is through structural design, which not only enhances the flexibility of intrinsic soft materials, but also gives flexibility to materials that are intrinsically rigid. Methods include separating rigid thin film materials into small islands, introducing serpentine, wavy, buckled interconnects, integrating rigid materials with soft substrates, etc. [42,43].

The research on silicon nanomembrane (Si NM) dissolution behavior greatly promotes the development of transient electronics, as it can leverage existing well-established Si semiconductor technology and realize high-performance biodegradable electronics. The dissolution rates of Si NMs in solutions with different ionic types and relevant concentrations [23,24], temperatures [24], pH values [23], concentrations of protein [44], as well as doping levels [22] have been investigated, all of which play an important role during the silicon dissolution process. The dissolution rates of Si NMs under different conditions are tabulated in Table 2. For example, dissolution rates have been observed for Si NMs (slightly p-doped 10^{-17} cm^{-3}, 100 orientation) in aqueous solutions containing various chloride and phosphate concentrations at different temperatures. Higher temperatures and concentrations of chlorides and phosphates can greatly promote Si dissolution, probably through a nucleophilic dissolution process [24]. The underlying mechanism regarding the influence of chlorides and phosphates has been evaluated through density functional theory (DFT) and molecular dynamics (MD) simulations [24]. Dissolution rates of Si are found to be sensitive to calcium and magnesium ions as well [44]; e.g., the addition of 1 mM of Ca^{2+} and Mg^{2+} can slightly increase the rates in phosphate buffered saline solutions. As shown in Table 2, the presence of albumin decelerates the dissolution rates, probably due to the absorption of the protein onto the Si surface [44]. In addition, the types and concentrations of dopants for Si NMs can affect the dissolution rate significantly, and a sharp decrease in dissolution rate can be found when dopant concentrations exceed a certain level, i.e., 10^{20} cm^{-3}.

Similarly, dissolution rates of poly-Si, a-Si, alloys of silicon, SiGe, and Ge show great dependence on the pH, temperatures, proteins, and type of ions [26]. For instance, the rates of these materials at physiological temperatures (37 °C) are higher than those at room temperature. At similar pHs, bovine serum leads to dissolution rates at 37 °C that are 30–40 times higher than those of a phosphate buffer solution for poly-Si, a-Si, and nano-Si. For SiGe, the dissolution rate exhibits an even more strongly accelerated rate (~185 times) in bovine serum. Besides Si and SiGe, dissolution rates of Ge and two-dimensional (2D) MoS_2 materials have also been evaluated in physiological solutions, and the dissolution rates are summarized in Table 3. The dissolution of monolayer MoS_2 crystals in PBS occurs as a defect-induced etching progress, in which the grain boundaries dissolve first, followed by the crystalline regions. Moreover, the increased concentrations of Na^+ and K^+ accelerate the degradation, because the existence of Na^+ or K^+ leads to lattice distortions of MoS_2 and the formation of Na_2S.

Table 2. The dissolution behavior of silicon nanomembranes (Si NMs) under different conditions [22–24,26,44].

Functional Materials	Temperature °C	Aqueous Solution	pH	Doping Type cm^{-3}	Dissolution Rate nm day^{-1}
Mono-Si NMs [24]	37	Phosphate 0.05 M	7.5	10^{17}(p)	2.512
		Phosphate 0.1 M			25.119
		Phosphate 0.5 M			50.119
		Phosphate 1 M			63.096
		Chloride 0.05 M			1.259
		Chloride 0.1 M			6.309
		Chloride 0.5 M			63.096
		Chloride 1 M			63.096
	50	Phosphate 0.05 M	7.5	10^{17}(p)	3.162
		Phosphate 0.1 M			31.623
		Phosphate 0.5 M			125.893
		Phosphate 1 M			251.189
		Chloride 0.05 M			5.012
		Chloride 0.1 M			15.849
		Chloride 0.5 M			199.526
		Chloride 1 M			398.107

Table 2. *Cont.*

Functional Materials	Temperature °C	Aqueous Solution	pH	Doping Type cm^{-3}	Dissolution Rate $nm\ day^{-1}$
Mono-Si NMs [22]	37	Buffer solution 0.1 M	7.4	10^{17}(p) 10^{19}(p) 10^{20}(p)	3.162 3.162 0.501
	37	Buffer solution 0.1 M	7.4	10^{17}(b) 10^{19}(b) 10^{20}(b)	3.162 3.162 0.251
	Room temperature (RT)	Coke	2.6	-	0.600
	RT	Milk	6.4	-	23.300
	RT	PBS 0.1 M	7.4	-	1.820
Mono-Si NMs [23]	37	Bovine serum	7.4	-	100.800
		Sea water	7.8	-	4.115
Mono-Si NMs [44]	37	Albumin phosphate buffered saline (PBS) Na$^+$ Albumin PBS Mg^{2+} Albumin PBS Ca^{2+}	7.4	10^{15}(b)	42.100 45.010 51.000
	20	Purified water	5.5	10^{15}(b) 10^{20}(b)	<0.010 <0.010
	20	Tap water	7.5	10^{15}(b) 10^{20}(b)	0.710 0.420
	37	Serum	7.4	10^{15}(b) 10^{20}(b)	21.020 0.500
	37	Hank's balanced salt solution (HBSS)	7.6	10^{15}(b) 10^{20}(b)	58.010 7.010
	37	HBSS w/Ca, Mg	7.6	10^{15}(b) 10^{20}(b)	66.020 8.020
	37	HBSS	8.2	10^{15}(b) 10^{20}(b)	129.030 58.000
	37	HBSS w/Ca, Mg	8.2	10^{15}(b) 10^{20}(b)	178.000 69.010
	20	Purified water Tap water Serum	5.5 7.5 7.4	10^{15}(b)	0.010 0.720 3.500
	37	Purified water Tap water Sweat Serum HBSS HBSS w/Ca, Mg HBSS HBSS w/Ca, Mg	5.5 7.5 4.5 7.4 7.6 7.6 8.2 8.2	10^{15}(b)	0.210 2.620 0.530 21.000 58.210 66.010 129.020 178.000
poly-Si NMs [26]	RT	Buffer solution	7 7.4 8 10	-	1.020 1.585 10.010 398.107
	37	Buffer solution	7 7.4 8 10	-	1.259 3.162 19.953 562.341
a-Si NMs [26]	RT	Buffer solution	7 7.4 8 10	-	1.778 3.981 15.849 501.187
	37	Buffer solution	7 7.4 8 10	-	1.585 5.011 31.623 630.957

Note: p stands for phosphate doping, and b stands for boron doping.

Table 3. The dissolution behavior of Ge and 2D MoS_2 under different conditions [26,45].

Functional Materials	Temperature °C	Aqueous Solution	pH	Dissolution Rate nm day^{-1}
Ge [26]	RT	Aqueous Buffer solution	7	0.794
			7.4	1.995
			8	15.849
			10	501.187
	37	Aqueous Buffer solution	7	1.259
			7.4	3.162
			8	19.953
			10	562.341
Poly-MoS$_2$ [45]	40	1.0 M PBS	7.4	0.010
			12	0.010
	60	1.0 M PBS	7.4	0.070
			12	0.160
	75	1.0 M PBS	7.4	0.200
			12	0.270
	85	1.0 M PBS	7.4	0.270
			12	0.400

Metals related to trace elements that are normally found in human body, such as Mg, Zn, W, Fe, Mo, and their oxides, are great candidates for interconnects and dielectric materials [23,29,46]. Strain-tolerant metallic thin films can be fabricated by electron-beam deposition, pulsed-laser deposition, or magnetron sputtering, following photolithography. Among them, Mg and Zn are utilized more frequently, owing to the easy processing property and better concentration tolerance for patients, which means lower costs and safer resorbable properties. However, the degradation rates of Mg and Zn are relative fast; metals with slower rates (W, Mo) are, therefore, more desirable if a longer life time is needed [29]. Fe thin films become rusted easily, and they are converted to iron oxides and hydroxides, which have extremely lower solubilities in neutral solutions, and slightly acidic environments are probably more desirable for inducing complete degradation [29].

Moreover, dielectric materials, including magnesium oxide (MgO), silicon dioxide (SiO_2), silicon nitride (Si_3N_4), and spin-on-glass (SOG), are also dissolvable in aqueous solutions. The dissolution rates of these materials depend not only on pHs, temperatures, and ion concentrations, but also on the physical and chemical properties of the films, which are affected by the deposition condition [10,14,47]. For example, the dissolution rates of oxides deposited by electron-beam (e-beam) evaporation are 100 times slower compared to those deposited by plasma-enhanced chemical vapor deposition (PECVD). For nitrides, the dissolution rate of a low-pressure chemical vapor deposition (LPCVD) nitride is slower than that of a PECVD nitride. The degradation rates of metals and dielectric materials are summarized in Tables 4 and 5, respectively.

Table 4. Dissolution behavior of metals [47–51].

Functional Materials	Test Conditions	Dissolution Rate nm day^{-1}	Dissolution Product
Mg [48]	Deionized water, RT	1680.000	$Mg(OH)_2$
Zn [49]	Deionized water, RT	168.000	$Zn(OH)_2$
Fe [47]	Simulated body fluids, 37 °C	5.000–80.000	$Fe(OH)_2$, $Fe(OH)_3$
Mo [50]	Deionized water, RT	7.200	H_2MoO_4
W [51]	Deionized water, RT	7.200–3.000–40.800	H_2WO_4

Table 5. Dissolution behaviors of dielectric materials in buffer solution at 37 °C [10,47].

Functional Materials	Fabrication Methods	Test Conditions	Dissolution Rate nm day^{-1}	Dissolution Product
SiO$_2$ [10]	E-beam	37 °C	10.000	Si(OH)$_4$
	PECVD	37 °C	0.100	
	Thermally grown	37 °C	0.003	
Si$_3$N$_4$ [10]	LPCVD	pH 7.4	0.158	Si(OH)$_4$ + NH$_3$
	LPCVD	pH 8	0.251	
	LPCVD	pH 10	0.316	
	LPCVD	pH 12	0.631	
	PECVD-LF	pH 7.4	0.794	
	PECVD-LF	pH 8	1.585	
	PECVD-LF	pH 10	1.995	
	PECVD-LF	pH 12	3.981	
	PECVD-HF	pH 7.4	0.794	
	PECVD-HF	pH 8	2.512	
	PECVD-HF	pH 10	6.310	
	PECVD-HF	pH 12	25.119	
Spin-on glass (SOG) [47]	cured at 300 °C	PBS, pH 7.4	50.000	Si(OH)$_4$
	cured at 800 °C	PBS, pH 7.4	6.000	

Figure 1a shows the representative flexible circuit based on dissolvable inorganic Si electronic materials on silk substrate, including transistors made by Si/MgO/Mg, diodes made by Si, and inductors and capacitors made by Mg/MgO, as well as resistor and connection wires made by Mg. The related transience properties in the operational characteristics of n-channel transistors are shown on the left side, which are comparable with transistors that are built with non-dissolvable materials. Logic circuits can be built based on the transistor unit cells, which provide a promising path to achieving soft and biodegradable multi-functional Si electronics [14]. Figure 1b illustrates a transient circuit composed of Ga$_2$O$_3$/In$_2$O$_3$/ZnO thin film transistors (TFTs), with transfer performance with widths (W)/lengths (L) (=30/10 µm). The output feature corresponds to a 0 to 10 V gate bias, with a step of 2 V, for 0 to 5 V drain bias (V$_{DS}$) [27], which represents an alternative inorganic semiconductor for soft transient electronics. In Figure 1c, W powders are integrated onto a flexible sodium carboxymethyl cellulose (Na–CMC) substrate to print a temperature sensor circuit with a sensing performance that is closed to the weather report, which indicates an alternative method for quickly achieving biodegradable circuits [28]. Two-dimensional materials, such as MoS$_2$, with attractive optical, electrical, and mechanical properties, have also been explored, to form biodegradable electronics. Figure 1d shows a transient pressure sensor that is integrated with Mo and MoS$_2$ as the functional materials, which can be utilized to prepare a temperature sensor in vivo. Meanwhile, the literature suggests that MoS$_2$ can gradually dissolve in PBS solution (pH = 7.4) at 75 °C, which may be adjusted by changing the grain size [45]. This investigation offers new insights incorporating ultrathin 2D materials for bioresorbable devices.

The biocompatibility of the materials and the products of their dissolution are important for applications in bioresorbable electronics. In vitro cytotoxicity studies on mono-Si, poly-Si, α-Si, SiGe, and Ge, with both neighboring stromal fibroblast cells and infiltrating immune cells, suggest that both of these materials and their dissolution products are biocompatible [26]. In addition, in vivo evaluations of Si NMs implanted into the subdermal regions of an albino, laboratory-bred strain of the house mouse (BALB/c mice), show that following five weeks of implantation, immunoprofiling of lymphocytes from the peripheral blood and draining lymph nodes revealed no significant differences in the percentages of CD4+ and CD8+ T cells for implanted animals and sham-operated controls, which suggests long-term immunological and tissue biocompatibility [23]. Furthermore, an in vitro assessment of cytotoxicity on a patterned array of Si NMs using cells from a metastatic breast cancer cell line (MAD-MB-231), and in vivo toxicity studies by implanting Si NMs on silk in the subdermal region of BALB/c mice, suggest this material is biocompatible, and that it has the potential to be used for long-term implantation [43]. Recently, in vitro cytotoxicity explored on 2D MoS_2 films with L-929 cells and mouse fibroblast cells showed that there is no adverse effect on cell adherence and proliferation in vitro for 24 days. In vivo long-term cytotoxicity and biocompatibility studies with MoS_2 layers implanting subcutaneously into BALB/c mice suggests that MoS_2 does not cause any serious immunological or inflammatory reactions, and that it is, therefore, suitable for long-term biomedical use.

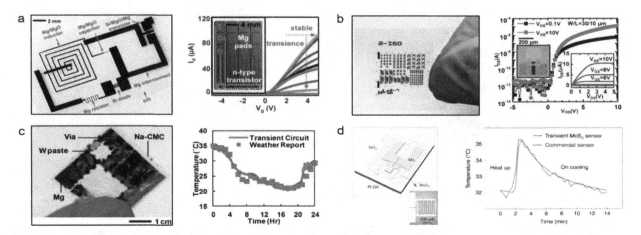

Figure 1. Different functional materials for soft and biodegradable devices. (**a**) Left: The circuit includes Si/MgO/Mg transistors, Si diodes, Mg/MgO inductors, and capacitors, as well as Mg resistors and interconnectors. Right: The transience of the operational characteristics of n-channel transistors. (**b**) Left: Schematic illustrations of transient $Ga_2O_3/In_2O_3/ZnO$ thin film transistors (TFTs) and circuits. Right: Transfer characteristics for $Ga_2O_3/In_2O_3/ZnO$ TFTs with widths (W)/lengths (L) (=30/10 μm). (**c**) Left: A transient printed circuit board (PCB) device with W and Mg for the temperature sensor; Right: Comparison for environmental temperatures measured by a transient circuit and the meteorological system. (**d**) Left: A multifunctional sensor using Mo and MoS_2; Right: Measurement of the intracranial temperature with transient MoS_2 and commercial sensors. Reproduced with permission from [14,27,28,45].

2.2. Organic Functional Materials

Conducting, semiconducting, and dielectric polymers are natural bridges between electronics and soft matter, because the vast chemical design space for polymers allows for the tunability of electronic, mechanical, and transient properties. A general strategy to create dielectric polymers is to incorporate high dielectric constant fills (e.g., SiO_2, aluminum oxide (Al_2O_3), hafnium oxide (HfO_2)) into a polymer matrix [12]. To circumvent the use of inorganic fillers, plant-based fibers (e.g., cotton, jute, bamboo, and banana fibers), sugars (e.g., glucose and lactose), and DNA and its precursors are promising natural polymers that intrinsically possess practical dielectric properties [52–58].

For conducting polymers, conjugated polymers that have been doped into a conducting state are used for device interconnectors and contacts. Common conducting polymers are polypyrrole (PPy), polyanniline (PANI), and poly(3,4-ethylenedioxythiophene) (PEDOT) [59]. One strategy for fabricating biodegradable conducting polymers is to blend conjugated polymers with biodegradable, insulating polymers. It has to be noted that these composites fabricated in this way are partially degradable, which means they are disintegrable, but the conductive polymers parts cannot be fully broken down to their monomers. Fully biodegradable conductive polymers might be obtained by conjugation breaking, but the conductivity of the materials is relatively lower than the partially degradable conductive polymers [12]. In addition, typical semiconducting polymers are polythiophenes (e.g., poly(3-hexylthiophene), P3HT), and diketopyrrolopyrroles (DPP) [60,61].

As with conducting polymers, blending has been utilized to generate partially degradable semiconducting polymers, e.g., by blending poly(3-thiophene methyl acetate) (P3TMA), a derivative of P3HT, with thermoplastic polyurethane (TPU) [62]. Fully degradable polymeric semiconductors have been achieved recently by introducing reversible imine bonds between DPP and p-phenylenediamine [63]. Conjugated molecules found in nature could also be utilized to build biodegradable electronics, including the natural dye indigo from the plants *Indigofera tinctorial* and *Isatis tinctorial* [64], natural pigment melanins [65,66], and β-carotene and anthraquinone derivatives [54,67].

2.3. Substrate Materials

Compared with functional materials, often with thicknesses of a few hundreds of nanometers, substrate materials with thicknesses at the micrometer scale contribute to the majority of the weight. As for soft electronics, substrate materials are a critically important consideration, because their mechanical properties can dominate that of the integrated system. Polymeric materials are often used as flexible substrate materials. Candidate materials need to be compatible with device fabrication processes, which usually involves high temperatures, water, and harsh solvents and, therefore, considerations of material properties centering around thermal stability and solvent compatibility are necessary. Degradation times, swelling rates, mechanical robustness, and the biocompatibility of the substrate materials are also critical to guiding the selection of substrates and, thus, achieving devices with controlled operational timeframes, as well as characteristics that match tissue environments. Although the properties of polymeric substrates vary greatly from material to material, these substrates tend to be flexible and biodegradable.

Based on these requirements, a series of substrate polymeric materials have been explored, which can be classified into natural materials and synthesized polymers. Materials that already exist in the natural environment have been applied as the substrates for biomedical electronics. These materials are biologically derived, which possess affinities and hypo-allergenicities to the human body, such as silk fibroin, cellulose, and chitosan, etc. Silk fibroin protein shows attractive properties that are related to biotechnology and biomedical fields [68–72], and possesses proper mechanical strength, a tunable life time, and minimum immune rejection. The n-channel metal-oxide-semiconductor field-effect transistors (MOSFETs) have been deposited onto thin silk film successfully, as shown in Figure 2a [20]. With similar characteristics, cellulose and chitosan are two other natural substrate materials, as shown in Figures 2b [63] and 2g [73], respectively. As a type of polysaccharide, cellulose is a richly-abundant substance in nature that composes of more than one-third of all plant components, and it even reaches an abundance of 90% in cotton [74]. Cellulose is a promising substrate for biomedical implants, as it takes advantage of attractive biocompatibility properties and degradation in a physiological environment [75–77]. Recently, a novel transistor system using Al_2O_3 as the dielectric layer and Fe as the electrodes, was prepared on ultrathin cellulose film to fabricate transient electronics [63]. In addition, as a derivative product of chitin by the deacetylation process, chitosan is another common substrate for temporary devices with proven biocompatibilities, as shown in Figure 2g [73]. Moreover, some other natural compounds such as potato starch, gelatin, or caramelized glucose have been used as substrates for designing biodegradable electronics [54]. Generally speaking, the dominant advantages of natural substrate materials are favorable, in terms of low-immunoreaction and great abundance, as well as low cost.

However, the intrinsic properties of natural materials limit their applications, as biodegradable electronics draw higher demands for substrates with specific properties relating to stability, mechanical strength, and degradation rate, etc., which promotes research for synthetic polymers [12]. Synthetic polymeric materials have been used in numerous biomedical applications for years, such as in bioresorbable stents and sutures [78–84]. Poly lactic-co-glycolic acid (PLGA) is a typical polymer that is used as a transient substrate, which is a copolymer of poly lactic acid (PLA) and poly glycolic acid (PGA). Compared to natural materials, the lifetime and mechanical strength of PLGA can be modified over a wide range by adjusting the ratio of PLA and PGA, which paves a promising path for biomedical implants with controllable working lives. In Figure 2d, transient complementary metal-oxide-semiconductors (CMOSs) are prepared on PLGA substrates with excellent operational characteristics [85]. Because of the different substrate requirements for biodegradable clinical devices, numerous polymers with different mechanical and disintegration performances are prepared and utilized as elastic substrate layers for soft and transient electronics, such as sodium carboxymethylcellulose (Na–CMC) [86], poly(caprolactone)–poly(glycerol sebacate)(PGS–PCL) [87], and poly(vinyl alcohol) (PVA) [27], etc., as shown in Figure 2c,e,f, respectively. Among them, PVA is a water-soluble polymer that forms flexible layers, which allows for the controlled transport rate of water through altering the crosslinking density of the chains and their subsequent swelling ratios. A recent report suggests that biodegradable elastomer poly (octamethylene maleate (anhydride) citrate) (POMaC) is an excellent candidate for applications in terms of its biocompatibility, mechanical properties, and degradation characteristics, which can be tuned by varying the polymerization conditions [88]. Besides, poly(1,8-octanediol-co-citrate) (POC) is a biodegradable elastomer that can take strains up to ~30% with linear elastic mechanical responses. Hydrogels as hydrophilic polymeric networks with 3D microstructures represent alternative options that are highly biocompatible and suitable for biomimetic applications, due to their water-rich natures and structural similarities to natural extracellular matrices. Moreover, they can be designed to degrade under controlled modes and rates by enzymatic hydrolysis, ester hydrolysis, photolytic cleavage, or a combination of these reactions.

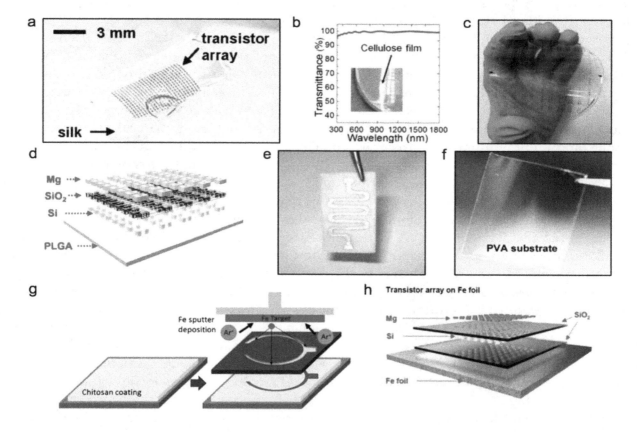

Figure 2. Various soft substrate materials for biodegradable electronics. (**a**) A silk substrate for transistor arrays. (**b**) A cellulose substrate for transistors. (**c**) A sodium carboxymethylcellulose (Na–CMC) bioresorbable substrate for Zn patterns. (**d**) A Poly lactic-co-glycolic acid (PLGA) substrate for transient electronic circuits. (**e**) An electrospun poly(caprolactone)–poly(glycerol sebacate) (PGS–PCL) sheet for a typical conductive pattern. (**f**) A PVA substrate for transient indium–gallium–zinc oxide (a-IGZO) TFTs. (**g**) A chitosan substrate for a biodegradable battery. (**h**) An Fe foil substrate for transistor arrays. Reproduced with permission from [20,27,47,63,85–87].

Although biodegradable polymeric substrates can often offer appropriate mechanical properties for soft and biodegradable electronics, direct device fabrication processed on polymer substrates is quite limited, as most types are sensitive to temperatures, solvents, or water. The swelling of most biodegradable polymers remains another challenge, as it can greatly shorten the functional lifetimes of electronic devices. Novel fabrication processes have been proposed to decouple polymeric substrates from the fabrication processes, which, however, introduce extra multiple fabrication steps; this will be discussed in the next section. Metal foils such as Mo, Fe, W, and Zn have also been proposed as alternatives to polymeric biodegradable substrates, to offer better compatibility with the fabrication process, because they are relatively temperature-resistant, and because they address swelling issues upon deployment in aqueous solutions, as illustrated in Figure 2h [47]. They can also show excellent electrical and thermal properties, favorable water and oxygen isolation performances, and they are relatively resistant to most solvents. However, the rigid properties of metal foils might limit their further applications.

2.4. Encapsulation Materials

Encapsulation materials, together with substrate materials, define the lifetimes of biodegradable electronics. Similarly, most polymeric substrate materials can be used to form strain-tolerant encapsulation layers, preventing rapid degradation of devices, such as PLGA, PCL, etc. [21,89]. Silk fibroin pockets have also been demonstrated to be useful for the controlled modulation of the device lifetime [90]. Similarly, POC can be used not only as the substrate layer, but also as the encapsulation layer, for transient biomedical devices, to protect them from the environment. However, water permeation resistance within biodegradable polymeric materials often cannot satisfy the requirements of devices when a longer lifetime is needed, e.g., an encapsulated Mg trace with silk fibroin could lose its conductivity within a few hours [14]. Encapsulation using a Si membrane (~1.5 μm) has been explored, and it can significantly extend the degradation times of dissolvable metals, e.g., Mg thin films with Si encapsulation result in a lifetime of 60 days in phosphate-buffered saline at 37 °C [44]. Bioresorbable electrocorticography electrodes based on Si encapsulation have demonstrated comparable recording results, compared to conventional standard electrodes, indicating the possibility of using a Si encapsulation layer for biodegradable electronics. In addition, alternating dielectric oxide layers of $SiO_2/Si_3N_4/SiO_2$ has also been proven to possess good water permeation resistance [30]. Further studies are needed to investigate biodegradable encapsulation materials with ultralow water permeation rates, as well as appropriate electrical properties and mechanical flexibilities, to achieve a wider range of operational time frames. Strategies include combining inorganic/organic multilayer materials to improve flexibility, and to introduce smart stimuli-responsive materials to precisely control the starting point of degradation.

3. Fabrication Schemes

Traditional device fabrication often involves photolithography, deposition, and etching processes. For the biomedical application, it is important to note that the implanted bioresorbable electronics require soft properties to realize their conformal contact with organs and tissues. In addition to that, the manufacturing process should not introduce any toxic materials or solvents, to guarantee favorable biocompatibilities. Consequently, novel fabrication techniques are needed to ensure material compatibility with the processing parameters.

For biodegradable devices, substrate materials with thicknesses at the micrometer scale contribute to the majority of the weight. Polymeric materials are often used as the substrates, because of their intrinsically soft and flexible properties, although metal foils have also been explored as an alternative [47]. Polymers are often dissolved into organic solvents and processed into a thin film format by drop casting, spin coating, or electrospinning methods. The thickness of the layer can be controlled by changing the relative solution concentrations, the speed of spin coating, or the electrospinning time [87,91]. The selections of proper solvents, spin-coating, or electrospinning parameters, and the surface treatments of handle substrates are critical to achieving free-standing polymer films with softness for the device fabrication.

The direct deposition of functional materials onto biodegradable and soft substrates, has been achieved through the use of shadow masks [14]. Decoupling fabrication processes from target biodegradable substrates through transfer-printing enables devices with a higher level of integration and more versatile material selections [85]. Figure 3a shows a transfer printing process utilizing foundry-based devices to achieve biodegradable 3D heterogeneous integrated circuits [21]. In order to obtain releasable micro-components from foundry-base wafers, a ~700 nm SiN$_x$ passive layer is deposited by plasma-enhanced chemical-vapor deposition (PECVD), followed by inductively-coupled plasma-reactive ion etching (ICP-RIE) process to form trenches. Poly(dimethylsiloxane) (PDMS) stamps are then utilized in a transfer printing process to remove and deliver the target collections (a total thickness of ~3 μm) onto target PLGA substrates. After that, a PLGA dielectric layer is prepared by the spin casting method, and a standard photolithography technology associated with RIE treatment, creates specific openings to make contact between the upper and lower layers. Another functional layer can then be prepared by applying a repeated procedure to finish the 3D integrated circuit. A combination of foundry-based Si wafers and transfer printing techniques provides a promising route towards high-performance and miniaturized biodegradable electronic systems.

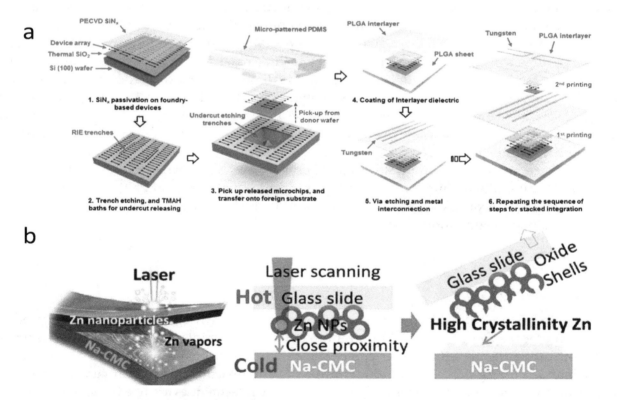

Figure 3. Fabrication schemes for soft and biodegradable electronics. (**a**) Preparation process of a 3D interconnected platform. Planarizing layers of PLGA serve as adhesives and interlayer dielectrics to facilitate 3D heterogeneous integration. (**b**) The schematic printing process for evaporation–condensation-mediated laser printing. Reproduced with permission from [21,86].

Printing techniques of biodegradable materials represent alternative methods to realize quick circuit patterns [46,86,89,92]. Figure 3b illustrates a fabrication approach to manufacture bioresorbable electronics. A continuous-wave (CW) fiber laser is utilized to supply sintering power, so as to crystalize Zn nanoparticles onto a soft Na–CMC substrate directly, with superior conductivity ($\sim$1.124 $\times$ 10^6 S m^{-1}) [86]. Such a fabrication technology offers a direct way for a roll-to-roll preparation platform to produce soft biodegradable electronics with high integration levels and low costs. In addition, highly conductive bioresorbable inks with an extended lifetime, consisting of polyanhydride and dispersed molybdenum microparticles, has also been reported. Such an ink can be applied to flexible wire and connection joints, as well as the antennas of bioresorbable devices [92]. These novel printing processes imply a fast and low-cost way to achieve biodegradable circuits.

4. Representative Soft and Biodegradable Devices for Biomedical Applications

Compared to conventional rigid implants, soft properties are favorable for biomedical implants to ensure conformally wrapping around biosystems that achieve intimate contact and minimize mechanical irritations, which are crucial and necessary for their applications, such as physiological signal detection and drug delivery. Combining biodegradable characteristics, devices can achieve fully bioresorption after usage, eliminating device retrieval. These devices could potentially serve as implantable diagnostic and therapeutic platforms, and they provide unprecedented physiological information and treatments, which are especially valuable for temporal biological processes, such as wound healing, neural network mapping, drug delivery, tissue regeneration, etc. Demonstrated soft and biodegradable electronic implants and pertinent power supply solutions will be reviewed in the following sections.

4.1. Diagnostic Platforms

For diagnostic purposes, because of their close connection with tissues and organs, soft transient electronics can detect abnormal physiological signals sensitively and precisely, even at the early stages of specific diseases, before they can be observed by conventional equipment, which is important for human healthcare and follow-up therapy. Figure 4 shows a soft and high-resolution recording system for electrocorticography (ECoG) based on Si devices [30], which offers a potential utility for treating neural disorders where biodegradation is required, to avoid tissue injury upon device removal. The flexible platform also enables the intimate contact of the device with the cerebral cortex, and allows for high-fidelity data recording. Figure 4a illustrates the structure of the device, consisting of a flexible PLGA substrate ($\sim$30 μm), a Si nanomembrane semiconductor, a Mo electrode ($\sim$300 nm), a SiO$_2$ gate dielectric, and SiO$_2$ ($\sim$300 nm)/Si$_3$N$_4$ ($\sim$400 nm)/SiO$_2$ ($\sim$300 nm) interlayer dielectrics. The device includes 128 metal oxide-semiconductor field-effect transistors (MOSFETs). Figure 4b exhibits the optical images of the unit cells of the device at different stages of fabrication, and a complete system. Figure 4c represents the linear (red) and log-scale (blue) transfer curves for representative n-channel MOSFET indication, with the mobility and on/off ratio of $\sim$400 cm^2 V^{-1} and $\sim$10^8, respectively. The device is implanted onto the whisker area, and Figure 4d reveals the schematic illustration of the whisker stimulation locations in a rat model. By stimulating the defined positions, the related evoked potential in a spatial distribution is recorded, as given in Figure 4e, indicating high resolution mapping of ECoG that matches or exceeds any existing devices. The sensing system can completely dissolve into an aqueous buffer solution gradually at pH = 12 and at 37 $^\circ$C, as shown in Figure 4f. The sensitive sensing and biodegradable features of this transient device offer a promising application for internal physiological signal collection, which is significantly important for disease diagnosis.

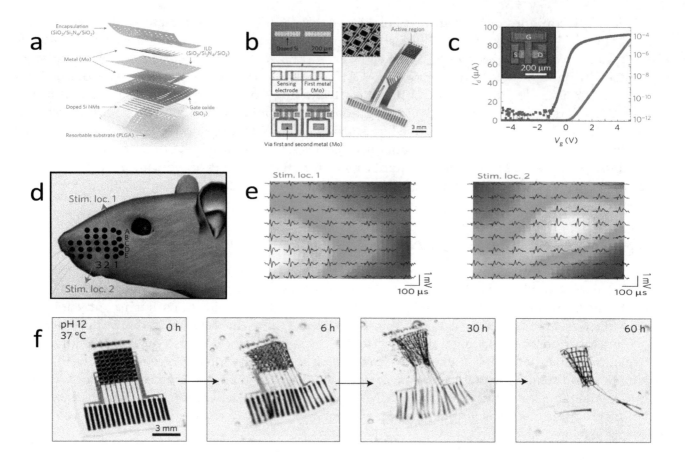

Figure 4. A soft and biodegradable neural electrode array sensor. (**a**) The schematic structure of an actively multiplexed sensing system for high-resolution electrocorticography. (**b**) Left: Optical micrograph images of a pair of subunits for the fabrication process. Right: The entire complete system. (**c**) Linear (red) and log scale (blue) transfer curves for a representative n-channel, MOSFET. (**d**) Schematic illustration of the whisker stimulation locations 1 and 2 (B1 and E3) in a rat model. (**e**) Left: Spatial distribution of the potentials evoked by the stimulation location B1. Right: Spatial distribution of the potentials evoked by stimulation location E3. (**f**) The degradation process at various stages of the sensor. Reproduced with permission from [30].

Stretchable and biodegradable pressure and strain sensors have also been reported for real-time monitoring for potential tendon recovery [88]. Figure 5a,b show the vertical structure and optical images of the sensor, respectively. The entire sensor is divided into four parts, including bottom and top encapsulation layers, as well as strain- and pressure-sensing areas, with Mg as the electrode, POMaC as the stretchable packaging layer, Poly(lactic acid) (PLLA) as the substrate, and PGS as the stretchable dielectric layer. Such a design allows for independent measurements of the strain and pressure. The sensor is implanted onto the back of a Sprague Dawley rat, as shown in Figure 5c. Figure 5d,e illustrate the collected pressure and strain signals after implantation for 2 and 3.5 weeks; the similar curves indicate a stable working performance. The biocompatibility of the sensor is demonstrated in Figure 5f, with CD68 positive cells decreasing gradually as the implantation period extends, suggesting that the inflammatory reaction is mitigated and, therefore, that excellent biocompatibility is reached. After more than two weeks of implantation, this sensor begins to degrade gradually. This research demonstrates the potential use of biodegradable devices for orthopedic applications.

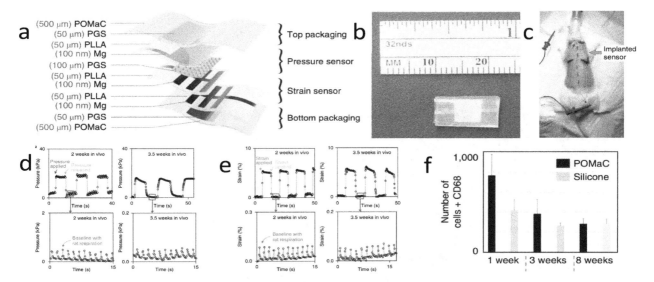

Figure 5. A stretchable and biodegradable strain and pressure sensor for orthopedic application. (**a**) Schematic diagram of the sensor space structure. (**b**) Optical image of the sensor. (**c**) The location of the implantable sensor. (**d**) Pressure signal detection two and 3.5 weeks after sensor implantation. (**e**) Strain signal detection two and 3.5 weeks after sensor implantation. (**f**) Results of immunohistochemistry. Reproduced with permission from [88].

4.2. Therapeutic Devices

In addition to diagnostic functions, soft and biodegradable electronics could also play an important role in therapeutic processes. For therapeutic platforms, flexible and biodegradable devices can offer personalized and precision treatments based on controlled performance and degradation rates. Bioresorbable devices can combine with drug delivery vehicles to achieve controlled drug release systems, which are critical for disease treatments.

The soft format of the sensor is favorable for controlled drug release with precise doses to specific areas, because of the conformal contact with tissues, which can improve treatment efficacy. Figure 6a displays the structure of a drug delivery system with a 2 × 2 array, consisting of inductive coupling coils and serpentine thermal heaters on a PLGA substrate [93]. The device allows for heating of the drug storage area through external wireless controls by inductive coupling. Drug release is thermally triggered by the phase transition of lipid layers imbedded with drugs. Figure 6b (left) shows the total cumulative percentage of doxorubicin released as a function of time from a device that is immersed in deionized water (12 mL) when it is activated by wireless external power between 0.1 to 1.3 W at 12.5 MHz and a distance of 2 mm. The release rate of the drug can be adjusted by adjusting the supplied power. Figure 6b (right) represents cumulative amounts of doxorubicin that are released wirelessly once a day, indicating good temperature-controlled drug release.

Wireless thermal therapy of bacterial management has also been demonstrated to assist with wound healing. Previous studies have revealed that some bacteria are highly sensitive to environmental changes, and that an increase in temperature lowers their survival [94–96]. Figure 6c (left) shows a transient radio frequency (RF) device for thermal therapy based on the Mg heater, embedded between silk fibroin layers [97]. Figure 6c (right) reveals related implantation processes for rats. The rats are infected by *Staphylococcus aureus* (*S. aureus*) with a subcutaneous injection (~5 μL) at the device implantation site, to mimic surgical site infections. The experimental rats are divided into untreated, low power (100 mW), and high power (500 mW) groups. Figure 6d (left) shows a thermal image of a rat with a high power supply after 10 min heat treatments, with the temperature reaching 49 °C. The infected tissues were collected after 24 h, and assessed by counting the normalized number of colony-forming units in the homogenates (n = 3) using standard plate-counting methods, and the related results are shown in Figure 6d (right). It is obvious that thermal treatment achieves a better bactericidal effect with higher temperatures. The concept of a biodegradable thermal therapy device can be widely applied to eliminate temperature-sensitive bacteria, which could be crucial to promoting the wound healing process.

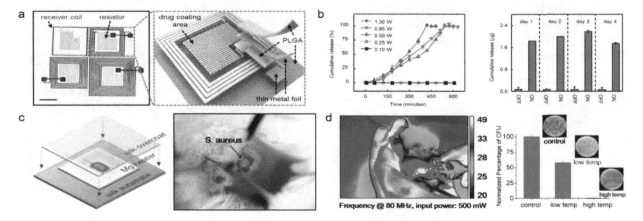

Figure 6. A thermally triggered drug delivery transient device and a radio frequency-controlled thermal therapy platform. (**a**) Images of the device structure. (**b**) Left: Cumulative release of doxorubicin from the device, operated with wireless power. Right: Controllable doxorubicin release from the device over 1 day on/off cycles. (**c**) Left: The schematic illustration of the radio frequency thermal therapy platform. Right: Photo of a device implanted in BALB/c mice. (**d**) Left: The thermal image of the device position while wirelessly powering the device. Right: The normalized number of colony-forming units after 24 h with different levels of input power. Reproduced with permission from [93,97].

4.3. Power Supply

Power supply is an essential component for biodegradable electronic systems, and great efforts have been made to explore biodegradable power sources, including batteries [98–102], supercapacitors [9], photovoltaic devices [103], radio frequency (RF) power scavengers [104], piezoelectric harvesters [25], etc. For biomedical applications, the power device should be flexible, stretchable, and miniaturized, to realize conformal contact and to minimize mechanical irritation.

A flexible and biodegradable RF wireless energy harvester appears in Figure 7a–d. Figure 7a,b illustrates the schematic structure of a wireless RF power transmitter, which consists of an RF antenna, an inductor, six capacitors, a resistor, and eight diodes [104]. By integrating with an Mg antenna, the RF system is capable of transmitting enough power to light up a red LED, as shown in Figure 7c. The entire system degrades rapidly in deionized water, as shown in Figure 7d. The demonstrated system provides a route for wireless energy harvesting for biodegradable implants; however, the current device volume limits its usage, and it needs further improvement. Figure 7e exhibits a flexible and biodegradable piezoelectric energy harvester based on ZnO on a silk substrate [25]. By bending the integrated film repeatedly, an output potential of 1.14 V, and curves of 0.55 nA are obtained, as shown in Figure 7f. Figure 7g illustrates the theoretical shape for the buckling of a device under compression. Although the piezoelectric energy harvester does not rely on an external device such as that for an RF energy scavenger, mechanical deformation inside the body is limited and, therefore, this limits the available power that can be obtained.

In summary, although various power solutions have been proposed, the performance of soft and biodegradable power supplies still remains an obstacle. The power density and the working life of the device should be further improved to satisfy the requirements of various biodegradable electronic systems. Materials and fabrication methods for power devices should also be advanced to achieve miniaturized, flexible, and stretchable platforms that are suitable as biomedical implants.

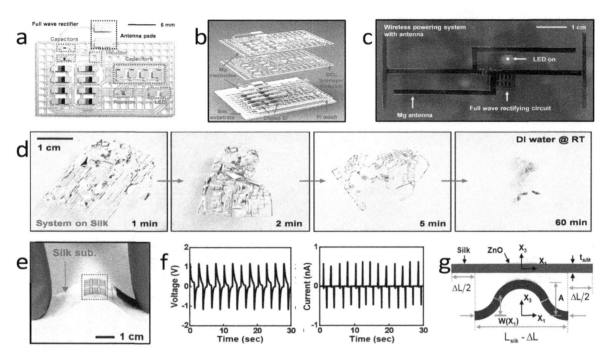

Figure 7. Flexible and biodegradable power harvesters. (**a**) A schematic illustration of transient RF power scavenging circuits. (**b**) A schematic illustration of an exploded view of the device. (**c**) An image of the device powered wirelessly with an RF transmitter and an Mg-receiving antenna. (**d**) Degradation process of the RF power harvester (**e**) Image of a soft and transient ZnO mechanical energy harvester on a silk substrate. (**f**) Output voltage and current ability during cycles of bending. (**g**) The theoretical shape for the buckling of a device under compression. Reproduced with permission from [25,104].

5. Summary and Outlook

As an emerging field, soft and biodegradable electronics have attracted more and more research interest because of their foreseeable applications for clinical implants, eco-friendly devices, and security hardware. For biodegradable biomedical devices, favorable biocompatibility, appropriate degradable rates, and robust mechanical properties, as well as superior performance, are desirable. Many studies have been made, to achieve remarkable progress towards biomedical applications.

However, there are still many issues that need to be addressed. More versatile materials with both biodegradable and soft properties need to be explored, to further broaden potential applications. For example, biodegradable functional materials that are highly stretchable and flexible could expand suitable implantation locations and significantly improve data recording sensitivities and accuracies, and minimize the irritation and inflammation that are associated with implantation. This could be achieved by developing composite structures that integrate hard and soft components, as well as through appropriate mechanical structure designs. Moreover, encapsulation materials with superior water resistance and soft properties are critical for waterproof sealing, to avoid the potential rupture of the encapsulation layer causing water leakage. Different from the fabrication methods for rigid biodegradable devices, novel fabrication technologies should be further explored to produce soft electronics with low costs and easy manufacturing procedures, as well as high levels of integration. In addition, the performance of soft devices, such as fast response and excellent sensitivity, as well as high accuracy, needs further improvement, and multifunctional electronics should be fabricated to meet the requirements of clinical standards. A comprehensive investigation of the device/tissue interface, and the metabolic processes of degradation products are also necessary to clarify the safety issues of biodegradable devices. These studies will improve the overall performance of soft and biodegradable devices, and they will promote the development of transient electronics, which could potentially make disease diagnosis and treatments more precise, effective, and intelligent.

Author Contributions: Literature search, R.L. & L.W.; Figures, R.L.; Tables, L.W.; Writing-Review & Editing, R.L. & L.W.; R.L. and L.W. contributed equally to the paper. Conceptualization & Writing, L.Y.

Acknowledgments: This work was supported by the National Natural Science Foundation of China (NSFC) 51601103 (L.Y.), 1000 Youth Talents Program in China (L.Y.), and the China Postdoctoral Science Foundation 2017M620769 (R.L.).

References

1. Dubal, D.P.; Chodankar, N.R.; Kim, D.H.; Gomez-Romero, P. Towards flexible solid-state supercapacitors for smart and wearable electronics. *Chem. Soc. Rev.* **2018**, *47*, 2065–2129. [CrossRef] [PubMed]
2. Annapureddy, V.; Na, S.M.; Hwang, G.T.; Kang, M.G.; Sriramdas, R.; Palneedi, H.; Yoon, W.H.; Hahn, B.D.; Kim, J.W.; Ahn, C.W.; et al. Exceeding milli-watt powering magneto-mechano-electric generator for standalone-powered electronics. *Energy Environ. Sci.* **2018**, *11*, 818–829. [CrossRef]
3. Salauddin, M.; Toyabur, R.M.; Maharjan, P.; Park, J.Y. High performance human-induced vibration driven hybrid energy harvester for powering portable electronics. *Nano Energy* **2018**, *45*, 236–246. [CrossRef]
4. Wang, S.H.; Xu, J.; Wang, W.C.; Wang, G.J.N.; Rastak, R.; Molina-Lopez, F.; Chung, J.W.; Niu, S.M.; Feig, V.R.; Lopez, J.; et al. Skin electronics from scalable fabrication of an intrinsically stretchable transistor array. *Nature* **2018**, *555*, 83–99. [CrossRef] [PubMed]
5. Falco, A.; Rivadeneyra, A.; Loghin, F.C.; Salmeron, J.F.; Lugli, P.; Abdelhalim, A. Towards low-power electronics: Self-recovering and flexible gas sensors. *J. Mater. Chem. A* **2018**, *6*, 7107–7113. [CrossRef]
6. Li, R.F.; Wang, L.; Kong, D.Y.; Yin, L. Recent progress on biodegradable materials and transient electronics. *Bioact. Mater.* **2018**, *3*, 322–333. [CrossRef] [PubMed]
7. Gao, Y.; Zhang, Y.; Wang, X.; Sim, K.; Liu, J.S.; Chen, J.; Feng, X.; Xu, H.X.; Yu, C.J. Moisture-triggered physically transient electronics. *Sci. Adv.* **2017**, *3*, e1701222. [CrossRef] [PubMed]
8. Yoon, J.; Lee, J.; Choi, B.; Lee, D.; Kim, D.H.; Kim, D.M.; Moon, D.I.; Lim, M.; Kim, S.; Choi, S.J. Flammable carbon nanotube transistors on a nitrocellulose paper substrate for transient electronics. *Nano Res.* **2017**, *10*, 87–96. [CrossRef]
9. Lee, G.; Kang, S.K.; Won, S.M.; Gutruf, P.; Jeong, Y.R.; Koo, J.; Lee, S.S.; Rogers, J.A.; Ha, J.S. Fully Biodegradable Microsupercapacitor for Power Storage in Transient Electronics. *Adv. Energy Mater.* **2017**, *7*, 1700157. [CrossRef]
10. Kang, S.-K.; Hwang, S.-W.; Cheng, H.; Yu, S.; Kim, B.H.; Kim, J.-H.; Huang, Y.; Rogers, J.A. Dissolution Behaviors and Applications of Silicon Oxides and Nitrides in Transient Electronics. *Adv. Funct. Mater.* **2014**, *24*, 4427–4434. [CrossRef]
11. Khanra, S.; Cipriano, T.; Lam, T.; White, T.A.; Fileti, E.E.; Alves, W.A.; Guha, S. Self-Assembled Peptide-Polyfluorene Nanocomposites for Biodegradable Organic Electronics. *Adv. Mater. Interfaces* **2015**, *2*, 1500265. [CrossRef]
12. Feig, V.R.; Tran, H.; Bao, Z.N. Biodegradable Polymeric Materials in Degradable Electronic Devices. *ACS Cent. Sci.* **2018**, *4*, 337–348. [CrossRef] [PubMed]
13. Kang, S.K.; Koo, J.; Lee, Y.K.; Rogers, J.A. Advanced Materials and Devices for Bioresorbable Electronics. *Acc. Chem. Res.* **2018**, *51*, 988–998. [CrossRef] [PubMed]
14. Hwang, S.W.; Tao, H.; Kim, D.H.; Cheng, H.Y.; Song, J.K.; Rill, E.; Brenckle, M.A.; Panilaitis, B.; Won, S.M.; Kim, Y.S.; et al. A Physically Transient Form of Silicon Electronics. *Science* **2012**, *337*, 1640–1644. [CrossRef] [PubMed]
15. Kang, S.K.; Murphy, R.K.J.; Hwang, S.W.; Lee, S.M.; Harburg, D.V.; Krueger, N.A.; Shin, J.H.; Gamble, P.; Cheng, H.Y.; Yu, S.; et al. Bioresorbable silicon electronic sensors for the brain. *Nature* **2016**, *530*, 71. [CrossRef] [PubMed]
16. Irimia-Vladu, M.; Glowacki, E.D.; Voss, G.; Bauer, S.; Sariciftci, N.S. Green and biodegradable electronics. *Mater. Today* **2012**, *15*, 340–346. [CrossRef]

17. Park, C.W.; Kang, S.K.; Hernandez, H.L.; Kaitz, J.A.; Wie, D.S.; Shin, J.; Lee, O.P.; Sottos, N.R.; Moore, J.S.; Rogers, J.A.; et al. Thermally Triggered Degradation of Transient Electronic Devices. *Adv. Mater.* **2015**, *27*, 3783–3788. [CrossRef] [PubMed]

18. Hernandez, H.L.; Kang, S.K.; Lee, O.P.; Hwang, S.W.; Kaitz, J.A.; Inci, B.; Park, C.W.; Chung, S.J.; Sottos, N.R.; Moore, J.S.; et al. Triggered Transience of Metastable Poly(phthalaldehyde) for Transient Electronics. *Adv. Mater.* **2014**, *26*, 7637–7642. [CrossRef] [PubMed]

19. Kim, D.H.; Lu, N.S.; Ma, R.; Kim, Y.S.; Kim, R.H.; Wang, S.D.; Wu, J.; Won, S.M.; Tao, H.; Islam, A.; et al. Epidermal Electronics. *Science* **2011**, *333*, 838–843. [CrossRef] [PubMed]

20. Hwang, S.W.; Kim, D.H.; Tao, H.; Kim, T.I.; Kim, S.; Yu, K.J.; Panilaitis, B.; Jeong, J.W.; Song, J.K.; Omenetto, F.G.; et al. Materials and Fabrication Processes for Transient and Bioresorbable High-Performance Electronics. *Adv. Funct. Mater.* **2013**, *23*, 4087–4093. [CrossRef]

21. Chang, J.K.; Chang, H.P.; Guo, Q.; Koo, J.; Wu, C.I.; Rogers, J.A. Biodegradable Electronic Systems in 3D, Heterogeneously Integrated Formats. *Adv. Mater.* **2018**, *30*, 1704955. [CrossRef] [PubMed]

22. Hwang, S.-W.; Park, G.; Edwards, C.; Corbin, E.A.; Kang, S.-K.; Cheng, H.; Song, J.-K.; Kim, J.-H.; Yu, S.; Ng, J.; et al. Dissolution Chemistry and Biocompatibility of Single-Crystalline Silicon Nanomembranes and Associated Materials for Transient Electronics. *ACS Nano* **2014**, *8*, 5843–5851. [CrossRef] [PubMed]

23. Hwang, S.W.; Park, G.; Cheng, H.; Song, J.K.; Kang, S.K.; Yin, L.; Kim, J.H.; Omenetto, F.G.; Huang, Y.G.; Lee, K.M.; et al. 25th Anniversary Article: Materials for High-Performance Biodegradable Semiconductor Devices. *Adv. Mater.* **2014**, *26*, 1992–2000. [CrossRef] [PubMed]

24. Yin, L.; Farimani, A.B.; Min, K.; Vishal, N.; Lam, J.; Lee, Y.K.; Aluru, N.R.; Rogers, J.A. Mechanisms for hydrolysis of silicon nanomembranes as used in bioresorbable electronics. *Adv. Mater.* **2015**, *27*, 1857–1864. [CrossRef] [PubMed]

25. Dagdeviren, C.; Hwang, S.W.; Su, Y.W.; Kim, S.; Cheng, H.Y.; Gur, O.; Haney, R.; Omenetto, F.G.; Huang, Y.G.; Rogers, J.A. Transient, Biocompatible Electronics and Energy Harvesters Based on ZnO. *Small* **2013**, *9*, 3398–3404. [CrossRef] [PubMed]

26. Kang, S.K.; Park, G.; Kim, K.; Hwang, S.W.; Cheng, H.Y.; Shin, J.H.; Chung, S.J.; Kim, M.; Yin, L.; Lee, J.C.; et al. Dissolution Chemistry and Biocompatibility of Silicon- and Germanium-Based Semiconductors for Transient Electronics. *ACS Appl. Mater. Interfaces* **2015**, *7*, 9297–9305. [CrossRef] [PubMed]

27. Jin, S.H.; Kang, S.K.; Cho, I.T.; Han, S.Y.; Chung, H.U.; Lee, D.J.; Shin, J.; Baek, G.W.; Kim, T.I.; Lee, J.H.; et al. Water-Soluble Thin Film Transistors and Circuits Based on Amorphous Indium-Gallium-Zinc Oxide. *ACS Appl. Mater. Interfaces* **2015**, *7*, 8268–8274. [CrossRef] [PubMed]

28. Huang, X.; Liu, Y.H.; Hwang, S.W.; Kang, S.K.; Patnaik, D.; Cortes, J.F.; Rogers, J.A. Biodegradable Materials for Multilayer Transient Printed Circuit Boards. *Adv. Mater.* **2014**, *26*, 7371–7377. [CrossRef] [PubMed]

29. Yin, L.; Cheng, H.; Mao, S.; Haasch, R.; Liu, Y.; Xie, X.; Hwang, S.-W.; Jain, H.; Kang, S.-K.; Su, Y.; et al. Dissolvable Metals for Transient Electronics. *Adv. Funct. Mater.* **2014**, *24*, 645–658. [CrossRef]

30. Yu, K.J.; Kuzum, D.; Hwang, S.W.; Kim, B.H.; Juul, H.; Kim, N.H.; Won, S.M.; Chiang, K.; Trumpis, M.; Richardson, A.G.; et al. Bioresorbable silicon electronics for transient spatiotemporal mapping of electrical activity from the cerebral cortex. *Nat. Mater.* **2016**, *15*, 782. [CrossRef] [PubMed]

31. Institute of Medicine (US) Panel on Micronutrients. *Dietary Reference Intakes for Vitamin A, Vitamin K, Arsenic, Boron, Chromium, Copper, Iodine, Iron, Manganese, Molybdenum, Nickel, Silicon, Vanadium, and Zinc*; A Report of the Panel on Micronutrients, Subcommittees on Upper Reference Levels of Nutrients and of Interpretation and Uses of Dietary Reference Intakes, and the Standing Committee on the Scientific Evaluation of Dietary Reference Intakes; National Academy Press: Washington, DC, USA, 2001.

32. Ysart, G.; Miller, P.; Crews, H.; Robb, P.; Baxter, M.; De L'Argy, C.; Lofthouse, S.; Sargent, C.; Harrison, N. Dietary exposure estimates of 30 elements from the UK Total Diet Study. *Food Addit. Contam.* **1999**, *16*, 391–403. [CrossRef] [PubMed]

33. Millour, S.; Noel, L.; Chekri, R.; Vastel, C.; Kadar, A.; Sirot, V.; Leblanc, J.C.; Guerin, T. Strontium, silver, tin, iron, tellurium, gallium, germanium, barium and vanadium levels in foodstuffs from the Second French Total Diet Study. *J. Food Compos. Anal.* **2012**, *25*, 108–129. [CrossRef]

34. Tao, S.H.; Bolger, P.M. Hazard assessment of germanium supplements. *Regul. Toxicol. Pharm.* **1997**, *25*, 211–219. [CrossRef] [PubMed]

35. James, B.; Zhang, W.L.; Sun, P.; Wu, M.Y.; Li, H.H.; Khaliq, M.A.; Jayasuriya, P.; James, S.; Wang, G. Tungsten (W) bioavailability in paddy rice soils and its accumulation in rice (*Oryza sativa*). *Int. J. Environ. Health Res.* **2017**, *27*, 487–497. [CrossRef] [PubMed]

36. Institute of Medicine (US) Standing Committee on the Scientific Evaluation of Dietary Reference Intakes. *Dietary Reference Intakes for Calcium, Phosphorus, Magnesium, Vitamin D, and Fluoride*; National Academy Press: Washington, DC, USA, 1997.

37. Rogers, J.A.; Lagally, M.G.; Nuzzo, R.G. Synthesis, assembly and applications of semiconductor nanomembranes. *Nature* **2011**, *477*, 45–53. [CrossRef] [PubMed]

38. Hofmann, S.; Ducati, C.; Neill, R.J.; Piscanec, S.; Ferrari, A.C.; Geng, J.; Dunin-Borkowski, R.E.; Robertson, J. Gold catalyzed growth of silicon nanowires by plasma enhanced chemical vapor deposition. *J. Appl. Phys.* **2003**, *94*, 6005–6012. [CrossRef]

39. Guo, X.L.; Tabata, H.; Kawai, T. Pulsed laser reactive deposition of p-type ZnO film enhanced by an electron cyclotron resonance source. *J. Cryst. Growth* **2001**, *223*, 135–139. [CrossRef]

40. Schropp, R.E.I.; Feenstra, K.E.; Molenbroek, E.C.; Meiling, H.; Rath, J.K. Device-quality polycrystalline and amorphous silicon films by hot-wire chemical vapour deposition. *Philos. Mag. B* **1997**, *76*, 309–321. [CrossRef]

41. Lee, W.J.; Park, W.T.; Park, S.; Sung, S.; Noh, Y.Y.; Yoon, M.H. Large-Scale Precise Printing of Ultrathin Sol-Gel Oxide Dielectrics for Directly Patterned Solution-Processed Metal Oxide Transistor Arrays. *Adv. Mater.* **2015**, *27*, 5043–5048. [CrossRef] [PubMed]

42. Kim, D.H.; Ghaffari, R.; Lu, N.S.; Rogers, J.A. Flexible and Stretchable Electronics for Biointegrated Devices. *Annu. Rev. Biomed. Eng.* **2012**, *14*, 113–128. [CrossRef] [PubMed]

43. Ahn, J.H.; Kim, H.S.; Lee, K.J.; Jeon, S.; Kang, S.J.; Sun, Y.G.; Nuzzo, R.G.; Rogers, J.A. Heterogeneous three-dimensional electronics by use of printed semiconductor nanomaterials. *Science* **2006**, *314*, 1754–1757. [CrossRef] [PubMed]

44. Lee, Y.K.; Yu, K.J.; Song, E.M.; Farimani, A.B.; Vitale, F.; Xie, Z.Q.; Yoon, Y.; Kim, Y.; Richardson, A.; Luan, H.W.; et al. Dissolution of Monocrystalline Silicon Nanomembranes and Their Use as Encapsulation Layers and Electrical Interfaces in Water-Soluble Electronics. *ACS Nano* **2017**, *11*, 12562–12572. [CrossRef] [PubMed]

45. Chen, X.; Park, Y.J.; Kang, M.; Kang, S.K.; Koo, J.; Shinde, S.M.; Shin, J.; Jeon, S.; Park, G.; Yan, Y.; et al. CVD-grown monolayer MoS2 in bioabsorbable electronics and biosensors. *Nat. Commun.* **2018**, *9*, 1690. [CrossRef] [PubMed]

46. Mahajan, B.K.; Yu, X.W.; Shou, W.; Pan, H.; Huang, X. Mechanically Milled Irregular Zinc Nanoparticles for Printable Bioresorbable Electronics. *Small* **2017**, *13*, 1700065. [CrossRef] [PubMed]

47. Kang, S.-K.; Hwang, S.-W.; Yu, S.; Seo, J.-H.; Corbin, E.A.; Shin, J.; Wie, D.S.; Bashir, R.; Ma, Z.; Rogers, J.A. Biodegradable Thin Metal Foils and Spin-On Glass Materials for Transient Electronics. *Adv. Funct. Mater.* **2015**, *25*, 1789–1797. [CrossRef]

48. Kirkland, N.T.; Birbilis, N.; Staiger, M.P. Assessing the corrosion of biodegradable magnesium implants: A critical review of current methodologies and their limitations. *Acta Biomater.* **2012**, *8*, 925–936. [CrossRef] [PubMed]

49. Bowen, P.K.; Drelich, J.; Goldman, J. Zinc Exhibits Ideal Physiological Corrosion Behavior for Bioabsorbable Stents. *Adv. Mater.* **2013**, *25*, 2577–2582. [CrossRef] [PubMed]

50. Badawy, W.A.; Al-Kharafi, F.M. Corrosion and passivation behaviors of molybdenum in aqueous solutions of different pH. *Electrochim. Acta* **1998**, *44*, 693–702. [CrossRef]

51. Patrick, E.; Orazem, M.E.; Sanchez, J.C.; Nishida, T. Corrosion of tungsten microelectrodes used in neural recording applications. *J. Neurosci. Meth.* **2011**, *198*, 158–171. [CrossRef] [PubMed]

52. Hemstreet, J.M. Dielectric constant of cotton. *J. Electrost.* **1982**, *13*, 345–353. [CrossRef]

53. Jayamani, E.; Hamdan, S.; Rahman, M.R.; Bin Bakri, M.K. Comparative Study of Dielectric Properties of Hybrid Natural Fiber Composites. *Procedia Eng.* **2014**, *97*, 536–544. [CrossRef]

54. Irimia-Vladu, M.; Troshin, P.A.; Reisinger, M.; Shmygleva, L.; Kanbur, Y.; Schwabegger, G.; Bodea, M.; Schwodiauer, R.; Mumyatov, A.; Fergus, J.W.; et al. Biocompatible and Biodegradable Materials for Organic Field-Effect Transistors. *Adv. Funct. Mater.* **2010**, *20*, 4069–4076. [CrossRef]

55. Singh, T.B.; Sariciftci, N.S.; Grote, J.G. Bio-Organic Optoelectronic Devices Using DNA. *Org. Electron.* **2010**, *223*, 189–212.

56. Yumusak, C.; Singh, T.B.; Sariciftci, N.S.; Grote, J.G. Bioorganic field effect transistors based on crosslinked deoxyribonucleic acid (DNA) gate dielectric. *Appl. Phys. Lett.* **2009**, *95*, 263304. [CrossRef]

57. Singh, B.; Sariciftci, N.S.; Grote, J.G.; Hopkins, F.K. Bioorganic-semiconductor-field-effect-transistor based on deoxyribonucleic acid gate dielectric. *J. Appl. Phys.* **2006**, *100*, 024514. [CrossRef]

58. Wang, L.; Yoshida, J.; Ogata, N.; Sasaki, S.; Kajiyama, T. Self-Assembled Supramolecular Films Derived from Marine Deoxyribonucleic Acid (DNA)—Cationic Surfactant Complexes: Large-Scale Preparation and Optical and Thermal Properties. *Chem. Mater.* **2001**, *13*, 1273–1281. [CrossRef]

59. Worfolk, B.J.; Andrews, S.C.; Park, S.; Reinspach, J.; Liu, N.; Toney, M.F.; Mannsfeld, S.C.; Bao, Z.N. Ultrahigh electrical conductivity in solutionsheared polymeric transparent films. *Proc. Natl. Acad. Sci. USA* **2015**, *112*, 14138–14143. [CrossRef] [PubMed]

60. Qiao, Y.L.; Guo, Y.L.; Yu, C.M.; Zhang, F.J.; Xu, W.; Liu, Y.Q.; Zhu, D.B. Diketopyrrolopyrrole-Containing Quinoidal Small Molecules for High-Performance, Air-Stable, and Solution-Processable n-Channel Organic Field-Effect Transistors. *J. Am. Chem. Soc.* **2012**, *134*, 4084–4087. [CrossRef] [PubMed]

61. Chen, H.J.; Guo, Y.L.; Yu, G.; Zhao, Y.; Zhang, J.; Gao, D.; Liu, H.T.; Liu, Y.Q. Highly p-Extended Copolymers with Diketopyrrolopyrrole Moieties for High-Performance Field-Effect Transistors. *Adv. Mater.* **2012**, *24*, 4618–4622. [CrossRef] [PubMed]

62. Madrigal, M.M.P.; Giannotti, M.I.; Oncins, G.; Franco, L.; Armelin, E.; Puiggali, J.; Sanz, F.; del Valle, L.J.; Aleman, C. Bioactive nanomembranes of semiconductor polythiophene and thermoplastic polyurethane: Thermal, nanostructural and nanomechanical properties. *Polym. Chem.* **2013**, *4*, 568–583. [CrossRef]

63. Lei, T.; Guan, M.; Liu, J.; Lin, H.C.; Pfattner, R.; Shaw, L.; McGuire, A.F.; Huang, T.C.; Shao, L.L.; Cheng, K.T.; et al. Biocompatible and totally disintegrable semiconducting polymer for ultrathin and ultralightweight transient electronics. *Proc. Natl. Acad. Sci. USA* **2017**, *114*, 5107–5112. [CrossRef] [PubMed]

64. Irimia-Vladu, M.; Glowacki, E.D.; Troshin, P.A.; Schwabegger, G.; Leonat, L.; Susarova, D.K.; Krystal, O.; Ullah, M.; Kanbur, Y.; Bodea, M.A.; et al. Indigo—A Natural Pigment for High Performance Ambipolar Organic Field Effect Transistors and Circuits. *Adv. Mater.* **2012**, *24*, 375–380. [CrossRef] [PubMed]

65. Mostert, A.B.; Powell, B.J.; Pratt, F.L.; Hanson, G.R.; Sarna, T.; Gentle, I.R.; Meredith, P. Role of semiconductivity and ion transport in the electrical conduction of melanin. *Proc. Natl. Acad. Sci. USA* **2012**, *109*, 8943–8947. [CrossRef] [PubMed]

66. Bettinger, C.J.; Bruggeman, P.P.; Misra, A.; Borenstein, J.T.; Langer, R. Biocompatibility of biodegradable semiconducting melanin films for nerve tissue engineering. *Biomaterials* **2009**, *30*, 3050–3057. [CrossRef] [PubMed]

67. Ramachandran, G.K.; Tomfohr, J.K.; Li, J.; Sankey, O.F.; Zarate, X.; Primak, A.; Terazono, Y.; Moore, T.A.; Moore, A.L.; Gust, D.; et al. Electron transport properties of a carotene molecule in a metal-(single molecule)-metal junction. *J. Phys. Chem. B* **2003**, *107*, 6162–6169. [CrossRef]

68. Koh, L.D.; Yeo, J.; Lee, Y.Y.; Ong, Q.; Han, M.Y.; Tee, B.C.K. Advancing the frontiers of silk fibroin protein-based materials for futuristic electronics and clinical wound-healing. *Mater. Sci. Eng. C Mater.* **2018**, *86*, 151–172. [CrossRef] [PubMed]

69. Li, G.; Li, Y.; Chen, G.Q.; He, J.H.; Han, Y.F.; Wang, X.Q.; Kaplan, D.L. Silk-Based Biomaterials in Biomedical Textiles and Fiber-Based Implants. *Adv. Healthc. Mater.* **2015**, *4*, 1134–1151. [CrossRef] [PubMed]

70. Xie, M.B.; Li, Y.; Li, J.S.; Chen, A.Z.; Zhao, Z.; Li, G. Biomedical Applications of Silk Fibroin. In *Textile Bioengineering and Informatics Symposium Proceedings*; Textile Bioengineering & Informatics Society Ltd.: Hong Kong, China, 2014; Volumes 1 and 2, pp. 207–218.

71. Taddei, P.; Chiono, V.; Anghileri, A.; Vozzi, G.; Freddi, G.; Ciardelli, G. Silk Fibroin/Gelatin Blend Films Crosslinked with Enzymes for Biomedical Applications. *Macromol. Biosci.* **2013**, *13*, 1492–1510. [CrossRef] [PubMed]

72. Pal, R.K.; Farghaly, A.A.; Wang, C.Z.; Collinson, M.M.; Kundu, S.C.; Yadavalli, V.K. Conducting polymer-silk biocomposites for flexible and biodegradable electrochemical sensors. *Biosens. Bioelectron.* **2016**, *81*, 294–302. [CrossRef] [PubMed]

73. Edupuganti, V.; Solanki, R. Fabrication, characterization, and modeling of a biodegradable battery for transient electronics. *J. Power Sources* **2016**, *336*, 447–454. [CrossRef]

74. Jiang, L.; Zhang, J. Biodegradable and biobased polymers. In *Applied Plastics Engineering Handbook*, 2nd ed.; William Andrew Publishing: Oxford, UK, 2017; pp. 127–143.

75. Zhu, H.L.; Fang, Z.Q.; Preston, C.; Li, Y.Y.; Hu, L.B. Transparent paper: Fabrications, properties, and device applications. *Energy Environ. Sci.* **2014**, *7*, 269–287. [CrossRef]

76. Zhu, H.L.; Xiao, Z.G.; Liu, D.T.; Li, Y.Y.; Weadock, N.J.; Fang, Z.Q.; Huang, J.S.; Hu, L.B. Biodegradable transparent substrates for flexible organic-light-emitting diodes. *Energy Environ. Sci.* **2013**, *6*, 2105–2111. [CrossRef]

77. Jung, Y.H.; Chang, T.H.; Zhang, H.L.; Yao, C.H.; Zheng, Q.F.; Yang, V.W.; Mi, H.Y.; Kim, M.; Cho, S.J.; Park, D.W.; et al. High-performance green flexible electronics based on biodegradable cellulose nanofibril paper. *Nat. Commun.* **2015**, *6*, 7170. [CrossRef] [PubMed]

78. Li, Z.Q.; Wang, H.C.; Lv, S.Z.; Liu, L.; Guo, W.Y.; Yuan, M.; Yan, H.B.; Zhao, H.J.; Lang, S.P. Clinical Comparative Study on Efficacy and Safety for Treatment of Coronary Heart Disease with Cobalt-Base Alloy Bio Absorbable Polymer Sirolimus-Eluting Stent and Partner Stent. *Heart* **2011**, *97*, A149. [CrossRef]

79. Wu, Y.T.; Gao, Y.C. Five Years Follow Up Result after Application of Biodegradable Polymer Sirolimus-Eluting Stent in Patients with Coronary Heart Disease and Diabetes Mellitus. *Heart* **2013**, *99*, E175.

80. Inigo-Garcia, L.A.; Martinez-Garcia, F.J.; Milan-Pinilla, A.; Valle-Alberca, A.; Fernandez-Lopez, L.; Traverso-Castilla, V.V.; Delgado-Aguilar, A.; Bravo-Marques, R.; Ramirez-Moreno, A.; Siles-Rubio, J.R. Biodegradable Polymer Drug Eluting Stent: Efficacy and Safety with Short Regimen of Antiplatelet Therapy. *Cardiology* **2016**, *134*, 48.

81. Pilgrim, T.; Heg, D.; Roffi, M.; Tuller, D.; Muller, O.; Vuilliomenet, A.; Cook, S.; Weilenmann, D.; Kaiser, C.; Jamshidi, P.; et al. Ultrathin strut biodegradable polymer sirolimus-eluting stent versus durable polymer everolimus-eluting stent for percutaneous coronary revascularisation (BIOSCIENCE): A randomised, single-blind, non-inferiority trial. *Lancet* **2014**, *384*, 2111–2122. [CrossRef]

82. Waksman, R.; Pakala, R.; Baffour, R.; Seabron, R.; Hellinga, D.; Chan, R.; Su, S.H.; Kolodgie, F.; Virmani, R. In vivo comparison of a polymer-free Biolimus A9-eluting stent with a biodegradable polymer-based Biolimus A9 eluting stent and a bare metal stent in balloon denuded and radiated hypercholesterolemic rabbit iliac arteries. *Catheter. Cardiovasc. Interv.* **2012**, *80*, 429–436. [CrossRef] [PubMed]

83. Balch, O.K.; Collier, M.A.; DeBault, L.E.; Johnson, L.L. Bioabsorbable suture anchor (co-polymer 85/15 D,L lactide/glycolide) implanted in bone: Correlation of physical/mechanical properties, magnetic resonance imaging, and histological response. *Arthroscopy* **1999**, *15*, 691–708. [CrossRef]

84. Im, S.H.; Jung, Y.; Kim, S.H. Current status and future direction of biodegradable metallic and polymeric vascular scaffolds for next-generation stents. *Acta Biomater.* **2017**, *60*, 3–22. [CrossRef] [PubMed]

85. Hwang, S.W.; Song, J.K.; Huang, X.; Cheng, H.Y.; Kang, S.K.; Kim, B.H.; Kim, J.H.; Yu, S.; Huang, Y.G.; Rogers, J.A. High-Performance Biodegradable/Transient Electronics on Biodegradable Polymers. *Adv. Mater.* **2014**, *26*, 3905–3911. [CrossRef] [PubMed]

86. Shou, W.; Mahajan, B.K.; Ludwig, B.; Yu, X.W.; Staggs, J.; Huang, X.; Pan, H. Low-Cost Manufacturing of Bioresorbable Conductors by Evaporation-Condensation-Mediated Laser Printing and Sintering of Zn Nanoparticles. *Adv. Mater.* **2017**, *29*, 1700172. [CrossRef] [PubMed]

87. Najafabadi, A.H.; Tamayol, A.; Annabi, N.; Ochoa, M.; Mostafalu, P.; Akbari, M.; Nikkhah, M.; Rahimi, R.; Dokmeci, M.R.; Sonkusale, S.; et al. Biodegradable Nanofibrous Polymeric Substrates for Generating Elastic and Flexible Electronics. *Adv. Mater.* **2014**, *26*, 5823–5830. [CrossRef] [PubMed]

88. Boutry, C.M.; Kaizawa, Y.; Schroeder, B.C.; Chortos, A.; Legrand, A.; Wang, Z.; Chang, J.; Fox, P.; Bao, Z. A stretchable and biodegradable strain and pressure sensor for orthopaedic application. *Nat. Electron.* **2018**, *1*, 314–321. [CrossRef]

89. Lee, Y.K.; Kim, J.; Kim, Y.; Kwak, J.W.; Yoon, Y.; Rogers, J.A. Room Temperature Electrochemical Sintering of Zn Microparticles and Its Use in Printable Conducting Inks for Bioresorbable Electronics. *Adv. Mater.* **2017**, *29*, 1702665. [CrossRef] [PubMed]

90. Brenckle, M.A.; Cheng, H.Y.; Hwang, S.; Tao, H.; Paquette, M.; Kaplan, D.L.; Rogers, J.A.; Huang, Y.G.; Omenetto, F.G. Modulated Degradation of Transient Electronic Devices through Multilayer Silk Fibroin Pockets. *ACS Appl. Mater. Interfaces* **2015**, *7*, 19870–19875. [CrossRef] [PubMed]

91. Pan, R.Z.; Xuan, W.P.; Chen, J.K.; Dong, S.R.; Jin, H.; Wang, X.Z.; Li, H.L.; Luo, J.K. Fully biodegradable triboelectric nanogenerators based on electrospun polylactic acid and nanostructured gelatin films. *Nano Energy* **2018**, *45*, 193–202. [CrossRef]

92. Lee, S.; Koo, J.; Kang, S.K.; Park, G.; Lee, Y.J.; Chen, Y.Y.; Lim, S.A.; Lee, K.M.; Rogers, J.A. Metal microparticle—Polymer composites as printable, bio/ecoresorbable conductive inks. *Mater. Today* **2018**, *21*, 207–215. [CrossRef]

93. Lee, C.H.; Kim, H.; Harburg, D.V.; Park, G.; Ma, Y.J.; Pan, T.S.; Kim, J.S.; Lee, N.Y.; Kim, B.H.; Jang, K.I.; et al. Biological lipid membranes for on-demand, wireless drug delivery from thin, bioresorbable electronic implants. *Npg Asia Mater.* **2015**, *7*, e227. [CrossRef] [PubMed]

94. White, M.D.; Bosio, C.M.; Duplantis, B.N.; Nano, F.E. Human body temperature and new approaches to constructing temperature-sensitive bacterial vaccines. *Cell. Mol. Life Sci.* **2011**, *68*, 3019–3031. [CrossRef] [PubMed]

95. Duplantis, B.N.; Bosio, C.M.; Nano, F.E. Temperature-sensitive bacterial pathogens generated by the substitution of essential genes from cold-loving bacteria: Potential use as live vaccines. *J. Mol. Med.* **2011**, *89*, 437–444. [CrossRef] [PubMed]

96. Hooke, A.M. Temperature-Sensitive Mutants of Bacterial Pathogens—Isolation and Use to Determine Host Clearance and In-Vivo Replication Rates. *Method Enzymol.* **1994**, *235*, 448–457.

97. Tao, H.; Hwang, S.W.; Marelli, B.; An, B.; Moreau, J.E.; Yang, M.M.; Brenckle, M.A.; Kim, S.; Kaplan, D.L.; Rogers, J.A.; et al. Silk-based resorbable electronic devices for remotely controlled therapy and in vivo infection abatement. *Proc. Natl. Acad. Sci. USA* **2014**, *111*, 17385–17389. [CrossRef] [PubMed]

98. Yin, L.; Huang, X.; Xu, H.X.; Zhang, Y.F.; Lam, J.; Cheng, J.J.; Rogers, J.A. Materials, Designs, and Operational Characteristics for Fully Biodegradable Primary Batteries. *Adv. Mater.* **2014**, *26*, 3879–3884. [CrossRef] [PubMed]

99. Bouhlala, M.A.; Kameche, M.; Tadji, A.; Benouar, A. Chitosan hydrogel-based electrolyte for clean and biodegradable batteries: Energetic and conductometric studies. *Phys. Chem. Liq.* **2018**, *56*, 266–278. [CrossRef]

100. Jia, X.T.; Wang, C.Y.; Ranganathan, V.; Napier, B.; Yu, C.C.; Chao, Y.F.; Forsyth, M.; Omenetto, F.G.; MacFarlane, D.R.; Wallace, G.G. A Biodegradable Thin-Film Magnesium Primary Battery Using Silk Fibroin-Ionic Liquid Polymer Electrolyte. *ACS Energy Lett.* **2017**, *2*, 831–836. [CrossRef]

101. Jia, X.T.; Wang, C.Y.; Zhao, C.; Ge, Y.; Wallace, G.G. Toward Biodegradable Mg-Air Bioelectric Batteries Composed of Silk Fibroin-Polypyrrole Film. *Adv. Funct. Mater.* **2016**, *26*, 1454–1462. [CrossRef]

102. Huang, X.Y.; Wang, D.; Yuan, Z.Y.; Xie, W.S.; Wu, Y.X.; Li, R.F.; Zhao, Y.; Luo, D.; Cen, L.; Chen, B.B.; et al. A Fully Biodegradable Battery for Self-Powered Transient Implants. *Small* **2018**, *14*, e1800994. [CrossRef] [PubMed]

103. Lu, L.Y.; Yang, Z.J.; Meacham, K.; Cvetkovic, C.; Corbin, E.A.; Vazquez-Guardado, A.; Xue, M.T.; Yin, L.; Boroumand, J.; Pakeltis, G.; et al. Biodegradable Monocrystalline Silicon Photovoltaic Microcells as Power Supplies for Transient Biomedical Implants. *Adv. Energy Mater.* **2018**, *8*, 1703035. [CrossRef]

104. Hwang, S.W.; Huang, X.; Seo, J.H.; Song, J.K.; Kim, S.; Hage-Ali, S.; Chung, H.J.; Tao, H.; Omenetto, F.G.; Ma, Z.Q.; et al. Materials for Bioresorbable Radio Frequency Electronics. *Adv. Mater.* **2013**, *25*, 3526–3531. [CrossRef] [PubMed]

An fMRI Compatible Smart Device for Measuring Palmar Grasping Actions in Newborns

Daniela Lo Presti [1], **Sofia Dall'Orso** [2,3], **Silvia Muceli** [2,3], **Tomoki Arichi** [3,4], **Sara Neumane** [3,5,6], **Anna Lukens** [4], **Riccardo Sabbadini** [1], **Carlo Massaroni** [1], **Michele Arturo Caponero** [7], **Domenico Formica** [8], **Etienne Burdet** [9] **and Emiliano Schena** [1,*]

[1]   Unit of Measurements and Biomedical Instrumentation, Università Campus Bio-Medico di Roma, Via Alvaro del Portillo, 00128 Rome, Italy; d.lopresti@unicampus.it (D.L.P.); r.sabbadini@unicampus.it (R.S.); c.massaroni@unicampus.it (C.M.)

[2]   Division of Signal Processing and Biomedical Engineering, Department of Electrical Engineering, Chalmers University of Technology, SE-412 96 Gothenburg, Sweden; dallorso@chalmers.se (S.D.); muceli@chalmers.se (S.M.)

[3]   Centre for the Developing Brain, School of Biomedical Engineering and Imaging Sciences, King's College London, London WC2R 2LS, UK; tomoki.arichi@kcl.ac.uk (T.A.); sara.neumane@kcl.ac.uk (S.N.)

[4]   Paediatric Neurosciences, Evelina London Children's Hospital, Guy's and St Thomas' NHS Foundation Trust, London SE1 7EH, UK; anna.lukens@gstt.nhs.uk

[5]   NeuroDiderot Unit UMR1141, Université de Paris, INSERM, F-75019 Paris, France

[6]   UNIACT, Université Paris-Saclay, CEA, NeuroSpin, F-91191 Gif-sur-Yvette, France

[7]   Photonics Micro- and Nanostructures Laboratory, ENEA Research Center of Frascati, 00044 Frascati (RM), Italy; michele.caponero@enea.it

[8]   Unit of Neurophysiology and Neuroengineering of Human-Technology Interaction (NeXt Lab), Università Campus Bio-Medico di Roma, Via Alvaro del Portillo, 00128 Rome, Italy; d.formica@unicampus.it

[9]   Department of Bioengineering, Imperial College London, London SW7 2AZ, UK; e.burdet@imperial.ac.uk

*   Correspondence: e.schena@unicampus.it

Abstract: Grasping is one of the first dominant motor behaviors that enable interaction of a newborn infant with its surroundings. Although atypical grasping patterns are considered predictive of neuromotor disorders and injuries, their clinical assessment suffers from examiner subjectivity, and the neuropathophysiology is poorly understood. Therefore, the combination of technology with functional magnetic resonance imaging (fMRI) may help to precisely map the brain activity associated with grasping and thus provide important insights into how functional outcomes can be improved following cerebral injury. This work introduces an MR-compatible device (i.e., smart graspable device (SGD)) for detecting grasping actions in newborn infants. Electromagnetic interference immunity (EMI) is achieved using a fiber Bragg grating sensor. Its biocompatibility and absence of electrical signals propagating through the fiber make the safety profile of the SGD particularly favorable for use with fragile infants. Firstly, the SGD design, fabrication, and metrological characterization are described, followed by preliminary assessments on a preterm newborn infant and an adult during an fMRI experiment. The results demonstrate that the combination of the SGD and fMRI can safely and precisely identify the brain activity associated with grasping behavior, which may enable early diagnosis of motor impairment and help guide tailored rehabilitation programs.

Keywords: fiber Bragg grating sensors (FBGs); functional magnetic resonance imaging (fMRI); grasping actions detection; motor assessment; MR-compatible measuring systems

1. Introduction

Human infants exhibit a range of spontaneous movements and primitive reflexes as they develop across the first few months following birth. Among these, the grasping reflex is considered a key behavior that enables their first interactions with their surroundings [1]. The absence of such a reflex during the first days after birth or its long-lasting persistence after sixth months of age is associated with underlying brain injury and considered to be predictive of later neuromotor impairment, e.g., cerebral palsy (CP) [2]. For this reason, clinical assessment tools for neurodevelopment disorders and brain abnormalities in the infant period (particularly for those born preterm or at high risk of developing later CP) usually incorporate a component that involves eliciting the grasp reflex [3,4].

Clinical assessment of palmar grasp is currently performed by applying light pressure on the infant's palm with an object or the examiner's finger to induce hand closure. This approach is entirely qualitative and based on the use of functional scales and the examiner's expertise [5] and is therefore potentially affected by inter-rater variability [6]. Furthermore, whilst clinicians and physiotherapists may develop discriminative experience about the quality of this reflex, they will still lack the sensitivity to identify subtle features not perceivable by a human observer (e.g., the discrimination of active/passive touch or the quantitative measurement of grasping strength and holding time). Therefore, a quantitative measure of grasping actions may provide new and valuable information about infant motor behavior. Consequently, there is a pressing need for new technologies that could enable the accurate measurement of grasping behavior and thus objectively evaluate sensorimotor function in the newborn. The use of such a technology could provide further insights into the relationship between motor behavior and underlying patterns of brain activity when combined with neuroimaging techniques [7]. This knowledge may be crucial in the context of early brain injury at a time when there is a high capacity for compensatory neural plasticity and thus the potential to improve functional outcome through patient-specific tailored therapies [8,9].

Functional magnetic resonance imaging (fMRI) allows for the non-invasive study of human brain function and has been successfully applied even with very young subjects [10–13]. In a typical fMRI experiment, brain responses when performing a task (which can be either an active action or passive stimulation) are identified by measuring temporal changes in the blood oxygen level dependent (BOLD) signal. However, a large challenge in performing fMRI studies with newborn infants is designing and effectively providing a task to this inherently uncooperative population. Technology can potentially resolve this difficulty and enable fMRI studies by allowing precise patterns of safe stimulation or accurate measures of spontaneous behavior while the subject is inside the scanner [6,8].

With the advance of sensor technology, several solutions have been proposed to quantitatively assess grasping behavior in infants and thus remove subjectivity. The majority of these studies have utilized technologies to assess grasping behavior in terms of strength and holding time, as well as to investigate the relationship between grasping pattern and intrinsic (e.g., infant gender, weight, premature births) and extrinsic factors (e.g., object shape and texture) [14,15]. The aforementioned measuring systems have used pressure transducers based on electrical components which are unusable inside the MRI scanner [6,16–19]. MR-compatible technology requires unconventional solutions to ensure safety due to the strong static magnetic field and avoid electromagnetic interference (EMI), with further attention required for successfully imaging infant subjects. Fiber Bragg gratings (FBGs) may be a solution to overcome this issue [20]. They are highly sensitive, small-sized, light, non-toxic, and immune to EMI [21]. Therefore, these features meet the technical and clinical requirements (e.g., MR-compatibility and safety) of devices for detecting and measuring grasping in preterm and term neonates both inside and outside the MRI scanner [6].

To date, only a few studies have systematically investigated functional brain activity in newborn infants using assistive technologies [8,9]. In [16], a customized robotic interface was used to passively move the limbs of preterm infants and identify the corresponding brain responses within the sensorimotor cortex. This study showed that the human brain is already functionally organized even at a very young age and paved the path for future investigations of task-related functional responses in preterm infants. Whilst the authors investigated the somatosensory response related to passive movements, they were unable to detect grasping actions.

The present study aims to develop an FBG-based measuring system (hereinafter called the smart graspable device (SGD)) to detect grasping actions in newborns. The SGD consists of an FBG sensor encapsulated into a soft silicone matrix. The FBG ensures that the device has EMI and the ideal safety profile for working with infants and inside the MRI environment. The device softness and cylindrical shape mimicking the ones of a finger additionally provides easy affordance and usability. Assessing grasp with the proposed device is based around the principle of the transduction of external forces (F_{ext}) applied by an infant's hand on the device into grating strain (ε) via squeezing and releasing of the silicone. In this paper we firstly described the design and fabrication of the proposed device so as to fulfill all technical and clinical requirements according to the target population (i.e., preterm and term newborns). Then, the sensitivity of the SGD to F_{ext} was estimated. Finally, two preliminary trials were carried out to investigate the performances of the proposed device when used by a preterm infant in the neonatal intensive care unit and an adult during an fMRI experiment.

2. Basic Requirements and Components of the Smart Graspable Device

2.1. Technological and Clinical Requirements

Designing a sensing device able to detect natural grasping actions and work simultaneously within an fMRI experiment is very challenging. Furthermore, there are additional constraints set by the target population (i.e., preterm and term newborn infants), which are not fulfilled by the majority of devices currently proposed in the literature [6,22]. In addition, the electromagnetic field inside the MRI environment can affect the working capability of most electronic devices proposed for grasp measurements and can induce currents in metal loops leading to infant contact burns [23,24]. In the same way, ferromagnetic elements widely used as components of electronic graspable devices may cause artefacts on the MRI images themselves, affecting diagnostic image quality [25].

As newborn infants are inherently uncooperative subjects, a further requirement of the device is that their natural movements can be safely measured under natural conditions [6,19]. To allow for handling by a newborn infant, the proposed tool should be small and lightweight, and its shape should be appropriate to improve engagement and encourage palmar grasping [26]. Moreover, high sensitivity to a low range of loads is necessary to detect the hand closure of a newborn infant, as well as being biocompatible and easily cleaned to reduce the risk of cross-infection between subjects [15,27].

To meet all of these technical and clinical requirements, an FBG sensor was chosen as the sensing element. A flexible and non-toxic silicone rubber (i.e., Dragon Skin™ 10) was used as a squeezable matrix to encapsulate the FBG sensor [28]. Lastly, a polylactic acid (PLA) structure characterized by a linkage mechanism filled with the soft silicone was designed according to the index finger dimensions of an adult human, as this is typically used to insert into the infant's palm to elicit the grasping reflex. The proposed solution is highly sensitive, robust, safe, affordable, and infant-friendly.

2.2. Fiber Bragg Gratings Working Principles

An FBG sensor is a distributed Bragg grating inscribed into a short segment of an optical fiber produced by creating a perturbation of the effective refractive index (η_{eff}) of the fiber core. In its simplest form, this periodic perturbation is sinusoidal with Λ, the constant grating pitch.

Generally, an FBG works in reflection as a notch filter; when a broadband spectrum of light is guided within the core and hits on the grating segment, a smooth Gaussian-shaped narrow spectrum is reflected and represents the output of the FBG. The center of the reflected Gaussian peak is known as the Bragg wavelength (λ_B) and satisfies the Bragg condition [29].

$$\lambda_B = 2\,\eta_{eff}\Lambda \tag{1}$$

Strain along the fiber longitudinal axis (ε) and temperature changes (ΔT) induce variations of Λ and η_{eff}, which result in a λ_B shift ($\Delta \lambda_B$) as in

$$\Delta \lambda_B = \lambda_B \left[(1 - P_e) \varepsilon + (\alpha_\Lambda + \xi) \Delta T \right] \tag{2}$$

The first term of Equation (2) represents the ε effect on the grating, with Pe the effective strain-optic constant; the second term represents the ΔT effect, with α_Λ and ξ denoting the thermal expansion and the thermo-optic coefficients of the fiber, respectively. When the effects of ΔT are negligible, Equation (2) in [29] can be rewritten as

$$\Delta \lambda_B = \lambda_B (1 - P_e) \varepsilon \tag{3}$$

In this work, the SGD is able to detect grasping forces applied by a newborn infant through the compression of the silicone encapsulation that allows transducing loads applied on the device into longitudinal ε experienced by the FBG.

Based on the need for a physical connection to a dedicated device (i.e., the FBG interrogator) for enlightening the gratings and reading their outputs, a patch cord can be used to connect the FBG-based device inside the MRI scanner to the interrogator placed in the control room. This connection allows separation of the SGD inside the MRI scanner room from the measuring circuitry located in the control room.

2.3. Dragon Skin™ Silicones

Dragon Skin™ materials (commercialized by Smooth On Inc., Macungie, PA, USA) are platinum care bicomponent silicone rubbers used in a variety of scenarios, including medical fields (e.g., in prosthetics as cushioning materials and in physiological monitoring for flexible sensor development [30,31]). They are highly compliant and highly flexible. Moreover, they are skin safe in compliance with ISO 10993-10 (Biological evaluation of medical devices—Part 10: Tests for irritation and skin sensitization) [28,32].

Dragon Skin™ silicones are commercialized as liquid silicone rubbers in the form of an elastomer kit containing two components (A and B). Part A contains the platinum catalyst, part B the crosslinker [33]. The manufacturer recommends mixing Dragon Skin™ silicones in the proportion of 1A:1B by weight and thinning the liquid formulation with Silicon Thinner™ to lower the viscosity of the mix for easier pouring and vacuum degassing [34]. Curing temperature and time are also defined in the technical bulletin. Dragon Skin™ silicones are commercialized in different hardnesses expressed in terms of Shore A Scale: 10 (Very Fast, Fast, Medium, Slow), 20, and 30, with curing time ranging from 4 min to 45 min according to the silicone hardness.

In this work, the mechanical properties of Dragon Skin™ 10 Medium, 20, and 30 were investigated in terms of stress–strain properties. To better quantify the compression behavior of Dragon Skin™ silicones, the Young modulus E (expressed in MPa) was calculated to facilitate the selection of the material that best satisfies all the requirements mentioned above. Considering the scenario of interest and target population, the application of low squeezing forces will induce a compression on the silicone rubber with ε values lower than 10% of the rubber sample (l_0). Thus, the stress–strain relationship can be described by Hooke's law [33]:

$$\sigma = E \, \varepsilon \tag{4}$$

where σ is the stress (i.e., the external force applied to the sample per its cross-sectional area) and ε is calculated as $(l - l_0)/l_0$.

The standard ISO 7743:2017 (Rubber, vulcanized or thermoplastic—Determination of compression stress–strain properties) was used for defining the dimensions of the cylindrical pieces used for the compression tests. The test piece B (method C) with a diameter of 17.8 ± 0.2 mm and a height of 25.0 ± 0.2 mm was chosen [35]. Dragon Skin™ 10 Medium, 20, and 30 were poured into a cylindrical mold designed in Solidworks (Dassault Systemes, Waltham, MA, USA) and 3D printed using PLA. As suggested by the technical bulletin, the curing process was carried out at room temperature for 5 h, 4 h, and 16 h for Dragon Skin™ 10, 20, and 30, respectively. A total of fifteen specimens were fabricated, five pieces for each hardness level.

Compression tests were carried out using a testing machine (Instron®, Norwood, MA, USA, model 3365, load cell with a range of measurement of ±10 N, an accuracy of 0.02 N, and a resolution of 10^{-5} N) to apply controlled ε values (from 0% to 25% of l_0 as suggested by the standard ISO 7743:2017) in a quasi-static condition (at a low displacement rate of 2 mm·min^{-1}). The static assessment of each specimen was executed by positioning the cylinder-shaped sample between the lower and the upper plates of the machine, as shown in Figure 1. A total of five repetitive compression tests were carried out at room temperature for a total of twenty tests per sample. The loads and the displacements applied by the compression machine to the specimen were recorded at a sampling frequency of 100 Hz using Instron® Bluehill Universal software.

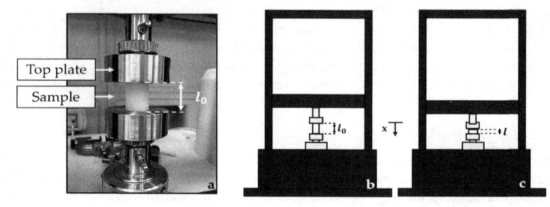

Figure 1. Set-up of the compression tests (**a**): the cylinder-shaped sample between the lower and the upper plates of the Instron machine and the initial sample length before (l_0) and during the compression (l) are illustrated ((**b**,**c**), respectively). The top plate moves at constant speed parallel to the *x*-axis (**c**).

The stress–strain relationships (σ vs. ε) of each Dragon Skin™ material were obtained by processing the collected data through a custom algorithm. The mean value of experimental σ (σ_{exp}) and the repeatability of the system response were determined by calculating the related uncertainty across the twenty tests by considering a t-Student reference distribution with 19 degrees of freedom and a level of confidence of 95% [36]. The best fitting line of the calibration curve was obtained, and its angular coefficient was calculated to estimate E. Lastly, the linearity error was calculated by using Equation (5) in terms of the maximum linearity error (% u_L^{max}).

$$\% \, u_L^{max} = \{max \, [\sigma_{exp} \, (\varepsilon) - \sigma_{th} \, (\varepsilon)] \cdot \sigma^{fs}_{exp}{}^{-1}\} \cdot 100 \qquad (5)$$

where σ^{fs}_{exp} is the full-scale output range, $\sigma_{exp}(\varepsilon)$ the experimental stress experienced by the sample at a specific ε, and $\sigma_{th}(\varepsilon)$ is the theoretical stress obtained by the linear model at the same ε value.

Results showed E values of 0.24 MPa, 0.47 MPa, and 0.74 MPa for Dragon Skin™ 10, 20, and 30, respectively (see Figure 2). R-square (R^2) values higher than 0.98 were found for all the responses, and linearity errors of 5.7%, 7.8%, and 8.9% were obtained for Dragon Skin™ 10, 20, and 30, respectively.

Our results quantified the mechanical properties of Dragon Skin™ in terms of compression behavior. As expected, Dragon Skin™ 10 was found to be more flexible than Dragon Skin™ 20 and Dragon Skin™ 30. In particular, the E value of Dragon Skin™ 10 was approximately half that of Dragon Skin™ 20 (i.e., 0.24 MPa vs. 0.47 MPa) and one-third that of Dragon Skin™ 30 (i.e., 0.24 MPa vs. 0.74 MPa). The high R^2 values (for all tests $R^2 > 0.98$) indicated good agreement between the experimental data and the linear model. Moreover, the Dragon Skin™ 10 response showed the best linear behavior as testified by the % u_L^{max} value (i.e., 5.7%), which was lower than those of Dragon Skin™ 20 (i.e., 7.8%) and Dragon Skin™ 30 (i.e., 8.9%), as shown in the respective plots in Figure 2.

Finally, Dragon Skin™ 10 showed the best results in terms of uncertainty (maximum uncertainty of 0.004 MPa) when compared to Dragon Skin™ 20 (i.e., 0.01 MPa) and Dragon Skin™ 30 (i.e., 0.007 MPa).

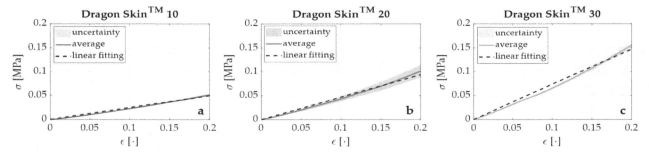

Figure 2. The σ–ε relationships for Dragon Skin™ 10, 20, and 30 are shown in blue (**a**), red (**b**), and green (**c**), respectively. In particular, the continuous lines represent the average σ_{exp} values, the shaded areas the related uncertainties, and the black dotted lines the σ_{th} values obtained by the best linear fitting model.

These findings demonstrated that Dragon Skin™ 10 is best suited to meet the technical requirements of the SGD, particularly given the expected low ranges of F_{ext} applied by newborn infants, which would likely require high flexibility; Dragon Skin™ 10 allows the SGD to be easily squeezed by a newborn for the F_{ext} transduction into grating ε.

3. The Smart Graspable Device

3.1. Design and Manufacturing of the Smart Graspable Device

The idea behind the system design and manufacturing was based on the need for it to be sensitive enough to detect F_{ext} applied by the infant and able to transduce F_{ext} into grating ε measured by the FBG sensor. At the same time, the device should be robust and safe enough to be handled and grasped by a newborn infant in a variety of settings.

The medium consists of a PLA-based structure characterized by a linkage mechanism and filled by flexible silicone (i.e., Dragon Skin™ 10). The transduction mechanism exploits four-bar linkages hinged to the PLA structure ends to convert the applied F_{ext} into ε via the silicone squeezing and releasing. When the newborn infant grasps the device, the silicone is squeezed and the FBG is strained; it is then unstrained once the SGD is released again (see Figure 3).

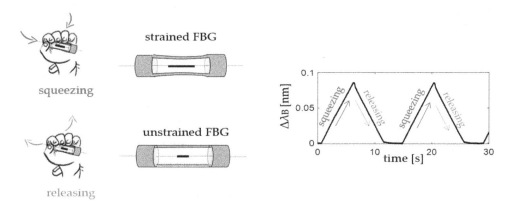

Figure 3. The smart graspable device (SGD) principle of working during grasping: squeezing (in red) and releasing (in blue) phases.

The PLA structure is a hollow cylinder made up of two semi-cylindrical pieces (see Figure 4A,B). Each piece is constituted of two end parts perpendicularly spaced by two bar linkages (40 mm of length, 4.2 mm of width, and 1 mm of depth). The bar linkages are hinged along the ends with a uniform interval of 60° to form a symmetrical structure (Figure 4A, top and front views). One semi-cylinder has a 10-mm long conduit to accommodate the jacket (yellow cable in Figure 4B). The jacket is the last layer of protection of the optical fiber from the end of the PLA structure to the interrogation unit.

The outer diameter of the PLA structure is 12 mm, and its overall length is 50 mm, which corresponds roughly to the dimensions of a human finger. The sensing element embedded into the PLA structure consists of an FBG sensor (λ_B of 1547 nm and grating length of 10 mm, commercialized by AtGrating Technologies, Shenzhen, China) configured with the middle part of the optical fiber encapsulated into a Dragon Skin™ 10 silicone matrix.

The encapsulation was fabricated as follows:

1.   the optical fiber was tightly suspended inside the PLA structure by firmly gluing its two ends inside the small grooves fabricated at the center of the structure ends. This configuration utilized pre-tension to keep the FBG in a stretched state in order to improve its resolution and sensitivity (stage 1 in Figure 4B);
2.   the PLA structure was placed inside a mold to allow cavity filling without any silicone spilling. The silicone rubber was synthesized by mixing A and B liquid components of Dragon Skin™ polymer at a ratio of 1:1; the mix was degassed and poured into the cavity (stage 2 in Figure 4B);
3.   a curing process of 5 h was carried out at room temperature, as suggested in the technical bulletin [28], to allow the silicone rubber vulcanization before extracting the SGD from the mold (stage 3 in Figure 4B).

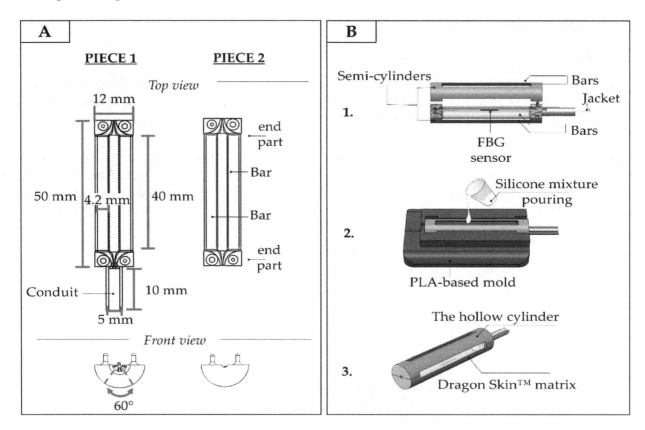

Figure 4. (**A**) The geometrical features of an SGD; (**B**) The main manufacturing steps: the FBG sensor positioning (step 1), the silicone mixture pouring (step 2), and the SGD removed from the mold after the rubber vulcanization (step 3).

Two nominally identical SGDs (from now on referred to as SGD^1 and SGD^2) were developed following the same manufacturing stages previously described.

To improve the SGDs usability during fMRI, both the devices were designed to also be able to instrument an already existing fMRI-compatible robotic interface for conducting experiments with newborn infants described in [8,9]. This interface was designed to accommodate the infant's forearm on a central non-sensitive platform and to passively guide the flexion and extension of the infant wrist while the hand was wrapped around a bar. The instrumentation of the robotic interface with the proposed SGD was performed by switching the non-sensorized handlebar with the SGD, thus allowing the investigation of brain activity related to grasping and spontaneous movements (Figure 5A,B). To fit the SGD to the robotic interface, two temporary PLA-based anchoring systems were fabricated (see Figure 5A). The anchoring mechanism was designed to allow quick and easy fitting of the SGD according to the fMRI investigation being performed.

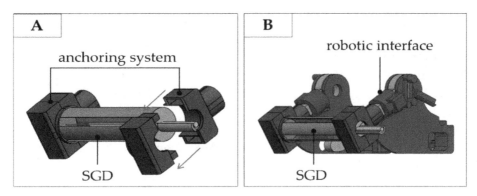

Figure 5. (**A**) A detail of the anchoring system elements designed to allow fitting of the SGD within an already existing robotic interface; (**B**) the SGD together with the robotic interface.

3.2. Metrological Characterization of the Smart Graspable Device

To estimate SGD sensitivity to F_{ext} (S_F), compression tests were performed by using a tensile testing machine (Instron, model 3365, load cell with a range of measurement of ± 10 N, an accuracy of 0.02 N, and a resolution of 10^{-5} N). The blocking system shown in Figure 6 was designed to avoid any axial rotation of SGD during the application of loads on the SGD bars. This system consisted of a support plate with two clamps to securely lock the SGD through M4 fixings.

Each sensor (i.e., SGD^1 and SGD^2) was placed on the lower base of the machine blocked to the support place by using the 3D-printed clamps. External loads in the range 0 N–2 N were applied on each bar of the SGD at a low compression rate of 2 mm·min^{-1} to simulate quasi-static conditions (see Figure 6).

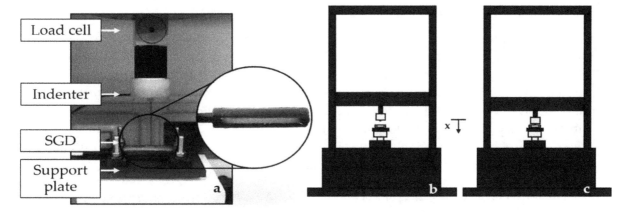

Figure 6. The SGD in the blocking system, the load cell, and the mechanical indenter are shown (**a**). A schematic representation of the SGD between the lower and the upper plates of the Instron machine is illustrated (**b**). The top plate moves at constant speed parallel to the x-axis (**c**).

The load was applied to the center of each bar by using a mechanical indenter (5 mm diameter). A total of five compression tests were performed on each of the four bars for a total of 20 tests. Once the five tests related to a single bar ended, the SGD was rotated 90° along its longitudinal axis, re-blocked to the support, and the second bar was loaded. The same procedure was repeated for the remaining two bars. The S_F value of each SGD was found averaging the twenty responses of all the bars to the applied loads.

During each test, the output from the tensile machine was collected at a sampling frequency of 100 Hz. The $\Delta\lambda_B$ values were simultaneously recorded using the optical spectrum interrogator (si255, Hyperion Platform, Micro Optics Inc., Atlanta, GA, USA) at the same sampling frequency.

The calibration curve ($\Delta\lambda_B$ vs. F_{ext}) was obtained by processing the collected data through a custom algorithm to evaluate the average value of $\Delta\lambda_B$ vs. F_{ext}. The first step was the synchronization of the experimental values of $\Delta\lambda_B$ and F_{ext}. Then, both the average value and the expanded uncertainty of $\Delta\lambda_B$ were calculated across the twenty tests. The expanded uncertainty was calculated by using a t-Student reference distribution (with 19 degrees of freedom and a level of confidence of 95%). Finally, a linear regression to find the equation of the line which best fits the experimental data (i.e., $\Delta\lambda_B$ vs. F_{ext}) was performed. Its slope represents the S_F value for SGD[1]. The same procedure was followed for SGD[2] (see Figure 7).

Results showed a S_F value of ~0.23 nm·N^{-1} for both devices, suggesting a good reproducibility of the fabrication process. Moreover, an $R^2 > 0.99$ indicated excellent agreement between the experimental data and the linear fitting model.

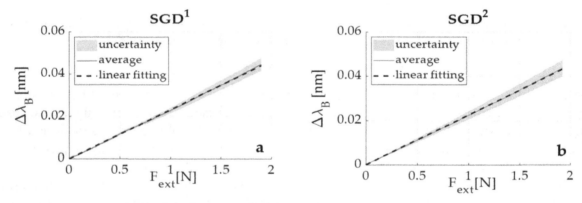

Figure 7. The $\Delta\lambda_B$ vs. F_{ext} of SGD[1] (**a**) and SGD[2] (**b**): in continuous magenta lines the average $\Delta\lambda_B$ vs. F_{ext} responses, in shaded magenta areas the related uncertainties, and in dotted black lines the best linear fitting.

4. Experimental Validation of the Smart Graspable Device

To assess the proposed SGDs performance in a real scenario, two explorative tests were performed with a newborn infant and an adult subject. Given the high agreement in S_F values between SGD[1] and SGD[2], SGD[1] was used for the following tests and for simplicity is now referred to as SGD. First, an explorative test was performed on a healthy newborn infant in the neonatal intensive care unit of St. Thomas Hospital (London, UK) to test compatibility of the SGD and assess its ability to detect a newborn infant's grasp. A further explorative trial within an fMRI experiment was then carried out to validate the device performances inside the MRI scanner and to confirm that activation within the brain areas associated with the grasping action detected by SGD could be identified with fMRI.

4.1. Experimental Trial on a Newborn: Protocol and Results

To assess the capability of SGD to detect grasping behavior in newborn infants, three healthy infants were recruited at St Thomas' Hospital (London, UK). Of them, only one infant (gestational age at birth: 36 weeks + 6 days, postmenstrual age at the time of recording: 37 weeks + 2 days) was in a suitable awake state at the time of the recording. The study was approved by the NHS research ethics committee (REC code: 12/LO/1247), and informed written consent was obtained from parents prior to participation. A neonatal physiotherapist under the supervision of a physician handled the SGD and applied light pressure on the infant's palm to induce hand closure around the device and elicit grasping behavior. Data from the SGD were collected using the FBG interrogator (si425, Micron Optics Inc., Atlanta, GA, USA) at a sampling frequency of 250 Hz, and a video used as reference was simultaneously recorded using a camera (Handycam, Sony, Minato-ku, Tokyo, Japan).

After data acquisition, the physiotherapist and the physician checked the recorded video to identify the time windows corresponding to the grasping action performed by the newborn infant. A total of five grasping events were identified (see Figure 8A).

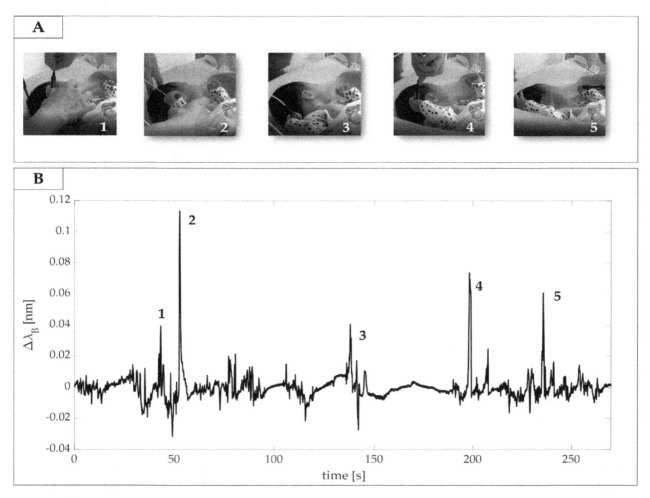

Figure 8. (**A**) Video frames of grasping actions identified by the clinicians; (**B**) the related signals collected by the SGD. Grasps actions are enumerated from 1 to 5.

Those time windows were then used to highlight changes in the SGD output associated with grasping actions. The signal showed evident peaks during the specific time windows related to presumed SGD squeezing and releasing actions (see Figure 8B). Results showed $\Delta\lambda_B$ values ranging from 0.04 nm to 0.11 nm that corresponded to forces ranging from ~0.17 N to ~0.48 N.

4.2. Experimental Trial on an Adult during fMRI: Protocol and Results

The second trial was performed on a healthy volunteer (32 years old, adult female volunteer) inside a 3 Tesla MRI scanner (Philips Achieva, Best, The Netherlands) located at St Thomas Hospital with a 32-channel receive head coil. High resolution structural T1-weighted and T2-weighted images were acquired for image registration purposes. BOLD contrast fMRI data with an EPI GRE sequence with parameters: x/y/z resolution: 3.5 mm × 3.5 mm × 6 mm; TR: 1500 ms; TE: 45 ms; FA 90°.

The subject was studied with her right hand fitted inside the instrumented robotic interface described in [8,9] with the right index and middle fingers strapped to the SGD on the handle bar.

The subject was then asked to use their two fingers to apply a brief force on the SGD at spontaneous and random times during an acquisition session lasting 225 s (corresponding to 150 images). The SGD signal was collected using the FBG interrogator (si425, Micron Optics Inc., Atlanta, GA, USA) at a sampling frequency of 250 Hz, and the recording started synchronously with the fMRI image acquisition so that the timing of task could be related to the fMRI timeseries. The task was designed to simulate a situation in which the experimenter is unaware of the timing of the task inside the scanner, as would be the case when studying spontaneous motor behavior in infants but can obtain this information from the output of the SGD. The experimental set-up and data flow are shown in Figure 9.

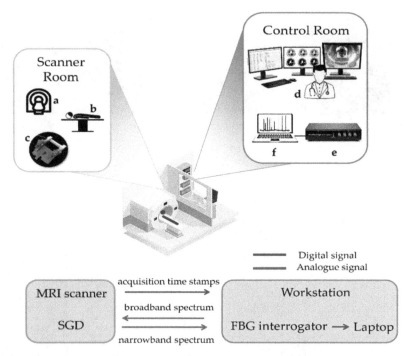

Figure 9. Experimental set-up of fMRI trial with the data flow: the MRI scanner (**a**), the patient (**b**), and the robotic interface instrumented by the SGD (**c**) in the scanner room, and the workstation (**d**), the FBG interrogator (**e**), and the laptop (**f**) in the control room. Digital and analogue data flows between the scanner and control rooms are shown using blue and red arrows, respectively.

The acquisition volume trigger markers (via a TTL pulse) were transmitted to the scanner workstation and used offline to synchronize the fMRI data with the signal recorded by the SGD. Data from the SGD were analyzed in the MATLAB R2019b environment (Mathworks, Natick, MA, USA). As shown in Figure 10A, the device was able to detect the force applied by the subject without prior knowledge of its timing (i.e., 26 actions in the SGD output across the period of acquisition) from which the event-related occurrence of the task could be defined for the fMRI data analysis.

In order to identify which voxels of the brain images were active during the task, it is possible to use a simple general linear model (GLM) to fit the BOLD time series within each voxel with a temporal model of the predicted activation, and the strength of each fit is used to generate a z-statistics map across the whole brain (z-score map in Figure 10). The predicted activation used as a model is built as the convolution of the experimental design (a vector that represents the timing of action vs. rest) and the hemodynamic response function (HRF) that act as a temporal smoothing kernel. The SGD-derived task pattern was then expressed in a binary vector form (with 1's representing action and 0's representing rest) where the events were identified using the *findpeaks* function on the normalized SGD signal in the MATLAB environment (see Figure 10A). Each event was represented by 8 ms centered at the peak of the action, and the binary vector was then convolved with the canonical hemodynamic response function (HRF) to generate the design model for the general linear model fMRI analysis (see Figure 10A). MRI data were processed using tools implemented in the FMRIB software library (FSL) in [37] following a standard pipeline which included high pass temporal filtering (with 0.02 Hz cut-off frequency), MCFLIRT rigid body motion correction, slice timing correction, brain extraction using BET, spatial smoothing (Gaussian of FWHM 5 mm), univariate general linear model (GLM) with additional 6 motion parameters derived from the rigid body motion correction as confound regressors, and cluster correction (p threshold 0.05). As predicted, significant clusters of positive BOLD activity were located in the primary contralateral (left) somatosensory and motor cortices and supplementary motor area correlating to the task performed by the subject, and the main cluster of activation was located at the hand knob on the precentral gyrus (see left (L) and right (R) lateral and top view on the 3D rendered brain images in Figure 10B).

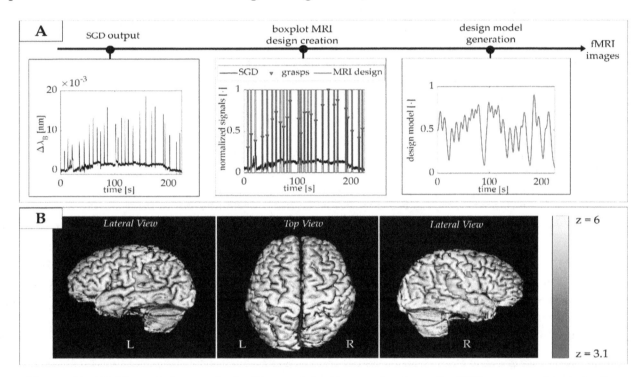

Figure 10. (**A**) Flow of data analysis. The peak in $\Delta\lambda_B$ coming from the SGD were used to infer the timing of the action and create a boxplot MRI design. This was convolved with the hemodynamic response function (HRF) to generate the design model for the general linear model (GLM); (**B**) Significant cluster of functional response to the task (in red and yellow) overlaid onto the subject's T1-weighted brain image with the z-score map.

5. Discussion

The key elements of the present study are the development of a novel smart device (i.e., the SGD), which can quantitatively measure the grasping behavior of newborn infants even within the MRI scanner environment. The design of the proposed device was guided by technical and clinical requirements predicated by the target population and with the intended use including small size, lightweight, high sensitivity, biocompatibility, and safety. In addition, the SGD was also designed to easily instrument an existing robotic interface used for fMRI studies of newborn infants.

To the best of our knowledge, the proposed SGD is the first fMRI-compatible device based on FBG able to detect and measure palmar grasp in preterm and term infants. The SGD is shaped and sized appropriately to be handled by a newborn infant's hand, easily squeezed, and able to detect low grasping F_{ext}. Furthermore, the FBGs' EMI compatibility ensures safety and working capability both outside and inside the MRI environment.

Two identical devices were fabricated (i.e., SGD[1] and SGD[2]). Both the responses of SGD[1] and SGD[2] to F_{ext} showed a linear behavior, which reached an average S_F value of ~0.23 nm·N^{-1}. This finding confirmed the high reproducibility of the manufacturing process as well as the capability of the SGD to detect the low ranges of F_{ext} applied by the target infant population. Two pilot tests were carried out to investigate the performance of the proposed SGD on a newborn infant in the neonatal intensive care unit and on an adult during an fMRI experiment. These preliminary validation experiments revealed that the SGD was capable of working in both cases, namely on a non-collaborative subject (i.e., the newborn infant) and within the MRI environment.

In the literature, pioneering work describing grasping behavior in infants began in the 1930s [38–40]. These first studies were based on functional scales or on the direct observation of infant responses to the application of light pressure on the palm [41]. These methods suffer from several limitations, including examiner subjectivity and incapability of quantifying grasping actions in terms of strength and duration. With the advancement of technological devices, novel methods emerged for assessing motor function in early infancy [7,14–16,18,19,42,43]. In particular, grasping behavior was studied in infants in terms of strength and holding time, with some studies proposing novel systems to investigate the relationship of these variables with intrinsic (e.g., infant sex [15], weight [27], preterm birth [1]) and extrinsic factors (e.g., object shape and texture [7]). Moreover, systems for objective assessment of grasping actions were developed to detect early abnormal neuromotor development and based on the premise that this could guide prompt intervention to improve functional outcome [43,44]. The main findings of the state-of-the-art showed a higher grasping strength and pronounced handedness symmetry in males more than females [15]; a decrease in holding time when the same object was repetitively put in the newborn infant's hand and an increase when its shape and smoothness changed [7]; and longer holding times in preterm in comparison to term neonates with significant differences related to sex [15].

Existing technological tools developed for measuring grasping in newborn infants can be grouped into devices worn on the examiner's finger [18] or those that are directly handled by an infant [16,18,19,43]. Very few of these systems were also specifically designed to be used by newborn infants in the first days following birth. All of these systems are based on pressure transducers with electrical components (i.e., piezoresistive sensors [16], force sensing resistors (FSR) [19], capacitive sensors [18], and conductive polymer layers [43]). These features do not allow their employment inside the MRI scanner. In contrast, our device is designed to be directly handled by a newborn infant and can be used in fMRI owing to the FBG sensor EMI immunity and the SGD's affordable shape.

In [16], as in our study, the device was designed to be directly grasped by a newborn infant without active involvement from the examiner during the experimental trial. An electrical sensing element (i.e., a piezoresistive pressure transducer) was used to develop a ring-shaped device consisting of a silicone-filled chamber hung within a rigid case and connected to the transducer (total diameter of 93 mm). This allowed for the measuring of infant grasping activity generated by chamber internal pressure changes due to the silicon squeezing. Our device is different, as the proposed SGD is based on optical technology instead of electrical components, is softer (10 A vs. 50 A), and is considerably lighter (8 g vs. 115 g). All of these features make our system more suitable for studying a wider range of infant populations including preterm and term infants.

Future studies will aim to investigate the feasibility of SGD assessment on a wider range of newborn infants both inside and outside the MRI scanner. Moreover, two SGDs can be used together in longitudinal studies to study the emergence of hand dominance and (bi)manual grasping to investigate developmental motor disorders resulting from localized brain injury. Further investigation may also be focused on optimizing the SGD for use with older infants, for instance across their first year as the transition to volitional prehension occurs. These studies will require a remodulation of system requirements (e.g., change in dimensions, FBG numbers, and silicone hardness) to optimize the SGD measuring properties for a different target population. Lastly, changes in grasping variables according to age, sex, and object texture could be performed to provide new insights into behavioral neurophysiology and neuropathology.

6. Conclusions

This paper described the first fMRI-compatible technological solution (SGD) based on FBG for detecting grasping actions in newborn infants. The use of such a device in conjunction with fMRI can shed new light on associated cerebral processes and may provide novel insight into the neuromotor impairments that result from neonatal brain injury. This knowledge may be crucial in the context of prompt diagnoses of atypical task-related brain activations and early brain injuries such as CP, at a time when there is a high capacity for compensatory neural plasticity. Furthermore, the technology-aided assessment of neurodevelopmental deviation from normal physiological development can provide useful biomarkers for establishing patient-tailored therapies and optimizing the rehabilitation outcomes.

Author Contributions: Conceptualization, D.L.P., S.D., S.M., R.S., T.A., D.F., E.B., E.S.; methodology, M.A.C., C.M., D.F., E.B., E.S.; software, D.L.P., S.D., R.S.; validation, D.L.P., S.D., T.A., S.N., A.L., E.S.; formal analysis, D.L.P., S.M., T.A., C.M., M.A.C., D.F., E.B., E.S.; investigation, D.L.P., S.D., T.A., S.N., A.L.; resources, T.A., M.A.C., C.M., E.B., E.S.; data curation, D.L.P., S.D., R.S.; writing—original draft preparation, D.L.P., S.D.; writing—review and editing, S.M., T.A., S.N., A.L., R.S., C.M., M.A.C., D.F., E.B., E.S.; visualization, D.L.P., S.D., S.M.; supervision, D.F., E.B., E.S.; project administration, D.L.P., D.F., B.E., E.S.; funding acquisition, D.L.P., S.M., T.A., D.F. All authors have read and agreed to the published version of the manuscript.

Ethical Statement: All subjects gave their informed consent for inclusion before they participated in the study. The study was conducted in accordance with the Declaration of Helsinki, and the protocol was approved by the UK NHS research Ethics Committee (12/LO/1247).

References

1. Lejeune, F.; Audeoud, F.; Marcus, L.; Streri, A.; Debillon, T.; Gentaz, E. The manual habituation and discrimination of shapes in preterm human infants from 33 to 34+6 post-conceptional age. *PLoS ONE* **2010**, *5*, e9108. [CrossRef] [PubMed]

2. Nelson, K.B.; Lynch, J.K. Stroke in newborn infants. *Lancet Neurol.* **2004**, *3*, 150–158. [CrossRef]

3. Mercuri, E.; Ricci, D.; Pane, M.; Baranello, G. The neurological examination of the newborn baby. *Early Hum. Dev.* **2005**, *81*, 947–956. [CrossRef] [PubMed]

4. Glick, T.H. Toward a more efficient and effective neurologic examination for the 21st century. *Eur. J. Neurol.* **2005**, *12*, 994–997. [CrossRef] [PubMed]

5. Moraes, M.V.M.; Tudella, E.; Ribeiro, J.; Beltrame, T.S.; Krebs, R.J. Reliability of the M-FLEX^{TM}: Equipment to measure palmar grasp strength in infants. *Infant Behav. Dev.* **2011**, *34*, 226–234. [CrossRef] [PubMed]

6. Allievi, A.G.; Arichi, T.; Gordon, A.L.; Burdet, E. Technology-aided assessment of sensorimotor function in early infancy. *Front. Neurol.* **2014**, *5*, 197. [CrossRef] [PubMed]

7. Molina, M.; Sann, C.; David, M.; Touré, Y.; Guillois, B.; Jouen, F. Active touch in late-preterm and early-term neonates. *Dev. Psychobiol.* **2015**, *57*, 322–335. [CrossRef] [PubMed]

8. Allievi, A.G.; Melendez-Calderon, A.; Arichi, T.; Edwards, A.D.; Burdet, E. An fMRI compatible wrist robotic interface to study brain development in neonates. *Ann. Biomed. Eng.* **2013**, *41*, 1181–1192. [CrossRef]

9. Dall'Orso, S.; Steinweg, J.; Allievi, A.G.; Edwards, A.D.; Burdet, E.; Arichi, T. Somatotopic mapping of the developing sensorimotor cortex in the preterm human brain. *Cereb. Cortex* **2018**, *28*, 2507–2515. [CrossRef]

10. Stippich, C.; Freitag, P.; Kassubek, J.; Sörös, P.; Kamada, K.; Kober, H.; Scheffler, K.; Hopfengärtner, R.; Bilecen, D.; Radü, E.; et al. Motor, somatosensory and auditory cortex localization by fMRI and MEG. *NeuroReport* **1998**, *9*, 1953–1957. [CrossRef]

11. Stippich, C.; Hofmann, R.; Kapfer, D.; Hempel, E.; Heiland, S.; Jansen, O.; Sartor, K. Somatotopic mapping of the human primary somatosensory cortex by fully automated tactile stimulation using functional magnetic resonance imaging. *Neurosci. Lett.* **1999**, *277*, 25–28. [CrossRef]

12. Moore, C.I.; Stern, C.E.; Corkin, S.; Fischl, B.; Gray, A.C.; Rosen, B.R.; Dale, A.M. Segregation of somatosensory activation in the human rolandic cortex using fMRI. *J. Neurophysiol.* **2000**, *84*, 558–569. [CrossRef] [PubMed]

13. Blatow, M.; Nennig, E.; Durst, A.; Sartor, K.; Stippich, C. fMRI reflects functional connectivity of human somatosensory cortex. *Neuroimage* **2007**, *37*, 927–936. [CrossRef] [PubMed]

14. Molina, M.; Jouen, F. Weight perception in 12-month-old infants. *Infant Behav. Dev.* **2003**, *26*, 49–63. [CrossRef]

15. Molina, M.; Jouen, F. Modulation of the palmar grasp behavior in neonates according to texture property. *Infant Behav. Dev.* **1998**, *21*, 659–666. [CrossRef]

16. Del Maestro, M.; Cecchi, F.; Serio, S.M.; Laschi, C.; Dario, P. Sensing device for measuring infants' grasping actions. *Sens. Actuators A Phys.* **2011**, *165*, 155–163. [CrossRef]

17. Baldoli, I.; Cecchi, F.; Guzzetta, A.; Laschi, C. Sensorized graspable devices for the study of motor imitation in infants. In Proceedings of the Annual International Conference of the IEEE Engineering in Medicine and Biology Society, EMBS, Milan, Italy, 25–29 August 2015; pp. 7394–7397.

18. Muhammad, T.; Lee, J.S.; Shin, Y.B.; Kim, S. A wearable device to measure the palmar grasp reflex of neonates in neonatal intensive care unit. *Sens. Actuators A Phys.* **2020**, *304*, 111905. [CrossRef]

19. Cecchi, F.; Serio, S.M.; Del Maestro, M.; Laschi, C.; Sgandurra, G.; Cioni, G.; Dario, P. Design and development of "biomechatronic gym" for early detection of neurological disorders in infants. In Proceedings of the 2010 Annual International Conference of the IEEE Engineering in Medicine and Biology Society, EMBC'10, Buenos Aires, Argentina, 31 August–4 September 2010; pp. 3414–3417.

20. Lo Presti, D.; Massaroni, C.; Leitao, C.S.J.; Domingues, M.F.; Sypabekova, M.; Barrera, D.; Floris, I.; Massari, L.; Oddo, C.M.; Sales, S.; et al. Fiber Bragg Gratings for medical applications and future challenges: A review. *IEEE Access* **2020**, *8*, 156863–156888. [CrossRef]

21. Othonos, A. Fiber Bragg gratings. *Rev. Sci. Instrum.* **1997**, *68*, 4309–4341. [CrossRef]

22. Gassert, R.; Burdet, E.; Chinzei, K. MRI-compatible robotics. *IEEE Eng. Med. Biol. Mag.* **2008**, *27*, 12–14. [CrossRef] [PubMed]

23. Dempsey, M.F.; Condon, B.; Hadley, D.M. MRI safety review. *Semin. Ultrasound CT MRI* **2002**, *23*, 392–401. [CrossRef]

24. Dempsey, M.F.; Condon, B. Thermal injuries associated with MRI. *Clin. Radiol.* **2001**, *56*, 457–465. [CrossRef] [PubMed]

25. Krupa, K.; Bekiesińska-Figatowska, M. Artifacts in magnetic resonance imaging. *Pol. J. Radiol.* **2015**, *80*, 93–106. [PubMed]

26. Hall, J.G.; Ursula, G.F.I.; Allanson, J.E. *Oxford Medical Publications: Handbook of Normal Physical*; Cambridge University Press: Cambridge, UK, 1989.

27. Molina, M.; Jouen, F. Manual cyclical activity as an explanatory tool in neonates. *Infant Behav. Dev.* **2004**, *27*, 42–53. [CrossRef]

28. Smooth-On Dragon Skin® High Performance Silicone Rubber. Available online: https://www.smooth-on.com/product-line/dragon-skin/ (accessed on 23 July 2020).

29. Erdogan, T. Fiber grating spectra. *J. Light. Technol.* **1997**, *15*, 1277–1294. [CrossRef]

30. Massaroni, C.; Zaltieri, M.; Lo Presti, D.; Tosi, D.; Schena, E. Fiber Bragg Grating Sensors for Cardiorespiratory Monitoring: A Review. *IEEE Sens. J.* **2020**. [CrossRef]

31. Lo Presti, D.; Carnevale, A.; D'Abbraccio, J.; Massari, L.; Massaroni, C.; Sabbadini, R.; Zaltieri, M.; Di Tocco, J.; Bravi, M.; Miccinilli, S.; et al. A multi-parametric wearable system to monitor neck movements and respiratory frequency of computer workers. *Sensors* **2020**, *20*, 536. [CrossRef]

32. BSI Biological Evaluation of Medical Devices Part 10: Tests for Irritation and Skin Sensitization. Available online: https://www.iso.org/standard/40884.html (accessed on 25 August 2020).

33. Mazurek, P.; Vudayagiri, S.; Skov, A.L. How to tailor flexible silicone elastomers with mechanical integrity: A tutorial review. *Chem. Soc. Rev.* **2019**, *48*, 1448–1464. [CrossRef]

34. Silicone Thinner® Product Information | Smooth-On, Inc. Available online: https://www.smooth-on.com/products/silicone-thinner/ (accessed on 25 August 2020).

35. ISO 7743:2011 Rubber, Vulcanized or Thermoplastic—Determination of Compression Stress-Strain Properties. Available online: https://www.iso.org/standard/72784.html (accessed on 25 August 2020).

36. Willink, R.; Willink, R. Guide to the Expression of Uncertainty in Measurement. In *Measurement Uncertainty and Probability*; Cambridge University Press: Cambridge, UK, 2013; pp. 237–244, ISBN 9267101889.

37. Jenkinson, M.; Beckmann, C.F.; Behrens, T.E.J.; Woolrich, M.W.; Smith, S.M. Review FSL. *Neuroimage* **2012**, *62*, 782–790. [CrossRef]
38. Halverson, H.M. An experimental study of prehension in infants by means of systematic cinema records. *Genet. Psychol. Monogr.* **1931**, *10*, 107–286.
39. Halverson, H.M. A further study of grasping. *J. Gen. Psychol.* **1932**, *7*, 34–64. [CrossRef]
40. Halverson, H.M. Studies of the grasping responses of early infancy: I. *Pedagog. Semin. J. Genet. Psychol.* **1937**, *51*, 371–392. [CrossRef]
41. Amiel-Tison, C.; Barrier, G.; Shnider, S.M.; Hughes, S.C.; Stefani, S.J. A new neurologic and adaptive capacity scoring system for evaluating obstetric medications in full-term newborns. *Anesthesiol. J. Am. Soc. Anesthesiol.* **1980**, *53*, S322. [CrossRef]
42. Forssberg, H.; Kinoshita, H.; Eliasson, A.C.; Johansson, R.S.; Westling, G.; Gordon, A.M. Development of human precision grip—II. Anticipatory control of isometric forces targeted for object's weight. *Exp. Brain Res.* **1992**, *90*, 393–398. [PubMed]
43. Cecchi, F.; Serio, S.M.; Perego, P.; Mattoli, V.; Damiani, F.; Laschi, C.; Dario, P. A mechatronic toy for measuring infants' grasping development. In Proceedings of the 2nd Biennial IEEE/RAS-EMBS International Conference on Biomedical Robotics and Biomechatronics, BioRob 2008, Scottsdale, AZ, USA, 19–22 October 2008; pp. 397–401.
44. Cioni, G.; Bos, A.F.; Einspieler, C.; Ferrari, F.; Martijn, A.; Paolicelli, P.B.; Rapisardi, G.; Roversi, M.F.; Prechtl, H.F.R. Early neurological signs in preterm infants with unilateral intraparenchymal echodensity. *Neuropediatrics* **2000**, *31*, 240–251. [CrossRef]

7

Spray Deposition of Ag Nanowire–Graphene Oxide Hybrid Electrodes for Flexible Polymer–Dispersed Liquid Crystal Displays

Yumi Choi [1], Chang Su Kim [2] and Sungjin Jo [1,*]

[1]   School of Architectural, Civil, Environmental, and Energy Engineering, Kyungpook National University,
      Daegu 41566, Korea; yums1026@gmail.com
[2]   Advanced Functional Thin Films Department, Korea Institute of Materials Science (KIMS),
      Changwon 51508, Korea; cskim1025@kims.re.kr
*   Correspondence: sungjin@knu.ac.kr

Abstract: We investigated the effect of different spray-coating parameters on the electro-optical properties of Ag nanowires (NWs). Highly transparent and conductive Ag NW–graphene oxide (GO) hybrid electrodes were fabricated by using the spray-coating technique. The Ag NW percolation network was modified with GO and this led to a reduced sheet resistance of the Ag NW–GO electrode as the result of a decrease in the inter-nanowire contact resistance. Although electrical conductivity and optical transmittance of the Ag NW electrodes have a trade-off relationship, Ag NW–GO hybrid electrodes exhibited significantly improved sheet resistance and slightly decreased transmittance compared to Ag NW electrodes. Ag NW–GO hybrid electrodes were integrated into smart windows based on polymer-dispersed liquid crystals (PDLCs) for the first time. Experimental results showed that the electro-optical properties of the PDLCs based on Ag NW–GO electrodes were superior when compared to those of PDLCs based on only Ag NW electrodes. This study revealed that the hybrid Ag NW–GO electrode is a promising material for manufacturing the large-area flexible indium tin oxide (ITO)-free PDLCs.

Keywords: silver nanowire; graphene oxide; polymer-dispersed liquid crystal; smart window; hybrid transparent conductive electrode

---

1. Introduction

Smart windows are controllable windows whose optical properties can be altered by applying an electric field. They are used for various applications including switchable privacy glasses, vehicle windows, and energy-saving windows [1–3]. Smart windows have recently attracted significant attention since they can minimize heating and cooling energies in buildings and transportation systems. Among the different electrooptically switchable active components available for smart windows such as polymer-dispersed liquid crystals (PDLCs), chromic materials, and suspended particles, PDLCs are an excellent candidate due to their high transmittance, wide viewing angle, high switching speed, and a relatively simple fabrication process [4,5].

The PDLCs consist of birefringent liquid crystal (LC) droplets that are uniformly dispersed in a solid polymer matrix. In order to fabricate smart windows based on PDLCs, the PDLC film is positioned between two transparent conductive electrodes (TCEs). The PDLC film can be switched from an opaque to a transparent state since the electric field between the TCEs aligns the directors of the LCs along the same direction. Therefore, TCEs with low sheet resistances and high transmittances are necessary in order to minimize the voltage drop across the electrode and ensure fast switching as well as smaller power consumption. Indium tin oxide (ITO) has been commonly used as a TCE for typical smart windows based on PDLCs. Although ITO has high conductivity and transmittance, its relatively high cost and fragile characteristics make it unsuitable for fabrication of large-area flexible smart windows.

There are several potential alternatives to ITO including conductive polymers, graphene, Ag nanowires (NWs), metal grids, and carbon nanotubes. Recently, conductive polymers, graphene, and Ag NWs have been successfully integrated into PDLC-based smart windows [6–8]. Although these emerging candidate materials are of primary interest, they suffer from lower electrical conductivities, complex fabrication processes, lower transmittances, and uneven distributions of the electric currents. In order to overcome the disadvantages of these individual TCE materials, hybrid TCEs such as Ag NW–graphene, Ag NW–conductive polymer, Ag NW–metal oxide, Ag NW–carbon nanotubes, and Ag NW–metal grids [9–13] have also been investigated. Even though these hybrid TCEs have been investigated for applications in various electronic devices including solar cells, organic light emitting diodes, flexible heaters, flexible sensors, and touch panels [14–18], no extensive studies have been reported on the application of hybrid electrodes for PDLC-based smart windows.

In this study, the hybrid Ag NW–GO electrode was used as a substitute for an ITO electrode in a PDLC. To the best of our knowledge, we report for the first time Ag NW–GO hybrid electrodes integrated into smart windows based on PDLCs. Because of the inverse relationship between optical transmittance and electrical resistivity of TCE, the optical properties of TCE deteriorate with increasing electrical conductivity. However, Ag NW–GO hybrid structure can reduce the resistances of Ag NW networks without affecting their transmittances. In this case, we have described the preparation of highly conductive and transparent Ag NW–GO hybrid electrodes by a simple spray-coating technique for the fast production of large-area flexible smart windows with a decreased production cost.

2. Materials and Methods

2.1. Ag NW–GO Hybrid Electrode Fabrication

A hybrid electrode was fabricated by using Ag NWs (Nanopyxis) dispersed in isopropyl alcohol (IPA) and GO (Uninanotech) dispersed in IPA. In order to fabricate the GO suspension, a 6.2 g/L GO suspension was diluted with IPA to 0.2 g/L and sonicated for 20 min. The polyethylene terephthalate (PET) substrates were cleaned with acetone, IPA, and deionized water. After drying, the PET films were treated with ultraviolet-ozone (UVO) for 5 min. Immediately after the UVO treatment, the Ag NW suspension was uniformly spray coated and annealed at 65 °C for 1 min. Lastly, in order to form Ag NW–GO hybrid electrodes, the GO suspension was spray coated onto the Ag NWs and dried at 65 °C for 5 min. For spray deposition, a fully automated spray coater was utilized.

2.2. PDLC Fabrication

The PDLCs, which is commercially available from Qingdao Liquid Crystal, were mixed with spacers at a weight ratio of 100:1 and stirred for 4 h to obtain a uniform thickness of the PDLC layer. The fully mixed solution was drop-dispersed on the substrate coated with Ag NW–GO. Subsequently, it was covered with another Ag NW–GO-coated substrate, which produced a sandwich structure (Figure S1). Lastly, the PDLC layer was photo-polymerized by using a mask aligner for 5 min.

3. Results and Discussion

In order to produce highly uniform, transparent, and conductive Ag NW networks by spray coating, various processing parameters such as dispensing pressure, spray pressure, nozzle–to–sample distance, scan speed, and substrate temperature should be simultaneously controlled [19]. We investigated the influence of each of these parameters on the morphology of the Ag NW network, which is known to affect their electro-optical properties. First, Ag NW networks were prepared at three different dispensing pressures: 0.1 psi, 0.5 psi, and 1 psi. Their optical transmittances (T) and sheet resistances (R_s) were measured and their morphologies were characterized by using scanning electron microscopy (SEM). Figure 1a shows a decrease in the T and R_s values with the increasing dispensing pressure. A higher dispensing pressure led to a higher flow rate of the Ag NW suspension, which affected the density of the Ag NW networks. As shown in Figure 2a,b and Figure S2a,b, the Ag NW density increased with the dispensing pressure. However, a high dispensing pressure could clog the nozzle, which leads to an irregular flow of the Ag NW suspension through the nozzle and, thus, to an irregular coating of Ag NWs. Ag NW-deficient areas were observed in Figure S2c due to the irregular deposition of Ag NWs at a dispensing pressure of 1 psi. In order to avoid this phenomenon, the dispensing pressure was maintained at 0.5 psi. Second, the nozzle–to–sample distance, which controls the mass of Ag NWs sprayed per unit area, was optimized to obtain uniform Ag NW networks [20]. The T and R_s values in Figure 1b show that the density of Ag NWs increased with a decreasing nozzle–to–substrate distance. The nozzle–to–substrate distance was chosen to be 6 cm since a smaller distance led to nonuniform Ag NW networks while a larger distance led to low-density Ag NW networks, which is shown in Figure 2d–f and Figure S2d–f. Lastly, we investigated the effect of the nozzle pressure on the electro-optical performance of the Ag NW network. The nozzle pressure was chosen to be as high as 35 psi because an increased nozzle pressure increased the Ag NW density, as shown in Figure 2g–i. The relationship between T and R_s of the Ag NW networks (Figure 1c) was consistent with the SEM results. A higher nozzle pressure led to large shear forces, which promoted the Ag NW suspension into smaller droplets that were beneficial for the deposition of more uniform films since small droplets tend to produce less prominent "coffee-staining" effects [21].

In order to enhance the electro-optical properties of the Ag NW networks, they were spray-coated with the GO suspension. Electrical conduction in an Ag NW network is dominated by the resistances at junctions of Ag NWs due to the percolative nature of conduction. The GO tends to bond with Ag NWs due to the strong electrostatic adhesion caused by the large number of oxygen-containing groups in GO [22]. The GO sheets adhered and wrapped around the Ag NWs, which led to the soldering of the inter-nanowire junctions and caused a significant reduction in the contact resistance of these junctions [23]. The optimized spray-coating parameters for the formation of Ag NW networks were also used for the spray coating of the GO suspension. As shown in Figure 3b and Figure S3, the Ag NW junctions were wrapped by the GO sheets and a small number of GO sheets were deposited in the optical pathway and unblocked by Ag NWs, which enhanced the electro-optical properties of the Ag NW–GO hybrid networks by reducing R_s while minimizing the loss of T. The transmittances, sheet resistances, and figures of merit (FoMs) of the Ag NW and Ag NW–GO hybrid networks are summarized in Table 1. The spray-coated Ag NW–GO hybrid networks exhibited excellent properties. A representative film had $T = 90.7\%$ and $R_s = 15.6 \, \Omega/\text{sq}$. Table 1 shows that the FoM was enhanced upon the formation of the Ag NW–GO hybrid network when compared to that of the Ag NW network.

Table 1. Sheet resistances, transmittances, and FoMs of the Ag NW and Ag NW–GO films.

Electrode	Sheet Resistance (Ω/sq)	Transmittance (%) (at 550 nm)	FoM ($10^{-3} \, \Omega^{-1}$)
Ag NW	22.8	92.0	19.1
Ag NW–GO	15.6	90.7	24.2

Furthermore, the uniformity of R_s of the Ag NW networks, which is one of the most important quality factors for large-area transparent conductive films, was improved upon the formation of the Ag NW–GO hybrid networks. The uniformities of large-area Ag NW and Ag NW–GO networks (200 mm × 200 mm) were estimated by measuring their R_s values at 81 points with intervals of 20 mm in the horizontal and vertical directions. Figure 4 shows the distribution of the R_s values of the Ag NW and Ag NW–GO networks. The standard deviation of R_s of the Ag NW and Ag NW–GO networks were 4.21 Ω/sq and 1.48 Ω/sq, respectively. Therefore, the improved electro-optical properties and high uniformity of the Ag NW–GO network fabricated by spray coating made it suitable for large-area smart window applications.

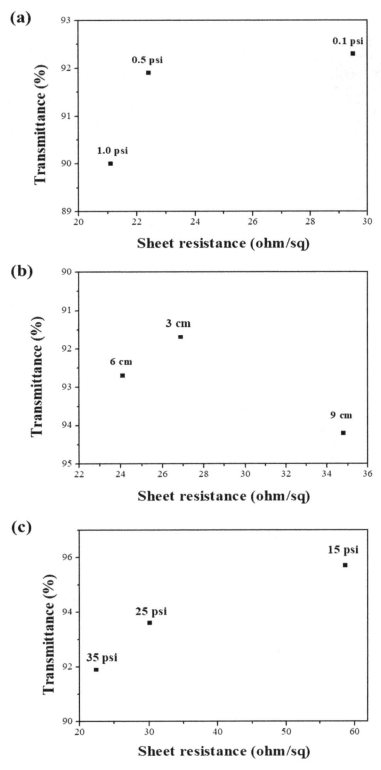

Figure 1. Transmittances at 550 nm and sheet resistances of the spray-coated Ag NW films as a function of the (**a**) dispensing pressure, (**b**) nozzle–to–substrate distance, and (**c**) nozzle pressure.

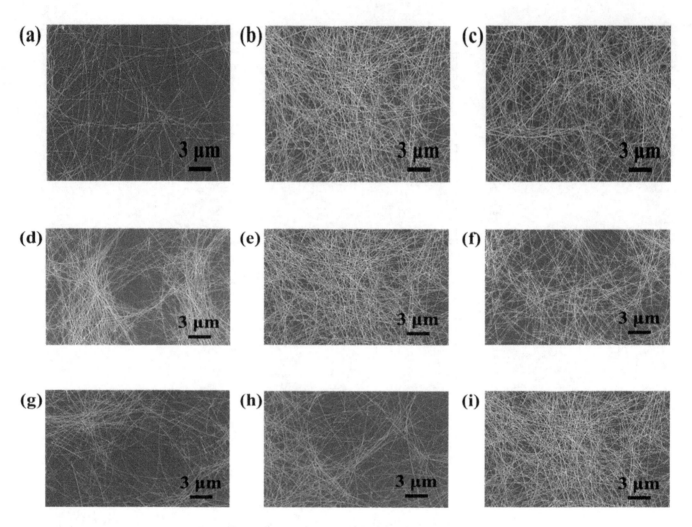

Figure 2. SEM images of Ag NW networks obtained with different spray-coating parameters including dispensing pressures of (**a**) 0.1 psi, (**b**) 0.5 psi, and (**c**) 1 psi, nozzle–to–substrate distances of (**d**) 3 cm, (**e**) 6 cm, and (**f**) 9 cm, and nozzle pressures of (**g**) 15 psi, (**h**) 25 psi, and (**i**) 35 psi.

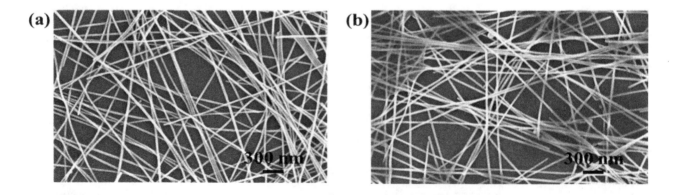

Figure 3. SEM images of the spray-coated (**a**) Ag NW network and (**b**) Ag NW network covered by GO nanosheets.

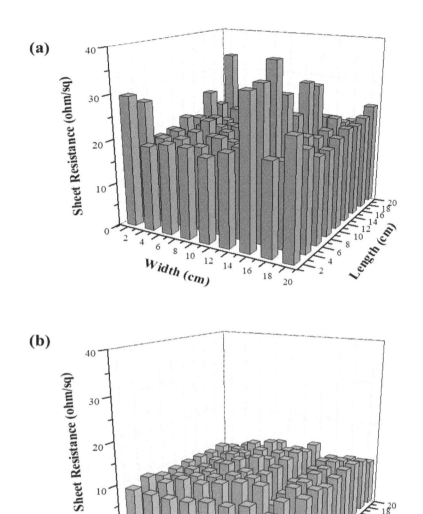

Figure 4. Histograms of the sheet resistances of the large-area, (**a**) Ag NW, and (**b**) Ag NW–GO hybrid electrodes.

The transmittances of the PDLC were measured at applied voltage amplitudes in the range of 0 to 80 V. Voltage–transmittance characteristics of PDLCs fabricated with Ag NW and Ag NW–GO hybrid electrodes are shown in Figure 5a. The difference in driving voltage between these two sets of PDLCs was clear. The driving voltage of the PDLC with Ag NW electrodes was larger than that of the PDLC fabricated by using Ag NW–GO electrodes. The transmittance of the PDLC based on the Ag NW–GO hybrid electrodes could reach 63% at 40 V while that of the Ag NW-based PDLC was only 53% at 40 V and the maximum transmittance was only 61% at 80 V. This result implied that the lower R_s of the Ag NW–GO electrodes than that of the Ag NW electrodes led to a lower driving voltage and lower energy consumption. Figure 5b shows the transmittances of the Ag NW and Ag NW–GO-based PDLCs in the on- (80 V) and off- (0 V) states as a function of the wavelength. The transmittance differences at 550 nm between the on-states and off-states for the Ag NW and Ag NW–GO-based PDLCs were 57% and 65%, respectively (Figure S4). Therefore, the Ag NW–GO-based PDLC was more desirable for use as a smart window since it was not only more transparent in the on state but could also be operated at a lower voltage.

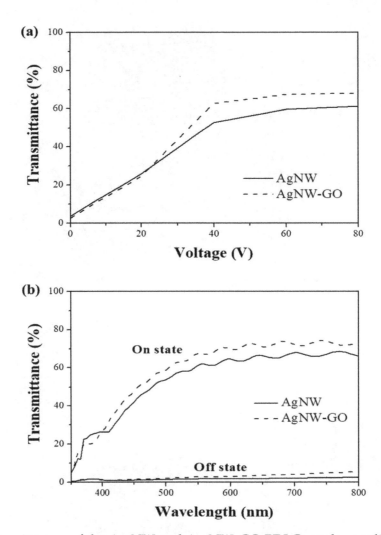

Figure 5. (a) Transmittances of the Ag NW and Ag NW–GO PDLCs under applied voltages in the range of 0 to 80 V at a wavelength of 550 nm. (b) Transmittance spectra of the Ag NW and Ag NW–GO PDLCs in the on- (80 V) and off- (0 V) states.

Photographs of the fabricated PDLCs in the on-states and off-states are shown in Figure 6. The difference in transmittance between the on-states and off-states was evident and in agreement with the results in Figure 5b. The fabricated PDLC was opaque in the off-state at which the printed text below the PDLC could hardly be observed. On the contrary, in the on-state, the printed text underneath the PDLC could be clearly observed since the PDLC was transparent. In the case of the Ag NW–GO-based PDLC, the printed text appears clearer than in the case of the Ag NW-based PDLC due to its high transmittance in the on-state. The high contrast between the on-states and off-states made the PDLC with Ag NW–GO suitable for smart windows.

Lastly, we aimed to fabricate a flexible large-area PDLC by utilizing the advantage of the PDLC based on the Ag NW–GO electrodes that were obtained by using the spray-coating technique. In order to fabricate a flexible large-area PDLC, Ag NW–GO was spray-coated on a PET substrate rather than on a glass substrate [24–26]. As shown in Figure 7a, the flexible PDLC operated perfectly and no damage was observed even though the PDLC was bent. The images of the large-area PDLC with the Ag NW–GO electrodes in Figure 7b,c show that the large-area PDLC operated uniformly in both on-states and off-states. This implied that the electric field between the Ag NW–GO electrodes was sufficiently uniform, which is consistent with the results illustrated in Figure 4b.

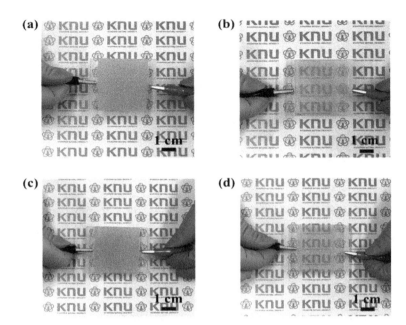

Figure 6. Photographs of the Ag NW PDLC in the (**a**) off-states and (**b**) on-states. Photographs of the Ag NW–GO PDLC in the (**c**) off-states and (**d**) on-states.

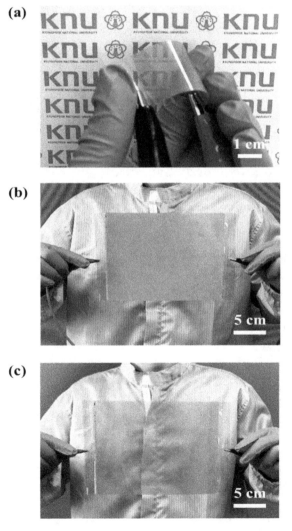

Figure 7. (**a**) Photograph of the flexible PDLC in the on-state. Photographs of the large-area PDLC in the (**b**) off-states and (**c**) on-states.

4. Conclusions

The spray-coating conditions were optimized for the fabrication of Ag NW–GO hybrid TCEs with high T and low R_s values, which can be used as superior alternatives to ITO TCEs. The PDLCs based on the Ag NW–GO electrodes exhibited a high transmittance of 63% in the on-state under a low driving voltage (40 V) due to the low R_s. The new class of flexible large-area PDLCs presented in this study demonstrate the promising potential of the spray-coated Ag NW–GO hybrid electrodes for PDLCs. This study provides a significant advancement toward the realization of flexible smart windows for future flexible optoelectronic applications.

Author Contributions: Y.C., C.S.K., and S.J. conceived and designed the experiments; Y.C., C.S.K., and S.J. performed the experiments and analyzed the data; Y.C. and S.J contributed to the manuscript preparation.

References

1. Lampert, C.M. Large-area smart glass and integrated photovoltaics. *Sol. Energ. Mater. Sol. Cells* **2003**, *76*, 489–499. [CrossRef]
2. Sol, J.A.; Timmermans, G.H.; van Breugel, A.J.; Schenning, A.P.; Debije, M.G. Multistate Luminescent Solar Concentrator "Smart" Windows. *Adv. Energy Mater.* **2018**, *8*, 1702922. [CrossRef]
3. Granqvist, C.G. Electrochromics for smart windows: Oxide-based thin films and devices. *Thin Solid Films* **2014**, *564*, 1–38. [CrossRef]
4. Cupelli, D.; Nicoletta, F.P.; Manfredi, S.; Vivacqua, M.; Formoso, P.; De Filpo, G.; Chidichimo, G. Self-adjusting smart windows based on polymer-dispersed liquid crystals. *Sol. Energ. Mater. Sol. Cells* **2009**, *93*, 2008–2012. [CrossRef]
5. Kim, Y.; Jung, D.; Jeong, S.; Kim, K.; Choi, W.; Seo, Y. Optical properties and optimized conditions for polymer dispersed liquid crystal containing UV curable polymer and nematic liquid crystal. *Curr. Appl. Phys.* **2015**, *15*, 292–297. [CrossRef]
6. Kim, Y.; Kim, K.; Kim, K.B.; Park, J.; Lee, N.; Seo, Y. Flexible polymer dispersed liquid crystal film with graphene transparent electrodes. *Curr. Appl. Phys.* **2016**, *16*, 409–414. [CrossRef]
7. Khaligh, H.H.; Liew, K.; Han, Y.; Abukhdeir, N.M.; Goldthorpe, I.A. Silver nanowire transparent electrodes for liquid crystal-based smart windows. *Sol. Energ. Mater. Sol. Cells* **2015**, *132*, 337–341. [CrossRef]
8. Chou, T.; Chen, S.; Chiang, Y.; Chang, T.; Lin, C.; Chao, C. Highly conductive PEDOT: PSS film by doping p-toluenesulfonic acid and post-treatment with dimethyl sulfoxide for ITO-free polymer dispersed liquid crystal device. *Org. Electron.* **2017**, *48*, 223–229. [CrossRef]
9. Lim, J.; Lee, S.; Kim, S.; Kim, T.; Koo, H.; Kim, H. Brush-paintable and highly stretchable Ag nanowire and PEDOT: PSS hybrid electrodes. *Sci. Rep.* **2017**, *7*, 14685. [CrossRef] [PubMed]
10. Ricciardulli, A.G.; Yang, S.; Wetzelaer, G.A.; Feng, X.; Blom, P.W. Hybrid Silver Nanowire and Graphene-Based Solution-Processed Transparent Electrode for Organic Optoelectronics. *Adv. Funct. Mater.* **2018**, *28*, 1706010. [CrossRef]
11. Chen, D.; Liang, J.; Liu, C.; Saldanha, G.; Zhao, F.; Tong, K.; Liu, J.; Pei, Q. Thermally stable silver nanowire–polyimide transparent electrode based on atomic layer deposition of zinc oxide on silver nanowires. *Adv. Funct. Mater.* **2015**, *25*, 7512–7520. [CrossRef]
12. Kim, C.; Jung, C.; Oh, Y.; Kim, D. A highly flexible transparent conductive electrode based on nanomaterials. *NPG Asia Mater.* **2017**, *9*, e438. [CrossRef]
13. Jang, J.; Im, H.; Jin, J.; Lee, J.; Lee, J.; Bae, B. A Flexible and Robust Transparent Conducting Electrode Platform Using an Electroplated Silver Grid/Surface-Embedded Silver Nanowire Hybrid Structure. *ACS Appl. Mater. Interfaces* **2016**, *8*, 27035–27043. [CrossRef] [PubMed]
14. Zhang, Q.; Di, Y.; Huard, C.M.; Guo, L.J.; Wei, J.; Guo, J. Highly stable and stretchable graphene–polymer processed silver nanowires hybrid electrodes for flexible displays. *J. Mater. Chem. C* **2015**, *3*, 1528–1536. [CrossRef]

15. Lee, J.; Lee, P.; Lee, H.B.; Hong, S.; Lee, I.; Yeo, J.; Lee, S.S.; Kim, T.; Lee, D.; Ko, S.H. Room-temperature nanosoldering of a very long metal nanowire network by conducting-polymer-assisted joining for a flexible touch-panel application. *Adv. Funct. Mater.* **2013**, *23*, 4171–4176. [CrossRef]

16. Zilberberg, K.; Gasse, F.; Pagui, R.; Polywka, A.; Behrendt, A.; Trost, S.; Heiderhoff, R.; Görrn, P.; Riedl, T. Highly Robust Indium-Free Transparent Conductive Electrodes Based on Composites of Silver Nanowires and Conductive Metal Oxides. *Adv. Funct. Mater.* **2014**, *24*, 1671–1678. [CrossRef]

17. Kim, D.; Zhu, L.; Jeong, D.; Chun, K.; Bang, Y.; Kim, S.; Kim, J.; Oh, S. Transparent flexible heater based on hybrid of carbon nanotubes and silver nanowires. *Carbon* **2013**, *63*, 530–536. [CrossRef]

18. Fan, Z.; Liu, B.; Liu, X.; Li, Z.; Wang, H.; Yang, S.; Wang, J. A flexible and disposable hybrid electrode based on Cu nanowires modified graphene transparent electrode for non-enzymatic glucose sensor. *Electrochim. Acta* **2013**, *109*, 602–608. [CrossRef]

19. Lee, J.; Shin, D.; Park, J. Fabrication of silver nanowire-based stretchable electrodes using spray coating. *Thin Solid Films* **2016**, *608*, 34–43. [CrossRef]

20. Scardaci, V.; Coull, R.; Lyons, P.E.; Rickard, D.; Coleman, J.N. Spray deposition of highly transparent, low-resistance networks of silver nanowires over large areas. *Small* **2011**, *7*, 2621–2628. [CrossRef] [PubMed]

21. Deegan, R.D.; Bakajin, O.; Dupont, T.F.; Huber, G.; Nagel, S.R.; Witten, T.A. Contact line deposits in an evaporating drop. *Phys. Rev. E* **2000**, *62*, 756. [CrossRef]

22. Ha, B.; Jo, S. Hybrid Ag nanowire transparent conductive electrodes with randomly oriented and grid-patterned Ag nanowire networks. *Sci. Rep.* **2017**, *7*, 11614. [CrossRef] [PubMed]

23. Liang, J.; Li, L.; Tong, K.; Ren, Z.; Hu, W.; Niu, X.; Chen, Y.; Pei, Q. Silver nanowire percolation network soldered with graphene oxide at room temperature and its application for fully stretchable polymer light-emitting diodes. *ACS Nano* **2014**, *8*, 1590–1600. [CrossRef] [PubMed]

24. Singh, A.; Salmi, Z.; Joshi, N.; Jha, P.; Decorse, P.; Lecoq, H.; Lau-Truong, S.; Jouini, M.; Aswal, D.; Chehimi, M. Electrochemical investigation of free-standing polypyrrole–silver nanocomposite films: A substrate free electrode material for supercapacitors. *RCS Adv.* **2013**, *3*, 24567–24575. [CrossRef]

25. Kim, Y.; Hong, J.; Lee, S. Fabrication of a highly bendable LCD with an elastomer substrate by using a replica-molding method. *J. Soc. Inf. Disp.* **2006**, *14*, 1091–1095. [CrossRef]

26. Kim, I.; Kim, T.; Lee, S.; Kim, B. Extremely Foldable and Highly Transparent Nanofiber-Based Electrodes for Liquid Crystal Smart Device. *Sci. Rep.* **2018**, *8*, 11517. [CrossRef] [PubMed]

8

Viscoelastic Hemostatic Assays: Moving from the Laboratory to the Site of Care—A Review of Established and Emerging Technologies

Jan Hartmann [1,*], Matthew Murphy [1] and Joao D. Dias [2]

[1] Haemonetics Corporation, Boston, MA 02110, USA; MMurphy@Haemonetics.com
[2] Haemonetics SA, Signy CH, 1274 Signy-Centre, Switzerland; joao.dias@haemonetics.com
* Correspondence: jan.hartmann@haemonetics.com

Abstract: Viscoelastic-based techniques to evaluate whole blood hemostasis have advanced substantially since they were first developed over 70 years ago but are still based upon the techniques first described by Dr. Hellmut Hartert in 1948. Today, the use of thromboelastography, the method of testing viscoelastic properties of blood coagulation, has moved out of the research laboratory and is now more widespread, used commonly during surgery, in emergency departments, intensive care units, and in labor wards. Thromboelastography is currently a rapidly growing field of technological advancement and is attracting significant investment. This review will first describe the history of the viscoelastic testing and the established first-generation devices, which were developed for use within the laboratory. This review will then describe the next-generation hemostasis monitoring devices, which were developed for use at the site of care for an expanding range of clinical applications. This review will then move on to experimental technologies, which promise to make viscoelastic testing more readily available in a wider range of clinical environments in the endeavor to improve patient care.

Keywords: blood; coagulation; hemostasis; point of care; ROTEM; TEG; thromboelastography; VHA; viscoelastic testing

1. Introduction

The use of techniques to evaluate hemostasis utilizing the viscoelastic properties of whole blood have been reported since the 1940s. The technology and clinical applications of viscoelastic hemostatic assays grew slowly over the next 40 years. In parallel, the use of today's standard hemostatic assays (prothrombin time, activated partial thromboplastin, international normalized ratio, etc.) became common. However, these assays only shed light on a small part of the overall hemostasis process. In the 1980s, the use of thromboelastography became more widespread during high blood loss procedures, such as cardiac surgery and liver transplantation [1,2], and in the management of major bleeding [3]. More recently, instrumentation quality and ease of use has improved dramatically. Viscoelastic hemostatic monitoring is now a rapidly growing field, drawing significant attention and investment. The current technological landscape has a host of new technologies being developed to improve the capability of the instrumentation and bring it closer to the site of care.

2. What Is Viscoelastic Testing?

Viscoelasticity is the characteristic of a material that behaves in both a viscous (permanent deformation) and elastic (temporary deformation) manner. Prior to clotting, whole blood is a purely viscous material and the response to shear stress will be permanent deformation. Once the shear stress is removed, the sample will not return to its original shape. As a blood sample begins to clot, the fluid becomes less viscous and more elastic in nature. The deformation induced by the shear stress becomes temporary as the fluid tries to return to its original shape. The primary measurement during viscoelastic hemostatic monitoring is the observation of the transition from a viscous to elastic state, and the measurement of the shear elastic modulus: a measure of the amount of force required to shear a material (also known as shear stiffness). The elastic modulus is defined as the ratio of shear stress to shear strain (Figure 1).

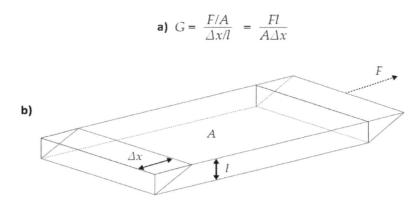

$$\text{a)}\quad G = \frac{F/A}{\Delta x/l} = \frac{Fl}{A\Delta x}$$

Figure 1. Shear elastic modulus. (**a**) Mathematical formula to express shear modulus; (**b**) Schematic representation of the shear principle. G = shear modulus; F = force; A = area; F/A = shear stress; Δx = transverse displacement; l = initial length. Reproduced with permission from [4].

3. History of Viscoelastic Testing

Viscoelastic hemostatic monitoring was first described in 1948 by Dr. Hellmut Hartert in Germany [5,6]. Dr. Hartert wanted a mechanism to quantify the dynamics of blood clot formation. He developed a mechanism that consisted of a cup with a concentric pin suspended within (Figure 2). The pin was suspended with a thin steel wire with a diameter of 0.2 mm, which acted as a torsional spring.

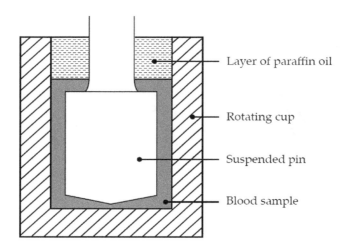

Figure 2. Dr. Hartert's cup and pin mechanism. Schematic drawing representing parts of the thromboelastograph that were in direct contact with the blood sample. The rotating cup was approximately 8 x 12 mm and made from stainless steel, the surface of which prevented detachment of the blood clot during cup rotation. The blood sample was covered by a layer of paraffin oil to prevent evaporation of the sample. Reproduced with permission from [4].

To perform a test, an activated sample of blood is placed in the cup and the pin lowered into place. The cup rotates in each direction by 1/24 radian, or 1/12 radian total rotation. The rotation occurs slowly, taking 3.5 s for one direction. The cup then comes to a stop for 1 s and then moves back in the other direction at the same speed. An entire "cycle" takes 9 s (two motion periods and two stationary periods). As the cup rotates with a viscous material (whole blood), the pin does not move. The shear between the rotating cup and stationary pin results in a permanent shear deformation of the blood. As the clot forms and grows in strength, the fluid within the cup begins its transition from a viscous to an elastic state. Energy is stored within the elasticity of the clot and the clot will try to return to its original shape, exerting a force on the pin, which causes the pin to rotate on its axis. The small rotations of the pin are transmitted to a film via a mirror coupled to the pin, which is illuminated by a slit lamp (Figure 3). The movement of the cup and pin after clotting is represented as a graphical chart in Figure 4.

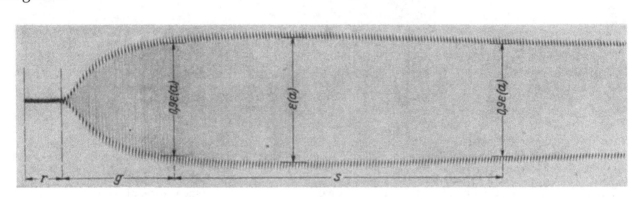

Figure 3. Output from Dr Hartert's cup and pin. Representation of the output from the entire cycle of the cup and pin system. The R period was described as the reaction time, g as the growth of the clot and s as the stable period clot strength. The amplitude of the waveform is proportional to the shear modulus of the clot within its elastic region and is analogous to clot strength. Reproduced with permission from [5].

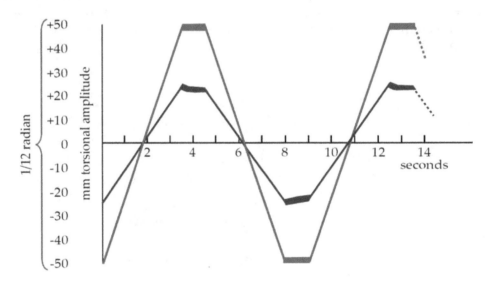

Figure 4. Chart representing the movement of Dr. Hartert's cup and pin after clotting of the blood sample. The red line represents the displacement of the cup and the blue line represents the displacement of the pin. The units on the x-axis represent the extent of the illuminated section of film by the rotating mirror. The units of mm amplitude on the y-axis remain today in many viscoelastic hemostatic assay systems. The units of mm to express a clot strength has been the source of confusion in this space. Reproduced with permission from [4].

Adoption of thromboelastography grew slowly following Dr. Hartert's initial work, limited primarily to research laboratories. It began to gain some momentum in the 1980s, particularly in high blood loss procedures such as liver transplantation [1] and cardiac surgery [7,8]. Two similar technologies were initially developed, Thromboelastography (Thrombelastograph® [TEG®] Hemostasis Analyzer) by Haemoscope, and Thromboelastometry (ROTEM®) by Tem International

GmbH. These two technologies defined the first 30 years of clinically adopted viscoelastic hemostatic assays. Both technologies were enhanced by the utilization of different assays to gain visibility on different aspects of clot formation. The assays and associated reagents have been developed to investigate different coagulation pathways, the contributions of platelets and fibrinogen to clot strength, and the effect of clot lysis.

As the use of viscoelastic hemostatic assays has grown into more applications, its clinical value has increased. This has attracted significant academic interest. As such, next-generation technologies are rapidly being developed. The remainder of this review will focus on the first-generation technologies that have pioneered this field, the next-generation devices that have more recently gained regulatory approval, and the experimental technologies on the horizon.

4. First-Generation Devices

4.1. TEG® 5000 (Haemoscope, Haemonetics)

The TEG® 5000 system was the first VHA device available, originally developed by Haemoscope and then acquired by Haemonetics. The system has a long clinical history and has been widely published in the literature [9–11]. The mechanism of the TEG® 5000 is very similar to what was originally developed by Dr. Hartert.

For TEG® 5000, the blood sample is placed in a heated cup and the cup is then oscillated through a 4°45′ rotation (Figure 5). A pin is suspended within the cup by a torsion wire. Before clotting, the shear that develops between the cup and pin results in a viscous shear of the test sample and therefore, no movement of the pin. As clot strength develops, the fluid gradually develops an elastic element, which results in movement of the pin. Instead of the light-based system used by Dr. Hartert, the TEG® 5000 uses an electromechanical proximity sensor to detect rotation of the pin. The total deflection of the pin is tracked and can be plotted as shown in Figure 6. A range of assays have been developed for the TEG® 5000 system, which includes those shown in Table 1.

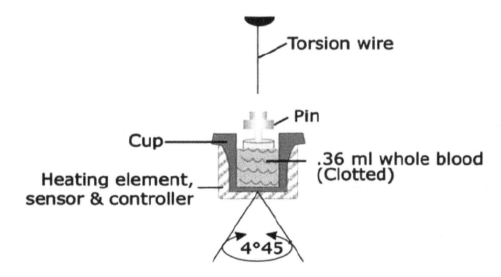

Figure 5. Schematic representation of the TEG® 5000 system. Thromboelastography conducted with the TEG® 5000 system uses approximately 0.36 mL of blood, which is placed into a cylindrical cup at 37 °C. A pin on a torsion wire is suspended in the blood, and the cup rotates in alternating directions (rotation angle 4°45′, cycle duration 10 s) to simulate venous flow. At the onset of each measurement, there is no torque between the cup and the pin, and the machine provides a reading of zero. As clotting occurs, fibrin fibers formed between the pin and the cup create a rotational force on the pin, which is measured via a torsion wire and an electromagnetic transducer; the readout line diverges from the baseline until it reaches a maximum value (maximum clot strength). With the onset of clot lysis, the readout converges back towards baseline. Reproduced with permission from Haemonetics [11].

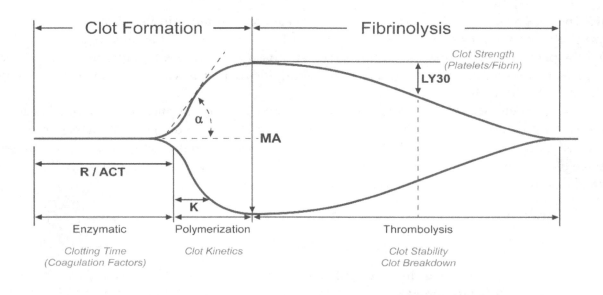

Figure 6. Plot of the total deflection of the pin from the TEG® 5000 system. The primary values that are derived from the resulting waveform are reaction time (R, or activated clotting time [ACT]), maximum amplitude (MA) and lysis at 30 minutes (LY30). R represents the time to the beginning of clot formation. MA is the maximum clot strength achieved. LY30 quantifies the reduction of clot strength, or the lysis (in the 30 min) following MA. K and α angle are also used to quantify the dynamics of clot formation. Reproduced from [12].

Table 1. Assays developed for the TEG® 5000 system.

TEG® Test	Description
Kaolin TEG®	Intrinsic pathway-activated assay.
Kaolin TEG® with Heparinase	Eliminates the effect of heparin. Used in conjunction with Kaolin TEG® to assess heparin effect.
RapidTEG™	Extrinsic and Intrinsic pathways to speed coagulation process and rapidly assess coagulation properties.
TEG® Functional Fibrinogen	Extrinsic pathway with platelet inhibitor to restrict platelet function. Allows for quantification of fibrinogen contribution to clot strength.
TEG® Platelet Mapping™	Utilises a platelet receptor-specific tracing in conjunction with Kaolin TEG®. Identifies level of platelet inhibition and aggregation.

4.2. ROTEM® Delta (Tem International GmbH)

The ROTEM® delta system was developed after the TEG® 5000 system and utilizes a similar approach with cups and pins making up the heart of the instrument. The difference lies in the actuation and detection of the cup and pin assembly. The cup is held stationary and heated, and a rotational force is applied to the pin. If there is no resistance to pin motion, the pin will rotate a full 4°75'. As the clot builds up, it restricts the rotation of the pin. The restriction of pin rotation is inversely proportional to the clot strength. Rotation of the pin is measured in a manner similar to that originally developed by Hartert; a collimated light beam from a light emitting diode is reflected off a mirror coupled to the pin. The motion of the pin is then tracked by a photosensor. As with the TEG® 5000, the ROTEM® delta system has a long clinical history. Various applications have been widely published [13,14] and a wide range of assays have been developed, including those shown below (Table 2).

Table 2. Assays developed for the ROTEM® delta system.

ROTEM® Test	Description
INTEM®	Contact activation with phospholipid and ellagic acid.
EXTEM®	Tissue factor activation.
HEPTEM®	Heparinase to neutralize heparin. Used in conjunction with INTEM® to assess heparin effect.
APTEM®	Inhibits fibrinolysis. Used in conjunction with EXTEM® to assess fibrinolysis.
FIBTEM®	Blocks platelet contribution to clot formation. Allows for quantification of fibrinogen contribution to clot strength.

4.3. Sonoclot® (Sienco)

Sonoclot® is another legacy device developed by Sienco. The Sonoclot® device differs from other legacy systems in that it is not a rotational-based system, but a linear motion system (Figure 7). A hollow, open-ended plastic probe is connected to the transducer head and immersed in a sample containing different coagulation activators or inhibitors, depending on the assay [15]. The probe oscillates vertically within the sample, with the oscillating motion modified as the blood sample begins to clot. The transducer outputs a signal that is proportional to the deflection of the test probe. The changes in the oscillatory pattern of the test probe are directly correlated to the viscoelastic properties of the sample. Measurements are taken over time and plotted along a time axis, similar to other legacy systems. The newest generation of the Sonoclot Analyzer is fully digitalized; however, it is not yet approved by the American Food and Drug Administration (FDA) and therefore is only utilized outside of the US.

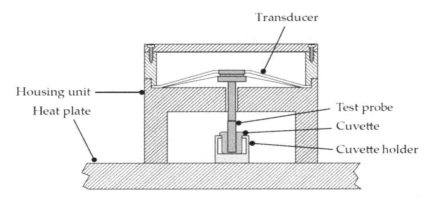

Figure 7. Schematic of the Sonoclot® system. The sample to be tested is placed in a cuvette within the housing unit. The linear test probe is then lowered into the cuvette and is in contact with the sample to be tested. An electric signal through the transducer produces a linear oscillatory motion of the test probe whilst a heat plate warms the sample to be tested through the cuvette holder. Adapted from US Patent 5,138,872 [16].

5. Towards Site of Care

The last two decades have seen rapid expansion of the use of viscoelastic hemostatic assays in an ever-expanding range of clinical applications. The devices described above did much to lay the groundwork for the clinical relevance of viscoelastic hemostatic assays. They offered a holistic view of the clotting process that simply was not available with traditional assay portfolios. However, the manual nature of performing the tests has limited the growth of its clinical utilization.

All of the first-generation devices require manual pipetting of blood samples and reagents. The open-nature of the systems limits their use in point-of-care applications. For many of the potential applications of this technology (cardiac surgery, trauma, etc.) speed and proximity to the patient are critical for success [17]. To overcome these limitations, the historic players in this market have developed next-generation systems. In addition, there are new entrants to this field with new technologies.

These next-generation technologies need to target several key factors to overcome the shortcomings of their predecessors.

- **Ease of use**—The ideal systems should decrease the overall number of manual transfer steps, or eliminate them altogether. Where possible, reagents should be dosed and reconstituted automatically. The user interface should be intuitive, with as little intervention as possible as the target users for these devices will extend beyond skilled medical laboratory technicians. Ideally, the systems would meet the requirements to be considered waived under Clinical Laboratory Improvement Amendments (CLIAs).

- **Size**—In order to optimize their use, the devices should be able to be utilized very close to the patient. This means they need to take up little valuable space in already crowded emergency rooms, cath labs and operating theatres. Taking up as little of this valuable real estate as possible is critical.

- **Resistance to ambient conditions**—Having a clear view of a patient's overall hemostasis as early as possible can be a lifesaving benefit in certain emergencies. In clinical scenarios such as stroke or massive trauma, getting feedback on the underlying hemostatic status of a patient as early as possible is critical. For this reason, next-generation devices may be used outside of traditional clinical settings. Environments such as ambulances, helicopters or even the battlefield should be considered. Fundamental technologies that may be sensitive to vibration or temperature may not be suitable for certain applications.

- **Remote viewing**—Fundamentally, these assays produce a sequence of results over a period of time and allow the entire clinical team to view results as they're being developed is important to timely intervention. Having the capability for readings to be displayed in real-time in the operating room may be critical. Allowing emergency department physicians to watch results develop whilst patients are being transported to the hospital will help prepare them for the arival of that patient.

Furthermore, unlike many of the first-generation devices that had significant inter-laboratory variance, with coefficients of variation >10% [18–20], these newer-generation devices have demonstrated reduced variance [21]. Whilst older-generation devices enabled users to focus on running channels of interest, newer devices detailed below require users to run entire cartridges. While this makes the assay process more streamlined and precise, it may be associated with increased cost.

5.1. TEG® 6s (Haemonetics)

To overcome the issues inherent with a manual device, Haemonetics released the TEG® 6s. The TEG® 6s is a cartridge-based system that automates all sample aliquoting, reagent mixing and testing. The system consists of a pneumatically controlled microfluidic cartridge that takes an initial blood sample and divides it across four distinct test channels. Each test channel includes a set of reagents to conduct four different assays simultaneously.

In order to bring the test methodology to a cartridge-based system, Haemonetics developed a new measurement technique. A fluid's shear modulus is proportional to its resonant frequency; the frequency at which a material will resonate when exposed to an excitation. The testing mechanism of the TEG® 6s consists of a droplet of fluid suspended between a light source and a photodetector (Figure 8). The droplet of fluid is excited by the displacement of a piezoelectric actuator. The piezoelectric actuator is driven with a function that includes all frequencies between 25 and 400 Hz, at increments of 0.25 Hz. When subjected to this range of frequencies, the sample will resonate at its resonant frequency. The optical sensors measure the displacement of the droplet and calculate the frequency of vibration with a Fourier transform.

The TEG® 6s system has gained regulatory clearance in the USA and Europe amongst other international markets and has been compared to first-generation thromboelastography systems in the literature [19,21–23]. The assays available with the TEG® 6s are similar to the TEG® 5000 and are available in three cartridge configurations. The Global Hemostasis cartridge includes Kaolin TEG® with Heparinase, RapidTEG™ and Functional Fibrinogen. It is also possible to have the Global Hemostasis cartridge without KaolinTEG® with Heparinase. The Platelet Mapping cartridge adds channels with adenosine diphosphate and arachidonic acid reagents to activate specific platelet activation pathways.

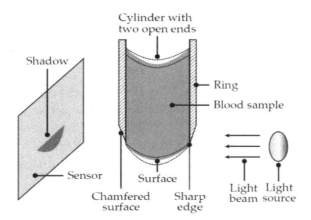

Figure 8. Schematic representation of the TEG® 6s. The diameter of the ring and cylinder is sized to allow the blood sample to be held within the cylinder by surface tension, without support at the bottom surface. The light source (light emitting diode) directs a beam of light at the blood sample, casting a shadow on the sensor. As the surface of the sample is excited by the light beam, the sample oscillates and the corresponding shadow becomes larger or smaller depending upon the elasticity of the blood sample. The resonant frequency of the blood sample is determined before, during and after coagulation. Changes in the resonant frequency of the sample are indicative of the hemostasis characteristics of the blood sample. Adapted from US Patent 7,879,615 B2 [24].

5.2. ROTEM® Sigma (Instrumentation Laboratories)

The ROTEM® sigma system is a transfer of the manual ROTEM® delta system to a cartridge-based system, which maintains the cup and pin methodology. The pins are embedded within the cartridge and actuated by the device when installed. The cartridge is capable of withdrawing a sample of blood from a tube and aliquoting it across four channels simultaneously. Fluid flow is controlled, and reagents are reconstituted automatically. The appropriate sample volume is deposited into each cup and the tests are initiated.

The ROTEM® sigma system offers two cartridges, the Sigma Complete and the Sigma Complete with Heparinase. Each cartridge provides the FIBTEM®, EXTEM®, INTEM® and APTEM® tests. The Heparinase cartridge allows for the neutralization of Heparin. The Sigma system has CE marking (Conformité Européene) for use in Europe, has been widely published, and been compared to the previous generation of thromboelastometry devices [23,25,26].

5.3. Quantra® (HemoSonics)

The Quantra® system developed by HemoSonics, which is CE marked and FDA cleared, utilizes Sonic Estimation of Elasticity via Resonance (SEER) technology [27]. This basic methodology has been used in the past in order to diagnose in vivo clots such as in deep vein thrombosis. Most diagnostic ultrasound devices use the echogenicity of a material in order to estimate its density. SEER technology analyzes the waveforms of the material and estimates the modulus of that material. By doing so, one can estimate if a clot has formed inside a vessel, and the extent of that clot. HemoSonics adapted this technology and refined it to get a more accurate estimate of the modulus of a fluid within a test chamber. The SEER technique has three distinct steps. The first step is data acquisition. This phase is broken up into a number of substeps. First, a low energy sensing pulse is sent into the test chamber. This sensing pulse provides a map of the location of acoustic scatterers within the sample. In the case of whole blood, the primary acoustic scatterers are red blood cells. Next, a higher energy forcing pulse is sent into the test chamber. This forcing pulse results in a displacement of the material within the test chamber. What follows is a series of sensing pulses to provide more maps of the acoustic scatterers. The next phase of the test is motion estimation. In order to estimate motion, a Finite Difference Time Domain model is utilized. This model outputs the relative motion of the acoustic scatterers. The output of this second phase is displacement vs. time waveform. The third phase of the test is to analyze the time displacement waveform for frequency. From this evaluation, the modulus of the fluid in the test chamber is estimated.

6. Emerging Technologies

Several emerging technologies are currently in development for point-of-care hemostatic testing, including microfluidics, fluorescent microscopy, electrochemical sensing, photoacoustic detection, and micro/nano electromechanical systems (MEMS/NEMS) [28]. In the section below, we outline several new devices/technologies that are currently under investigation for use as viscoelastic hemostatic assays; however, these technologies may also have other applications, such as monitoring microfluid dynamics and shear force in coagulation [29–34].

6.1. Laser Speckle Rheometry (Massachusettes General Hospital)

Laser Speckle Rheometry (Figure 9) is a technology being pioneered at the Wellman Center for Photomedicine at Massachusetts General Hospital and Harvard Medical School [35,36]. The technology has applications in a range of areas, including the catheter-based assessment of atherosclerotic plaques. One of the leading applications for the technology is as a viscoelastic hemostatic assay.

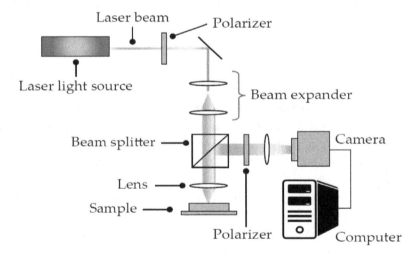

Figure 9. Schematic representation of the Laser Speckle Rheometry system. A laser light source shines a laser beam through a beam splitter onto a sample. The speckle pattern is detected by a camera and processed as described above. By analyzing the laser speckle pattern, the system can estimate the Brownian motion of the material. Brownian motion in such a sample is directly related to the viscoelastic properties of the material. During the blood clotting process, the change in viscoelastic properties can be evaluated and strongly correlated to parameters found in predicate viscoelastic hemostasis analyzers. Adapted from US Patent 8,772,039 B2 [35].

Laser speckle is a random intensity pattern that occurs by the interference of coherent light scattered from tissue. The technology uses a camera-based data acquisition system that detects the speckle pattern reflected from a material. A software algorithm detects changes in the speckle pattern over time. These changes are very sensitive to the passive Brownian motion of light scattering particles.

6.2. Mechanical Resonant Frequency (Abram Scientific)

Abram Scientific is developing a small, handheld approach to viscoelastic hemostatic monitoring [37]. The core technology is based on the concept that the resonant frequency of an object is affected by the medium that is surrounding that object. This can be described as viscoelastic damping. The measurement mechanism consists of a small vibrating element that is surrounded by the test sample. The vibrating element is actuated via an electric signal with a swept frequency. There is a detection mechanism that detects the resulting vibration frequency of the element. As the properties of the sample surrounding the vibrating element change, the frequency of vibration changes. In this way, the system is capable of detecting the viscoelastic properties of the sample. The Abrams Scientific device has the potential to be very compact with the vibrating element of the disposable device integrated into a layered microfluidic chip.

6.3. Ultrasonic Deformation (Levisonics)

Levisonics was formed with technology originally developed at Boston University and Tulane University [38]. This technology consists of an ultrasonic transducer that is positioned opposite a reflector. A standing ultrasonic wave is generated between the transducer and reflector. The radiation pressure generated is sufficient to balance the gravitational force on the sample, levitating it in position between a camera and light source. While the drop of blood is positioned at the pressure node of the standing wave, the amplitude can be modulated, which produces static or oscillatory shape deformations in the sample. These shape deformations are then recorded with a high-resolution digital camera or by laser scattering detection (Figure 10).

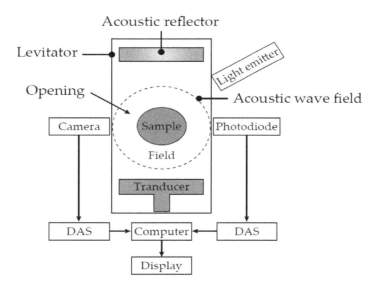

Figure 10. Schematic of the Levisonics ultrasonic transducer. The extent of shape deformations in the suspended blood droplet are directly correlated to the viscoelastic properties of the sample. As the amplitude of the standing wave is modulated, the shape of the sample will change from spherical to oblong. The camera system will track these shape changes and an algorithm converts them to viscoelastic properties. DAS = data acquisition system. Adapted from US Patent application 2017/0016878 A1 [38].

One potentially differentiating feature of this technology is the fact that the blood sample is able to be tested whilst not in contact with any artificial surfaces. This provides two potential benefits. First, there is no disruption to the fluid sample during the clotting process. This may eliminate any mechanical shear that could affect how the clot develops. Second, the absence of artificial surfaces being exposed to the sample during the clotting process may provide a more physiological environment.

6.4. Parallel Plate Viscometry (Entegrion)

Entegrion has developed a system that closely mimics traditional rheological test platforms used outside the medical industry [39]. In essence, they have developed a parallel plate viscometer (Figure 11). Their test cartridge consists of two parallel plates, each connected to a voice coil actuator. The sample to be tested lies between the two plates. Driving signals of various amplitudes and frequencies can elicit motion between the two plates. An optical system then detects the resulting motion on the sample. All the rheological information required to calculate the viscoelastic properties of the sample can be generated with this configuration. Entegrion has been able to integrate this technology into a small, point-of-care system. The resulting small footprint allows for applications in a range of clinical settings including pre-hospital emergency medicine.

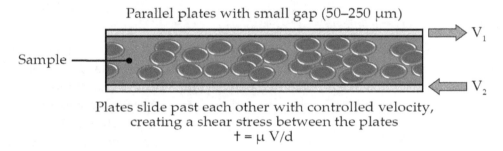

Figure 11. Parallel plate viscometry. Parallel plates slide past each other with controlled velocity to create a shear stress between the plates, which is represented as $t = \mu V/d$, where t = shear stress; μ = viscosity, $V = V_1 - V_2$, (relative linear velocity of the plates); d = gap between plates. Adapted from US Patent 8,450,078 B2 [39].

6.5. Traditional Viscoelastic Testing with "Active Tips" (Enicor)

Enicor has developed a novel solution for those who prefer the cost effectiveness and flexibility of an open system [40]. The measurement technology is very similar to the legacy devices such as TEG® and ROTEM®. With TEG®, the cup rotates and the resulting rotation on the pin is measured. With ROTEM®, the cup is held stationary and a rotational force is applied to the pin, which is then measured. With the ClotPro® system from enicor (Figure 12), the pin is held stationary and a rotational force is applied to the cup. The resulting rotation on the cup is measured.

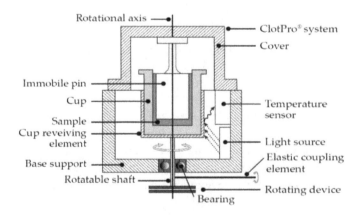

Figure 12. Schematic of the ClotPro® system. The ClotPro® system consists of a cup that contains the blood sample and a static pin, which is fixed to the cover. The cup rotates around the vertical axis, driven by an elastic coupling element, such as a spring wire, which is attached to the shaft. The light source (wavelength 1–3 μm) is placed within 75 mm of the shaft and cup-receiving element to act as a temperature control device. Adapted from International Patent WO,2018/137766,A1 [40].

With these legacy systems, multiple pipetting steps are required to meter and deliver the correct concentration of reagent into the sample cup. ClotPro® has simplified this by utilizing "Active Tips". Active tips are standard pipette tips that already contain the necessary amount of reagent. Blood is drawn into the tip and the reagent is automatically reconstituted in the correct dose. The blood is then dispensed into the cup and the test is initiated. The ClotPro® system also has a test menu similar to that of ROTEM®.

7. Conclusions

The field of viscoelastic hemostatic assays is rapidly growing and generating significant clinical studies, academic research, and industry funding. Whilst older devices have been available for several decades, new technologies are being introduced that promise to make viscoelastic testing more readily available in a wider range of clinical environments. New assays are being developed to give clinicians information about their patients' hemostasis that have never been available before. New indications that have been recently approved, or are currently under investigation, include trauma, interventional cardiology, extracorporeal cardiac assist, obstetrics and anti-coagulation therapy monitoring. The ability of viscoelastic hemostatic assays to deliver clear and readily actionable information about a patient's overall hemostatic status will continue to improve patient care in the years ahead; however, newer technologies and devices will have to demonstrate their clinical effectiveness.

Author Contributions: Initial literature search and review outline was generated by J.H. and M.M. M.M. drafted the initial manuscript with support from J.H. J.H., J.D.D. and M.M. reviewed the manuscript and provided substantial contributions to the final version. All authors have read and agreed to the published version of the manuscript.

Acknowledgments: The authors thank Meridian HealthComms, Plumley, UK for providing formatting and editorial assistance in the submission process, which was funded by Haemonetics, SA, Signy, Switzerland, in accordance with Good Publication Practice (GPP3).

References

1. Kang, Y.G.; Martin, D.J.; Marquez, J.; Lewis, J.H.; Bontempo, F.A.; Shaw, B.W., Jr.; Starzl, T.E.; Winter, P.M. Intraoperative changes in blood coagulation and thrombelastographic monitoring in liver transplantation. *Anesth. Analg.* **1985**, *64*, 888–896. [CrossRef]

2. Mallett, S.V. Clinical utility of viscoelastic tests of coagulation (TEG/ROTEM) in patients with liver disease and during liver transplantation. *Semin. Thromb. Hemost.* **2015**, *41*, 527–537. [CrossRef]

3. Curry, N.S.; Davenport, R.; Pavord, S.; Mallett, S.V.; Kitchen, D.; Klein, A.A.; Maybury, H.; Collins, P.W.; Laffan, M. The use of viscoelastic haemostatic assays in the management of major bleeding: A British Society for Haematology Guideline. *Br. J. Haematol.* **2018**, *182*, 789–806. [CrossRef]

4. Hochleitner, G.; Sutor, K.; Levett, C.; Leyser, H.; Schlimp, C.J.; Solomon, C. Revisiting Hartert's 1962 Calculation of the Physical Constants of Thrombelastography. *Clin. Appl. Thromb. Hemost.* **2017**, *23*, 201–210. [CrossRef]

5. Hartert, H. Coagulation analysis with thromboelastography, a new method. *Klin. Wochenschr.* **1948**, *26*, 577–658. [CrossRef]

6. Hartert, H.; Schaeder, J.A. The physical and biological constants of thrombelastography. *Biorheology* **1962**, *1*, 31–39. [CrossRef]

7. Martin, P.; Horkay, F.; Rajah, S.M.; Walker, D.R. Monitoring of coagulation status using thrombelastography during paediatric open heart surgery. *Int. J. Clin. Monit. Comput.* **1991**, *8*, 183–187. [CrossRef]

8. Spiess, B.D.; Gillies, B.S.A.; Chandler, W.; Verrier, E. Changes in transfusion therapy and reexploration rate after institution of a blood management program in cardiac surgical patients. *J. Cardiothorac. Vasc. Anesth.* **1995**, *9*, 168–173. [CrossRef]

9. McNicol, P.L.; Liu, G.; Harley, I.D.; McCall, P.R.; Przybylowski, G.M.; Bowkett, J.; Angus, P.W.; Hardy, K.J.; Jones, R.M. Patterns of coagulopathy during liver transplantation: Experience with the first 75 cases using thrombelastography. *Anaesth. Intensive Care* **1994**, *22*, 659–665. [CrossRef]

10. Zuckerman, L.; Cohen, E.; Vagher, J.; Woodward, E.; Caprini, J. Comparison of thrombelastography with common coagulation tests. *Thromb. Haemost.* **1981**, *46*, 752–756. [CrossRef]

11. Hartmann, J.; Mason, D.; Achneck, H. Thromboelastography (TEG) point-of-care diagnostic for hemostasis management. *Point Care* **2018**, *17*, 15–22. [CrossRef]

12. Dias, J.D.; Norem, K.; Doorneweerd, D.D.; Thurer, R.L.; Popovsky, M.A.; Omert, L.A. Use of thromboelastography (teg) for detection of new oral anticoagulants. *Arch. Pathol. Lab. Med.* **2015**, *139*, 665–673. [CrossRef]

13. Entholzner, E.K.; Mielke, L.L.; Calatzis, A.N.; Feyh, J.; Hipp, R.; Hargasser, S.R. Coagulation effects of a recently developed hydroxyethyl starch (HES 130/0.4) compared to hydroxyethyl starches with higher molecular weight. *Acta Anaesthesiol. Scand.* **2000**, *44*, 1116–1121. [CrossRef]

14. Novakovic-Anucin, S.; Kosanovic, D.; Gnip, S.; Canak, V.; Cabarkapa, V.; Mitic, G. Comparison of standard coagulation tests and rotational thromboelastometry for hemostatic system monitoring during orthotopic liver transplantation: Results from a pilot study. *Med. Pregl.* **2015**, *68*, 301–307. [CrossRef]

15. Ganter, M.T.; Hofer, C.K. Coagulation monitoring: Current techniques and clinical use of viscoelastic point-of-care coagulation devices. *Anesth. Analg.* **2008**, *106*, 1366–1375. [CrossRef]

16. Henderson, J.H. Fluid Viscoelastic Test Apparatus and Method. US Patent 5,138,872, 18 August 1992.

17. Evans, A.; Sutton, K.; Hernandez, S.; Tanyeri, M. Viscoelastic Hemostatic Assays - A Quest for Holy Grail of Coagulation Monitoring in Trauma Care. *Bioeng. Ann. J.* **2019**, *1*, 61–64.

18. Chitlur, M.; Sorensen, B.; Rivard, G.E.; Young, G.; Ingerslev, J.; Othman, M.; Nugent, D.; Kenet, G.; Escobar, M.; Lusher, J. Standardization of thromboelastography: A report from the TEG-ROTEM working group. *Haemophilia* **2011**, *17*, 532–537. [CrossRef]

19. Gurbel, P.A.; Bliden, K.P.; Tantry, U.S.; Monroe, A.L.; Muresan, A.A.; Brunner, N.E.; Lopez-Espina, C.G.; Delmenico, P.R.; Cohen, E.; Raviv, G.; et al. First report of the point-of-care TEG: A technical validation study of the TEG-6S system. *Platelets* **2016**, *27*, 642–649. [CrossRef]

20. Dias, J.D.; Pottgiesser, T.; Hartmann, J.; Duerschmied, D.; Bode, C.; Achneck, H.E. Comparison of three common whole blood platelet function tests for in vitro P2Y12 induced platelet inhibition. *J. Thromb. Thrombolysis* **2019**. [CrossRef]

21. Neal, M.D.; Moore, E.E.; Walsh, M.; Thomas, S.; Callcut, R.A.; Kornblith, L.Z.; Schreiber, M.; Ekeh, A.P.; Singer, A.J.; Lottenberg, L.; et al. A comparison between the TEG 6s and TEG 5000 analyzers to assess coagulation in trauma patients. *J. Trauma Acute Care Surg.* **2020**, *88*, 279–285. [CrossRef]

22. McCormack, D.; El-Gamel, A.; Gimpel, D.; Mak, J.; Robinson, S. A 'real-world' comparison of TEG® 5000 and TEG® 6s measurements and guided clinical management. *Heart Lung Circ.* **2019**, *28*, S79. [CrossRef]

23. Ziegler, B.; Voelckel, W.; Zipperle, J.; Grottke, O.; Schöchl, H. Comparison between the new fully automated viscoelastic coagulation analysers TEG® 6s and ROTEM® *sigma* in trauma patients: A prospective observational study. *Eur. J. Anaesthesiol.* **2019**, *36*, 834–842. [CrossRef] [PubMed]

24. Kautzky, H. Hemostasis Analyzer and Method. US Patent 7,879,615 B2, 1 February 2011.

25. Gillissen, A.; van den Akker, T.; Caram-Deelder, C.; Henriquez, D.D.C.A.; Bloemenkamp, K.W.M.; Eikenboom, J.; van der Bom, J.G.; de Maat, M.P.M. Comparison of thromboelastometry by ROTEM® *delta* and ROTEM® *sigma* in women with postpartum haemorrhage. *Scand. J. Clin. Lab. Investig.* **2019**, *79*, 32–38. [CrossRef]

26. Schenk, B.; Görlinger, K.; Treml, B.; Tauber, H.; Fries, D.; Niederwanger, C.; Oswald, E.; Bachler, M. A comparison of the new ROTEM® *sigma* with its predecessor, the ROTEM® *delta*. *Anaesthesia* **2019**, *74*, 348–356. [CrossRef]

27. Viola, F.; Kramer, M.; Walker, W.; Lawrence, M. Method and Apparatus for Characterization of Clot Formation. US Patent 7,892,188B2, 22 February 2011.

28. Mohammadi Aria, M.; Erten, A.; Yalcin, O. Technology Advancements in Blood Coagulation Measurements for Point-of-Care Diagnostic Testing. *Front. Bioeng. Biotechnol.* **2019**, *7*, 395. [CrossRef]

29. Colace, T.V.; Fogarty, P.F.; Panckeri, K.A.; Li, R.; Diamond, S.L. Microfluidic assay of hemophilic blood clotting: Distinct deficits in platelet and fibrin deposition at low factor levels. *J. Thromb. Haemost.* **2014**, *12*, 147–158. [CrossRef]

30. Colace, T.V.; Tormoen, G.W.; McCarty, O.J.; Diamond, S.L. Microfluidics and coagulation biology. *Annu. Rev. Biomed. Eng.* **2013**, *15*, 283–303. [CrossRef]

31. Jain, A.; Graveline, A.; Waterhouse, A.; Vernet, A.; Flaumenhaft, R.; Ingber, D.E. A shear gradient-activated microfluidic device for automated monitoring of whole blood haemostasis and platelet function. *Nat. Commun.* **2016**, *7*, 10176. [CrossRef]

32. Judith, R.M.; Fisher, J.K.; Spero, R.C.; Fiser, B.L.; Turner, A.; Oberhardt, B.; Taylor, R.M.; Falvo, M.R.; Superfine, R. Micro-elastometry on whole blood clots using actuated surface-attached posts (ASAPs). *Lab. Chip.* **2015**, *15*, 1385–1393. [CrossRef]

33. Maji, D.; De La Fuente, M.; Kucukal, E.; Sekhon, U.D.S.; Schmaier, A.H.; Sen Gupta, A.; Gurkan, U.A.; Nieman, M.T.; Stavrou, E.X.; Mohseni, P.; et al. Assessment of whole blood coagulation with a microfluidic dielectric sensor. *J. Thromb. Haemost.* **2018**, *16*, 2050–2056. [CrossRef]

34. Ting, L.H.; Feghhi, S.; Taparia, N.; Smith, A.O.; Karchin, A.; Lim, E.; John, A.S.; Wang, X.; Rue, T.; White, N.J.; et al. Contractile forces in platelet aggregates under microfluidic shear gradients reflect platelet inhibition and bleeding risk. *Nat. Commun.* **2019**, *10*, 1204. [CrossRef] [PubMed]

35. Nadkarni, S. Optical Thromboelastography System and Method for Evaluation of Blood Coagulation Metrics. U.S. Patent 8,772,039B2, 8 July 2014.

36. Nadkarni, S. Comprehensive coagulation profiling at the point-of-care using a novel laser-based approach. *Semin. Thromb. Hemost.* **2019**, *45*, 264–274. [CrossRef] [PubMed]

37. Abhishek, R.; Yoshimizu, N. Methods, Devices, and Systems for Measuring Physical Properties of Fluid. U.S. Patent 9,909,968B2, 6 March 2018.

38. Trustees of Boston University. Apparatus, Systems & Methods for Non-Contact Rheological Measurements of Biological Materials. U.S. Patent Application 2017/0016878A1, 19 January 2017.

39. Dennis, R.; Fischer, T.; DaCorta, J. Portable Coagulation Monitoring Device and Method of Assessing Coagulation Response. U.S. Patent 8,450,078B2, 28 May 2013.

40. Dynabyte Informationssysteme GmbH. Devices and Methods for Measuring Viscoelastic Changes of a Sample. International Patent WO 2018/137766,A1, 2 August 2018.

Optical Density Optimization of Malaria Pan Rapid Diagnostic Test Strips for Improved Test Zone Band Intensity

Prince Manta [1], Rupak Nagraik [2], Avinash Sharma [2], Akshay Kumar [3], Pritt Verma [4], Shravan Kumar Paswan [4], Dmitry O. Bokov [5], Juber Dastagir Shaikh [6], Roopvir Kaur [7], Ana Francesca Vommaro Leite [8], Silas Jose Braz Filho [8], Nimisha Shiwalkar [9], Purnadeo Persaud [10] and Deepak N. Kapoor [1,*]

[1] School of Pharmaceutical Sciences, Shoolini University of Biotechnology and Management Sciences, Solan 173212, India; princemanta@gmail.com

[2] School of Bioengineering and Food Technology, Shoolini University of Biotechnology and Management Sciences, Solan 173212, India; rupak.nagraik@gmail.com (R.N.); avinashsubms@gmail.com (A.S.)

[3] Department of Surgery, Medanta Hospital, Gurugram 122001, India; drakshay82@gmail.com

[4] Departments of Pharmacology, CSIR-National Botanical Research Institute, Lucknow 226001, India; preetverma06@gmail.com (P.V.); paswanshravan@gmail.com (S.K.P.)

[5] Institute of Pharmacy, Sechenov First Moscow State Medical University,8 Trubetskaya St., Moscow 119991, Russia; bokov_d_o@staff.sechenov.ru

[6] Department of Neurology, MGM Newbombay Hospital, Vashi, Navi Mumbai 400703, India; jubershaikh703@yahoo.com

[7] Department of Anesthesiology, Government Medical College, Amritsar 143001, India; roopvirsaini@gmail.com

[8] Department of Medicine, University of Minas Gerais, Passos 37902-313, Brazil; francescavommaroleite@gmail.com (A.F.V.L.); silasbrazf@gmail.com (S.J.B.F.)

[9] Department of Anesthesiology, MGM Hospital, Navi Mumbai 410209, India; dr.nimisha4u@gmail.com

[10] Department of Medicine, Kansas City University, Kansas City, MO 64106, USA; narpaulpersaud@hotmail.com

* Correspondence: deepakpharmatech@gmail.com

Abstract: For the last few decades, the immunochromatographic assay has been used for the rapid detection of biological markers in infectious diseases in humans and animals The assay, also known as lateral flow assay, is utilized for the detection of antigen or antibody in human infectious diseases. There are a series of steps involved in the development of these immuno-chromatographic test kits, from gold nano colloids preparation to nitrocellulose membrane coating (NCM). These tests are mostly used for qualitative assays by a visual interpretation of results. For the interpretation of the results, the color intensity of the test zone is therefore very significant. Herein, the study was performed on a malaria antigen test kit. Several studies have reported the use of gold nanoparticles (AuNPs) with varying diameters and its binding with various concentrations of protein in order to optimize tests. However, none of these studies have reported how to fix (improve) test zone band intensity (color), if different sized AuNPs were synthesized during a reaction and when conjugated equally with same amount of protein. Herein, different AuNPs with average diameter ranging from 10 nm to 50 nm were prepared and conjugated equally with protein concentration of 150 μg/mL with $K_D = 1.0 \times 10^{-3}$. Afterwards, the developed kits' test zone band intensity for all different sizes AuNPs was fixed to the same band level (high) by utilization of an ultraviolet-visible spectrophotometer. The study found that the same optical density (OD) has the same test zone band intensity irrespective of AuNP size. This study also illustrates the use of absorption maxima (λ max) techniques to characterize AuNPs and to prevent wastage of protein while developing immunochromatographic test kits.

Keywords: lateral flow assay; immuno-chromatographic; gold nanoparticles sensor; UV/Vis spectrophotometer; malaria pan rapid diagnostic strip; point-of-care

1. Introduction

Malaria is caused by parasites that are transmitted to humans via the bites of the infected female Anopheles mosquito. While preventable and curable, it still remains a paramount cause of morbidity and mortality in developing countries. Malaria is estimated to kill between 1.5 to 2.7 million people annually [1]. Malaria morbidity is estimated at about 300–500 million annually, and malaria clinical diagnosis is most effective at 50%. Malaria immunoassays use the inherent sensitivity, specificity and binding affinity of antibodies to respective antigens for the detection of antigens in a sample. In immunoassays, the sample tested includes whole blood, urine, saliva, serum, etc. [2]. In the Malaria Pan Antigen rapid test kit, the sample used is Red Blood cells containing specific antigens of *P. vivex and P. malariae/P. ovale* [3]. The red blood cells get lysed by a buffer solution to allow antigen–antibody binding at the test site. Immunoassay signals emanate from the gold-labeled antibody set for the antigen on a substratum at the binding site (Test line). Typical antibody labels include fluorescent molecules, nano- or microparticles, or enzymes. Gold nanoparticles (NPs) are the most widely used label [4]. Such immunoassays can be used in industry, clinical or laboratory settings, doctor's offices, or as over-the-counter tests [2]. At the test line, the naked eye will see a gold-labelled marker as a pink/red line [5]. In most countries, the diagnosis of malaria challenges multiple laboratories [3]. The laboratories require longer than one hour to analyze the findings, leading to less consistency in the analysis of the results.

1.1. Components of Immuno-Chromatographic Test Kits

The Immuno-Chromatographic kit is composed of components shown in Figure 1. The parts of the kits are attached on an inert polyvinyl chloride (PVC) backing material and further packed in a plastic cassette with a specimen port and reaction window displaying the capture and control zones [2]. The Immunochromatographic Test Kit has a sample pad, conventionally composed of glass fibres. The sample pad is selected to have zero cross-reactivity with the specimen. The sample pad is pretreated with a buffer for specimen pH adjustment and extraction of unspecific antigen form specimens [6]. One of the vital parts of the strip is nitrocellulose membrane (NCM). In this, the interaction between antigen and antibody takes place. Typically, a hydrophobic nitrocellulose membrane is used on which anti-target analyte antibodies are immobilized in a line that crosses the membrane to act as a capture zone on the test line [2]. The NCM membrane should be chosen based upon pore size [7]. Other parts of test strips are glass fibres or non-woven fibres based conjugate pads which can be pre-treated to avoid any cross-reactivity [8]. Conclusively, the conjugate pad is prepared by dipping the glass fibers into a colloidal solution of gold protein and then used after drying. In addition, an absorbent pad is present in the kit, which is designed to collect extra specimen samples passing the reaction membrane [9].

1.2. The Protein

In the Malaria Pan immunoassay, antibody protein is used for AuNP conjugation. Plasmodium lactate dehydrogenase (pLDH) and goat anti-mouse (GAM) protein are used for binding at test and control lines, respectively. An ultraviolet-visible spectrophotometer optimization technique was demonstrated in this work by formulating an immuno-chromatographic detection kit for Malaria Pan using AuNPs as an indicator. Various research works attempted to optimize the AuNP size [10–13], and the AuNPs of about 30–40 nm were reported to be optimal [11,12]. Khlebtsov and Byzova et al. also tried to determine the optimum concentration of protein required for AuNP conjugation [14,15].

In present research, gold nanoparticles (AuNPs) were utilized as labels, and the concentration of AuNPs with conjugate antibodies was tailored to a fine-tuned optical density (OD). The gold nanoparticles of various sizes (10 nm to 50 nm) were prepared, by quantifying λ max (absorption maxima) and dynamic light scattering (DLS). The relationship of AuNP diameters with a concentration of target protein was monitored to develop a better test kit. Finally, the developed immuno-chromatographic test kit test zone band intensity was tested using RGB and HSV color models. The reason to select a malaria test kit for the study is to create a more cost-effective rapid diagnostic test kits because malaria cases are found in countries where cost-effectiveness is significant. The study aim to improve test band intensity irrespective of AuNP size using a fixed quantity of protein while optimizing the optical density.

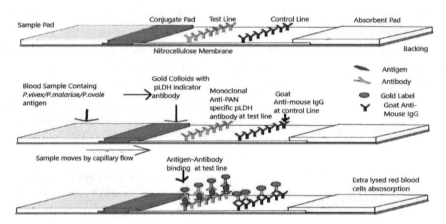

Figure 1. Presentation of lateral flow strip that works on sandwich assay. Blood sample lysed with buffer solution is added to the sample pad. *P. vivex/P. malariae/P. ovale* malaria antigens attach to antibodies in the red colored gold conjugate pad and the complex formed attaches to test line monoclonal anti-PAN specific pLDH antibodies. The excess labeled antibodies bind with Goat anti-mouse IgG antibodies in the control line. The extra lysed red blood cells get absorbed in the absorbent pad.

2. Materials and Methods

2.1. Reagents, Instruments and Other Support Materials

For the fabrication of immunochromatographic strip assay, sodium hydrogen phosphate, sucrose, disodium hydrogen phosphate, sodium chloride and bovine serum albumin (BSA) were purchased from Merck, Darmstadt, Germany. The gold chloride used for the synthesis of gold nanoparticles was purchased from Sigma-Aldrich, Tokyo, Japan. The Plasmodium lactate dehydrogenase (pLDH) antibodies' molecules and control line Goat anti-mouse protein were purchased from Fapon Biotech, Shenzhen, China. All the other chemicals and reagents used in the present study were of analytical grade reagents. The Delsa™ Nano Submicron Particle Size Zeta Potential instrument of Beckman Coulter, Brea, CA, USA was used for analyzing AuNP diameters. An ultraviolet-visible spectrophotometer 1900i of Shimadzu, Kyoto, Japan was used to measure optical density and absorbance maxima. The nitro cellulose membrane was coated with XYXYZ3210™ dispense platform of Bio-dot, Irvine, CA, USA. The centrifuge of Remi RM-12C, Mumbai, India was utilized for AuNP–protein conjugate centrifugation, and the magnetic stirrer of Remi, Mumbai, India was also used in the study. The nitrocellulose membrane was purchased form Nupore System Pvt. Ltd., Ghaziabad, India and Glass fibre sample pad and conjugate pad were purchased from Advanced Micro Devices, Ambala, India.

2.2. Experimental

2.2.1. Preparation of Gold Nanoparticles (AuNPs)

The gold nanoparticles were prepared by classical classical Turkevich and Fern methods by citrate reduction. In general, the Turkevich and Fern process reaction leads to formation of AuNPs of size range 10 nm to 100 nm [16,17]. Utilizing raw gold chloride ($AuHCl_4$) [18], the 1% light yellowish color solution was prepared by dissolving 1 gm of gold chloride in 100 mL of ultra-mili-Q water. The aforementioned 1% gold solution was furthermore dissolved into ultra-milli-Q water in order to obtain the optical density between 0.7 and 0.9 at λ max (absorption maxima) by taking a solution spectrum scan at wavelength between 700 nm and 400 nm. Now, the final gold solution had been refluxed for 30 min at 100 °C. The above-diluted gold solution was reduced by adding 1% (1 g of sodium citrate in 100 mL of water) sodium citrate solution of pH 7.80 ± 0.5 with refluxing until bright red color develops. Initially, the addition of a 1% solution of sodium citrate turns the color of the solution black. The color change from mildly yellowish to brick red confirms the synthesis of nanoparticles. The change in colour solution is due to the surface plasmon resonance effect (SPR) in which electrons excited to its higher state and produces a colour change. During the reduction mechanism, metal salts get converted into their ionic form when it combines with water. Different chemical functional groups of reducing agents combine with metal ions whether they are bivalent or monovalent and reduce it into a zerovalent state of small size [19].

The color transforms from red to pink to blue as the reaction proceeds. As the solution color turns pink, the reaction was stopped by decreasing the temperature to room temperature in the ice bath. Particle size distribution of synthesized nanoparticles was analysed by dynamic light scattering.

The five gold nanoparticles of the sizes 10 nm, 20 nm, 30 nm, 40 nm and 50 nm were chosen for protein conjugation after AuNP characterisation. The prepared pink-colored gold solution was characterized by spectrophotometric absorbance maxima (λ max) by scanning in a visible wavelength range of 700 nm to 400 nm.

2.2.2. Protein Conjugation with Gold NPs

For all the above-prepared AuNPs of size 10 nm to 50 nm, pH was adjusted separately to 7.00 ± 0.1 with 0.2 M Potassium Carbonate solution of pH 12.00 ± 0.5. The pH adjustment is predicated on the protein's isoelectric point, which varies from protein to protein. The pH was measured with the help of pH paper. The antibody pLDH (Plasmodium lactate dehydrogenase) reagents have been diluted to 150 μg/mL from the stock solution with 10 mM of Sodium Dihydrogen Phosphate buffer of pH 8.50 ± 0.1. Afterwards, the protein pLDH of 150 μg/mL concentration was conjugated to all five AuNPs (10 nm to 50 nm). Conjugation of the AuNPs and protein was achieved by stirring the solution to 10 ± 2 min. Following this, 1% BSA (Bovine Serum Albumin) was added into the gold conjugate solution and stirred for 30 ± 2 min for stabilisation and abstraction of unbound protein. For all five sizes of AuNPs, the single tuned protein concentration was used to detect the effect of gold nanoparticle size on the band intensity of developed kits.

2.2.3. Centrifugation

The above five separately prepared AuNP–protein conjugate solutions were centrifuged. The centrifugation was performed with a Relative Centrifugal Force (RCF) of 7000× g for 45 min at 4 °C to 8 °C temperature. The centrifugation of an AuNPs–protein conjugate solution at a force higher than 7000× g RCF can sometimes shows aggregation while centrifugation at a force slower than 7000× g RCF may give less residue with a dark supernatant. Centrifugation at 7000× g RCF gives a stable and good yield of the residue or pellet. The supernatant's aspiration was performed in a different beaker, and gold pellets were resuspended in the phosphate-buffered saline (PBS) buffer. The absorbance of the supernatant was measured at a 520 nm wavelength. If the OD was greater than 0.05, then the supernatant's re-centrifugation is performed one more time. The supernatant was discarded if the OD was less than 0.05. This will enable conjugate recovery and prevent wastage. The supernatant aspiration is performed in a separate beaker, accumulating the AnNP–protein pellets. Carefully, the supernatant aspiration and the residue re-suspension was accomplished in a re-suspension buffer. Figure 2 represents the protein conjugation and centrifugation procedure.

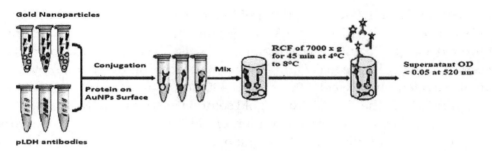

Figure 2. The diagrammatical representation of the protein conjugation and centrifugation methodology.

2.2.4. Conjugate Pad Prepration

All five separately re-suspended AuNPs—protein conjugate above solutions were diluted (ultra-pure mili-Q water) to a constant OD of 3.00 at 520 nm wavelength.

Following the dilution, five conjugate pads were prepared by dipping the glass fibre pad into the conjugate solution. In comparison, the other changes through the entire development of the kit was held constant, e.g., test line concentration and control line protein.

2.2.5. Membrane Coating

The five nitrocellulose membranes were coated at the test (Pan) and control line (C). The test and control line coating on the nitrocellulose membrane (NCM) was achieved with the use of a Bio-dot dispensing machine. First of all, the bio-dot machine stripping system (tubing and jets) was flushed with de-ionized water over ten cycles. The control and test solutions were then coated on NCMs. For drying, membrane sheets were kept in the oven at 30 °C for 30 min after coating. The concentrations of test and control line reagents were as follows:

2.2.6. Test Line Reagents Concentration

To obtain the final test solution, the pLDH (Plasmodium lactate dehydrogenase) antibody was diluted from the stock solution to 50 µg/mL with 1% sucrose solution in the PBS buffer. The antibody protein mixing in PBS buffer was performed with a magnetic stirrer, and a 0.22-micron filter was used to eliminate the suspended particles.

2.2.7. Control Line Reagents Concentration

To obtain the final control line solution, Goat Anti Mouse IgG was diluted from stock solution to 400 µg/mL with a 0.5 percent sucrose in the PBS buffer. To extract the suspended particles, mixing and filtration were achieved using a 0.22-micron filter.

3. Results and Discussion

3.1. Gold NP Characterization

Firstly, we prepared the most stable AuNPs of an average of of 10 nm to 50 nm in diameter. The AuNPs with absorbance maxima (λ max) ranging between 520 to 570 wavelengths were considered for the development of the Malaria Pan Antigen detection test kit. In this range of λ max, the AuNP size ranges from 10 nm to 50 nm as determined by the particle sizer. Figure 3A–E represent the AuNP size measured in dynamic light scattering (DLS). AuNPs of this range were selected due to their smaller particle size and lower polydispersity index (PDI). It has been observed that smaller sized nanoparticles have better conjugation with the protein [10–12,20]. The size of gold NPs depends on the sodium citrate content used [18]. The concentration of sodium citrate in gold solution affects the size of AuNPs, which can be controlled by measuring absorbance maxima (λ max). The sodium citrate of viz 0.2, 0.4, 0.6, 0.75 and 0.90 mg/mL in gold solutions produces nanoparticles (NPs) with average diameters of 10 nm (size distribution of 8 to 12 nm), 20 nm (size distribution of 17 to 23 nm),

30 nm (size distribution of 26 to 35 nm), 40 nm (size distribution of 32 to 50 nm) and 50 nm (size distribution of 36 to 80 nm), respectively (Figure 3). AuNPs shows λ max at varying wavelengths of 520 (10 nm), 530 (20 nm), 540 (30 nm), 560 (40 nm) and 570 (60 nm). Figure 4A–E represent the λ max of AuNPs. The optical density of prepared AuNPs at λ max ranges between 8.0 to 9.0. When sodium citrate concentration increases in AuNP solution, AuNP size does too. When the size of the gold NPs increases, the absorbance maxima (λ max) shift to higher wavelengths (Figure 5), and the color of the solution turns from pink to blue, reflecting nanoparticles' instability.

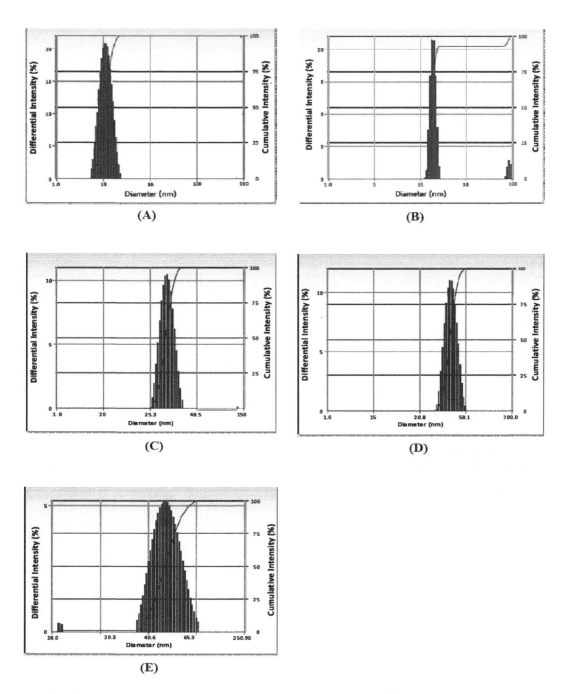

Figure 3. Synthesized gold nanoparticles' size distribution measured by the Zeta Seizer. The sodium citrate solutions of 0.2, 0.4, 0.6, 0.75 and 0.90 mg/mL in gold solutions' produced nanoparticles (NPs) with average diameters of (**A**) 10 nm (size distribution of 8 to 12 nm); (**B**) 20 nm (size distribution of 17 to 23 nm); (**C**) 30 nm (size distribution of 26 to 35 nm); (**D**) 40 nm (size distribution of 32 to 50 nm); and (**E**) 50 nm (size distribution of 36 to 80 nm).

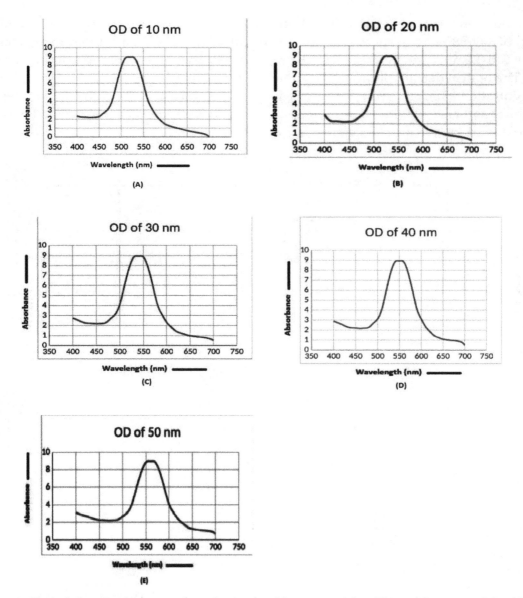

Figure 4. Optical density spectrum of synthesized gold nanoparticles. The gold nanoparticles (AUNPs) show different λ max (absorbance maxima) at different sizes; i.e., (**A**) λ max 520 nm at diameter of 10 nm; (**B**) λ max 530 nm at diameter of 20 nm; (**C**) λ max 540 nm at diameter of 30 nm; (**D**) λ max 560 nm at diameter of 40 nm; (**E**) λ max 570 nm at diameter of 50 nm.

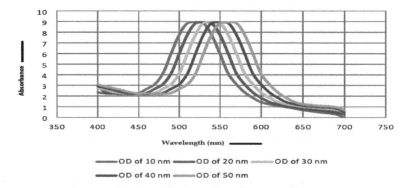

Figure 5. The graph shows a correlation of synthesized gold nanoparticles (10 nm, 20 nm, 30 nm, 40 nm and 50 nm) λ max (absorbance maxima) and Optical Density. With an increase in the size of the gold NPs, the absorbance maxima (λ max) shifts to higher wavelengths (520 nm to 570 nm), reflecting nanoparticle instability.

As the average diameters increase, the nanoparticles' size distribution increases, which causes the instability of AuNPs (Figure 3). This technique is widely used for the determination of particle size in colloidal solution, which, in turn, used to measure the thickness of capping or stabilizing agent along with its actual size of metallic core. These studies also determined the hydrodynamic diameter of the synthesized nanoparticles. These results also suggested that there is an absence of large aggregates when these nanoparticles were dispersed in aqueous medium [21].

3.2. Monitoring the Protein Loss

After centrifigation of AuNP–protein conjugate, a small portion of re-suspended solution was diluted (1 in 100) into ultra-pure mili-Q water to facilitate OD measurement at 520 nm. The OD values obtained are shown in Table 1.

Table 1. Optical density (OD) measurement results of synthesized gold nanoparticles–protein centrifuged re-suspension conjugate solution when diluted in 1–100.

S. No.	Gold Nanoparticles (AuNP) Size	Optical Density (OD) Observation
1	10 nm	0.301
2	20 nm	0.354
3	30 nm	0.368
4	40 nm	0.426
5	50 nm	0.385

Figure 6 and Table 1 indicate that 40 nm AuNPs have high OD, and thus AuNPs have maximum protein binding with AuNPs of 40 nm size. In contrast, the other AuNPs had less binding. This indicates that the supernatant lost extra unbound protein. This means that the additional unbound protein was lost in the supernatant. The protein depletion can also be checked with the use of UV/Vis spectrophotometer OD analysis.

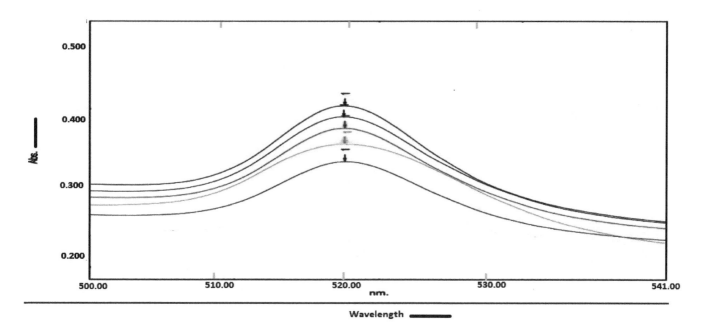

Figure 6. The spectrum overlay graph shows optical density of gold nanoparticles (10 nm, 20 nm, 30 nm, 40 nm and 50 nm) and protein conjugate solution (1–100 mL) measured at 520 nm of wavelength. The gold nanoparticles of average diameter of 40 nm have maximum optical density (0.426), which reflects the maximum protein binding.

3.3. Test Line Intensity Analysis

The developed kits were tested to find out the kit test zone band intensity (results) when equivalent protein ratios are conjugated with different AuNP sizes. The five immunochromatographic rapid test kits were formulated using a conjugate pad (10 nm to 50 nm) prepared above. Then, all five of the immunechromatographic test kits were assembled. Now, the five developed test kits were tested for band intensity using 5 μL of malaria (*P. vivax*) positive blood specimens of concentration 150 parasites/μL. The three specifications were given to test line viz. high test line intensity was ranked as +3, medium test line intensity was ranked as +2, and weak test line intensity was ranked as +1. Upon testing all kits with the same specimen samples, all kits showed an equal band intensity of +3 (high) as shown in Table 2. In this analysis, it was noticed that, if the final OD is tuned to one point, there will be no effects of AuNPs sizes on kit results (test zone intensity). OD-adjustment will refine the final test zone band intensity. Figure 7 is the systematic representation of the results. All five test kits developed after OD tuning to 3.0 were additionally verified for their specificity with 5 μL of Malaria Pf (Falciparum) antigen blood specimens of concentration 40 parasites/μL to find out test kit susceptibility for *P. Falciparum*. The specificity results of developed kits (Table 3) were found without any false positive indication (no Pan line appears), and the the control band intensity was high (+3).

Table 2. Test line intensity results of five Malaria Pan Ag immunochromatographic rapid test kits formulated using different diameter AuNPs. The kit final OD is tuned to one point (3.00) after conjugation with protein. Kit's test line intensity was tested using *P. vivax* positive blood specimen of a concentration of 150 parasites/μL. The band intensity for test (Pan) and control (C) line is ranked as: high test (+3), medium (+2) and weak (+1). Upon testing, all developed kits showed an equal sensitivity of +3 (high).

Test Zone Intensity of Kit Developed by 10 nm of AuNPs	Test Zone Intensity of Kit Developed by 20 nm of AuNPs	Test Zone Intensity of Kit Developed by 30 nm of AuNPs	Test Zone Intensity of Kit Developed by 40 nm of AuNPs	Test Zone Intensity of Kit Developed by 50 nm of AuNPs
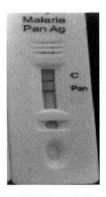	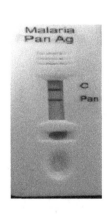	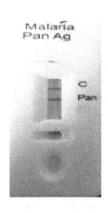	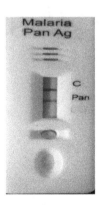	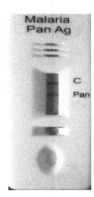
+3 (High) Intensity	+3 (High) Intensity	+3 (High) Intensity	+3 (High) Intensity	+3 (High) Intensity

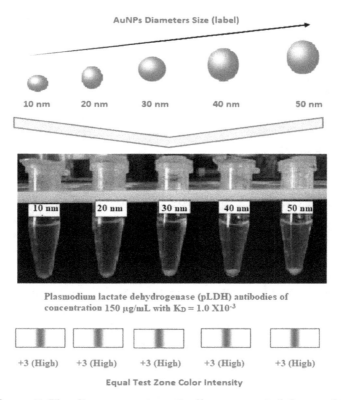

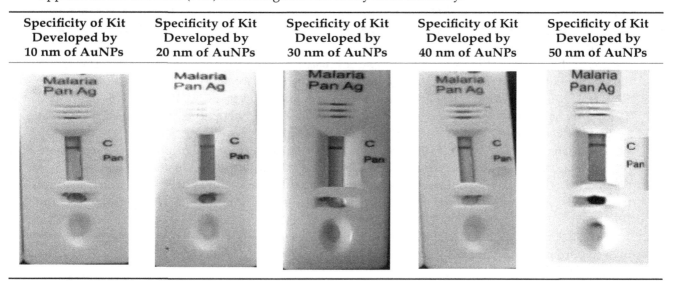

Figure 7. The diagram systematically represented the results.

Table 3. Specificity results of five Malaria Pan Ag immunochromatographic rapid test kits formulated using different sizes AuNPs. Kit's specificity was tested using *P. Falciparum* positive blood specimens of concentration 40 parasites/µL. The color band intensity for control (C) line was +3 (high) and no line appears on the test zone (Pan) indicating absence of any cross reactivity.

Specificity of Kit Developed by 10 nm of AuNPs	Specificity of Kit Developed by 20 nm of AuNPs	Specificity of Kit Developed by 30 nm of AuNPs	Specificity of Kit Developed by 40 nm of AuNPs	Specificity of Kit Developed by 50 nm of AuNPs

4. Conclusions

It can be concluded from the above study that the particle size of AuNPs has no effect on the test zone band intensity of Malaria Pan rapid diagnostic test kits if optical density of AuNP–protein conjugate is adjusted at 520 nm. The test zone band intensity was also observed to be maximum at 520 nm and optical density 3.0. It was found from the study that any quantity of protein can be utilized for AuNP conjugation, if the final optical density (OD) is adjusted correctly. It can also be concluded that, by optimizing the optical density, an enhanced test zone band intensity can be obtained while reducing the total number of trial and wastage of reagents.

Author Contributions: Conceptualization: P.M. and D.N.K.; Methodology: R.N and A.S.; Validation: A.K., J.D.S. and R.K.; Formal Analysis: A.F.V.L.; Investigation: S.J.B.F.; Data Curation: N.S.; Writing—Original Draft Preparation: P.M., R.N. and A.S.; Writing—Review and Editing: A.K.; Visualization: P.P.; Funding acquisition: D.O.B., S.K.P. and P.V.; Supervision: D.N.K. All authors have read and agreed to the published version of the manuscript.

References

1.   Mishra, M.N.; Misra, R.N. Immunochromatographic methods in malaria diagnosis. *Med. J. Armed Forces India* **2007**, *63*, 127–129. [CrossRef]
2.   Manta, P.; Agarwal, S.; Singh, G.; Bhamrah, S.S. Formulation, development and sensitivity, specificity comparison of gold, platinum and silver nano particle based HIV $\frac{1}{2}$ and hCG IVD rapid test kit (Immune chromatoghraphic test device). *World J. Pharm. Sci.* **2015**, *4*, 1870–1905.
3.   Maltha, J.; Gillet, P.; Jacobs, J. Malaria rapid diagnostic tests in endemic settings. *Clin. Microbes Infect.* **2013**, *19*, 399–407. [CrossRef] [PubMed]
4.   Koczula, K.M.; Gallotta, A. Lateral flow assays. *Essays Biochem.* **2016**, *60*, 111–120. [CrossRef] [PubMed]
5.   Gronowski, A.M. *Handbook of Clinical Laboratory Testing during Pregnancy*; Springer Science & Business Media: Berlin, Germany, 2004. [CrossRef]
6.   Benjamin, G.Y.; Bartholomew, B.; Abdullahi, J.; Labaran, L.M. Prevalence of Plasmodium falciparum and Haemoglobin Genotype Distribution among Malaria Patients in Zaria, Kaduna State, Nigeria. *South Asian J. Parasitol.* **2019**, *23*, 1–7. [CrossRef]
7.   Ramachandran, S.; Singhal, M.; McKenzie, K.G.; Osborn, J.L.; Arjyal, A.; Dongol, S.; Baker, S.G.; Basnyat, B.; Farrar, J.; Dolecek, C.; et al. A rapid, multiplexed, high-throughput flow-through membrane immunoassay: A convenient alternative to ELISA. *Diagnosis* **2013**, *3*, 244–260. [CrossRef] [PubMed]
8.   Tsai, T.T.; Huang, T.H.; Chen, C.A.; Ho, N.Y.; Chou, Y.J.; Chen, C.F. Development a stacking pad design for enhancing the sensitivity of lateral flow immunoassay. *Sci. Rep.* **2018**, *8*, 1–10. [CrossRef] [PubMed]
9.   Wong, R.; Tse, H. *Lateral Flow Immunoassay*; Springer Science & Business Media: Berlin, Germany, 2008. [CrossRef]
10. Lou, S.; Ye, J.Y.; Li, K.Q.; Wu, A. A gold nanoparticle-based immunochromatographic assay: The influence of nanoparticulate size. *Analyst* **2012**, *137*, 1174–1181. [CrossRef] [PubMed]
11. Kim, D.S.; Kim, Y.T.; Hong, S.B.; Kim, J.; Heo, N.S.; Lee, M.K.; Lee, S.J.; Kim, B.I.; Kim, I.S.; Huh, Y.S.; et al. Development of lateral flow assay based on size-controlled gold nanoparticles for detection of hepatitis B surface antigen. *Sensors* **2016**, *16*, 2154. [CrossRef] [PubMed]
12. Fang, C.; Chen, Z.; Li, L.; Xia, J. Barcode lateral flow immunochromatographic strip for prostate acid phosphatase determination. *J. Pharm. Biomed. Anal.* **2011**, *56*, 1035–1040. [CrossRef] [PubMed]
13. Safenkova, I.; Zherdev, A.; Dzantiev, B. Factors influencing the detection limit of the lateral-flow sandwich immunoassay: A case study with potato virus X. *Anal. Bioanal. Chem.* **2012**, *403*, 1595–1605. [CrossRef] [PubMed]
14. Banerjee, S.; Gautam, R.K.; Jaiswal, A.; Chattopadhyaya, M.C.; Sharma, Y.C. Rapid scavenging of methylene blue dye from a liquid phase by adsorption on alumina nanoparticles. *RSC Adv.* **2015**, *5*, 14425–14440. [CrossRef]
15. Kaur, K.; Forrest, J.A. Influence of particle size on the binding activity of proteins adsorbed onto gold nanoparticles. *Langmuir* **2012**, *28*, 2736–2744. [CrossRef]
16. Turkevich, J.; Stevenson, P.C.; Hillier, J. A Study of the nucleation and growth processes in the synthesis of colloidal gold. Discuss. *Faraday Soc.* **1951**, *11*, 55–75. [CrossRef]
17. Frens, G. Controlled Nucleation for the Regulation of the Particle Size in Monodisperse Gold Suspensions. *Nat. Phys. Sci.* **1973**, *241*, 20–22. [CrossRef]
18. Khlebtsov, B.N.; Tumskiy, R.S.; Burov, A.M.; Pylaev, T.E. Quantifying the Numbers of Gold Nanoparticles in the Test Zone of Lateral Flow Immunoassay Strips. *ACS Appl. Nano Mater.* **2019**, *2*, 5020–5028. [CrossRef]

19.   Byzova, N.A.; Safenkova, I.V.; Slutskaya, E.S.; Zherdev, A.V.; Dzantiev, B.B. Less is more: A comparison of antibody–gold nanoparticle conjugates of different ratios. *Bioconjugate Chem.* **2017**, *28*, 2737–2746. [CrossRef] [PubMed]

20.   Larm, N.E.; Essner, J.B.; Pokpas, K.; Canon, J.A.; Jahed, N.; Iwuoha, E.I.; Baker, G.A. Room-temperature turkevich method: Formation of gold nanoparticles at the speed of mixing using cyclic oxocarbon reducing agents. *J. Phys. Chem. C* **2018**, *122*, 5105–5118. [CrossRef]

21.   Sujitha, M.V.; Kannan, S. Green synthesis of gold nanoparticles using Citrus fruits (Citrus limon, Citrus reticulata and Citrus sinensis) aqueous extract and its characterization. *Spectrochim. Acta Part A Mol. Biomol. Spectrosc.* **2013**, *102*, 15–23. [CrossRef]

10

EEG-Brain Activity Monitoring and Predictive Analysis of Signals Using Artificial Neural Networks

Raluca Maria Aileni *, Sever Pasca and Adriana Florescu

Department of Applied Electronics and Information Engineering, Faculty of Electronics, Telecommunications and Information Technology, Politehnica University of Bucharest, 060042 Bucharest, Romania; pasca@colel.pub.ro (S.P.); adriana.florescu@upb.ro (A.F.)
* Correspondence: raluca.maria.aileni@gmail.com

Abstract: Predictive observation and real-time analysis of the values of biomedical signals and automatic detection of epileptic seizures before onset are beneficial for the development of warning systems for patients because the patient, once informed that an epilepsy seizure is about to start, can take safety measures in useful time. In this article, Daubechies discrete wavelet transform (DWT) was used, coupled with analysis of the correlations between biomedical signals that measure the electrical activity in the brain by electroencephalogram (EEG), electrical currents generated in muscles by electromyogram (EMG), and heart rate monitoring by photoplethysmography (PPG). In addition, we used artificial neural networks (ANN) for automatic detection of epileptic seizures before onset. We analyzed 30 EEG recordings 10 min before a seizure and during the seizure for 30 patients with epilepsy. In this work, we investigated the ANN dimensions of 10, 50, 100, and 150 neurons, and we found that using an ANN with 150 neurons generates an excellent performance in comparison to a 10-neuron-based ANN. However, this analyzes requests in an increased amount of time in comparison with an ANN with a lower neuron number. For real-time monitoring, the neurons number should be correlated with the response time and power consumption used in wearable devices.

Keywords: EEG; PPG; EMG; epilepsy; signal processing; brain monitoring; artificial neural network; predictive analysis

---

1. Introduction

1.1. Aim of the Work

Epilepsy is a disease that affects about 1% of the world's population. Crisis identification involves multi-channel EEG monitoring for 24–72 h. Crisis detection (grand mal) is essential for the diagnosis of epilepsy, the control of the crisis, and warning the patients in sufficient time before the seizure. Moreover, the observation and investigation of the biomedical signals values before an epileptic seizure are beneficial for developing prevention and support systems for patients because by informing the patient that an epilepsy seizure is about to occur, he or she can take his or her safety measures promptly. The correlations and covariance between the biomedical signals that EEG, PPG, and EMG collect from sensors are essential because, in the case of the patients with epilepsy, the heart rate increases, and uncontrolled tremors of the muscles or their stiffening may occur.

In the case of the patients with epilepsy, the real-time monitoring based on wearable devices with EEG, PPG, EMG integrated, and biomedical signals predictive analysis based on neural network systems with reduced processing time and low power computing is essential for warning before a seizure, and patients fall prevention.

1.2. State-of-the-Art

There are scientific studies that specify the use of artificial intelligence, using methods such as deep neural networks for patients' ECG-based authentication [1], ResNet-based signal recognition [2], arrhythmia detection [3,4], or learning feed-forward and recurrent neural networks [5]. The automatic signal detection was used in studies based on the discrete wavelet transform (DWT) for automated detection [4] or automated heartbeat classification [6].

The electrical activity of the brain monitoring by EEG (electroencephalogram) is useful to study the disease pathologies by analyzing the numerical distribution of data and correlating the brain signals (EEG) with other types of biomedical signals such as electrical activity of the heart obtained by electrocardiogram (ECG), heart rate monitoring by photoplethysmograph (PPG), and electrical activity produced by muscles by electromyography (EMG) [7–9].

To analyze the pathology of chronic diseases, the researchers also used the multivariate analysis of EEG, ECG, and PPG signals [10,11].

Mainly for predictive analysis of influence factors that generate a pathology or of the biomedical signal changes that could anticipate the existence of pathology are software applications for signal acquisition from sensors (EEG, ECG, PPG, or EMG), correlations [12], univariate, bivariate [13–15] or multivariate analyzes [16,17] of numerical data used, but computational methods [18] based on mathematical models are also used. Thus, computational models use studies on large populations (e.g., 274 patients [19]) and a large volume of data (e.g., 183 seizures recorded in 3565 h [20]). These analyses aim to find valid patterns [21] for a large population with similar independent variables (age, gender).

For the prediction of epileptic seizures, researchers used technologies such as machine learning, data mining, artificial neural networks [22] (backpropagation algorithm-for recognition and classification of EEG signals [23,24]), fuzzy systems [25], and predictive analysis statistics (multivariate [26], bivariate or univariate).

The study of the correlations between various electrical signals captured (e.g., EEG, ECG, PPG, and EMG) from the human body is essential because, in the case of patients with neurological disorders, the phenomenon of comorbidity exists and consists of overlapping of several diseases.

The electroencephalogram (EEG) represents a set of fluctuating field potentials produced by the simultaneous activity of a large number of neurons [27] and captured by electrodes located on the scalp. The EEG system consists of 10–20 metal electrodes distributed on the skin surface of the head and connected by 36 wires to the recording device. It measures the electrical potential detected by each electrode. EEG can be used in monitoring the brain during anesthesia [28], surgical procedures [29], and investigations of brain disorders (psychoses [30], meningoencephalitis [31], Parkinson [9], Alzheimer [32–37], dementia [38], epilepsy [39–42], central motor neuron syndrome [43], cerebral palsy [44–46], and muscular dystrophy [47]). Mainly, EEG systems are used to diagnose and monitor patients with neuropathology, especially in diagnosis of epilepsy and in studying the seizures, as well as the monitoring of treatment and evolution.

Electroencephalographic reactivity is evaluated using simple tests: eye-opening, hyperpnea (slow and full breathing), and intermittent light stimulation obtained with short and intense light discharges with gradually increasing frequency. The EEG assessment takes approximately 20 min and does not require hospitalization [48].

In the case of an electroencephalogram, the risks are minimal. Still, intermittent light stimulation or hyperventilation can produce epileptic seizures. Therefore, the examination is performed under the supervision of a physician who can recognize the crisis and immediately establish appropriate safety and therapeutic measures.

Epilepsy is a chronic disease of the brain that manifests through partial (focal) or generalized seizures due to spontaneous electrical discharges that occur in the brain.

Manifestations consist of involuntary movements of different body segments and abnormal neuro-vegetative sensations in the body. EEG analysis can be used to diagnose and monitor the patient in various stages of the disease (focal or generalized seizures, sleep) [38–41].

1.3. Contribution

In this paper, we present an efficient method for the detection of seizures based on artificial neural networks and correlations between biomedical signals.

Our study included 30 subjects from the CAP Sleep Database [49,50]. Our selected records were sampled at 160 Hz. The records consisted of both normal EEG and EEG spikes specific to epileptic seizures. The signals captured were from 13 EEG channels, submentalis and bilateral anterior tibialis EMG, and an earlobe PPG sensor. We used the artificial neural network and the Levenberg–Marquardt backpropagation optimization algorithm in MATLAB for implementing the classification and 3D plots. Data pre-processing and feature extraction were implemented using MATLAB 2019a (Mathworks, Santa Clara, CA, USA). All the experiments were carried out in Windows 8.1, 8 GB RAM, and 64-bit operating system.

The rest of the paper is structured as follows: the methods for signals decomposition, filtering, EEG biomedical signals, and theoretical methodology are presented in Section 2. Section 3 presents the predictive analysis of the signals using artificial neural networks. Aspects concerning the biomedical signals covariance are discussed in Section 4. The conclusions of the work are presented in Section 5.

2. Materials and Methods

The proposed method was tested using the CAP Sleep Database. The CAP Sleep Database comprises 40 recordings of patients (male and female) diagnosed with nocturnal frontal lobe epilepsy. The record duration is 8 h, approximately.

Our study included 30 subjects from the CAP Sleep Database. Our selected records were sampled at 160 Hz. The records consist of both normal EEG and EEG spikes specific to epileptic seizures. We analyzed 30 EEG recordings 10 min before a seizure and during the seizure in 30 patients with epilepsy. The signals analyzed are from 13 EEG channels, submentalis and bilateral anterior tibialis EMG, and an earlobe PPG sensor.

Within this research, the topic has used the detection of electrical signals from the brain using the EEG head with non-invasive electrodes (for the available biomedical signals in the PhysioNet databases).

In the discrete-time domain, digital filters (low-pass filter for signals with a frequency lower than a selected cutoff frequency and a high-pass filter that passes signals with a frequency higher than a cutoff frequency chosen) have been used for signal analysis.

Discrete wavelet transformation (DWT) [48] is calculated by additional high-pass and successive low-pass filters and sub-sampling using the Mallat algorithm [51]. Additional filtering applied to a real EEG signal leads to double the number of data from the original one being requested after each filtration to reduce the number of samples by sub-sampling of the EEG signal. DWT uses the dyadic variant. In the wavelet analysis, approximations (a (n)) and details (d (n)) are used (Figures 1 and 2):

1.   Approximations (a (n)) are the components at high scales and low frequencies;
2.   Details (d (n)) are components at low levels and high rates.

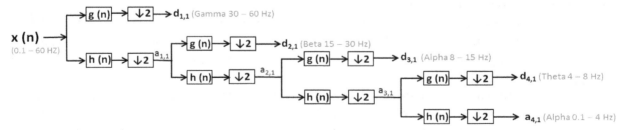

Figure 1. Electroencephalogram (EEG) from a patient with no seizure-signal filtering and decomposition using the discrete wavelet transform (DWT) method.

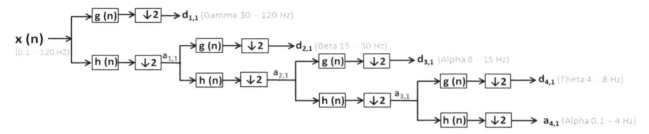

Figure 2. EEG from a patient with epileptic seizure-signal filtering and decomposition using the DWT method.

To reduce the continuous-time signal to a discrete-time signal, the EEG signals were sampled with a sampling frequency ($fs = 160$ Hz). EEG signals were filtered by a low-pass filter (60 Hz) and a high-pass filter (0.1 Hz) and decomposed using the discrete wavelet transform [52,53] for patients without epilepsy (Figure 1).

In the case of epilepsy, seizures detection consists of finding EEG segments with seizures and onset and offset points [53]. For pattern profiling, it is necessary to monitor a large population of patients with epilepsy for 24–48 h. Because gamma frequency oscillations (30–120 Hz) often precede interictal epileptiform spike discharges (IEDs) [54], we used DWT with Daubechies function, and we considered the low-pass filter 120 Hz to observe the gamma wave specific to an epileptic seizure. Some scientific papers report the values around 100–600 Hz for gamma waves—that is, not associated with IEDs, but occurring during epileptic seizures [54,55]. However, other researchers [54,56] reported the fluctuation of gamma wave values.

EEG signals were filtered by a low-pass filter (120 Hz) and a high-pass filter (0.1 Hz) and decomposed using the discrete wavelet transform for patients with epileptic seizures (Figure 2).

x (n)—signal (0.1–60 Hz), respective for patient with seizure x (n)—signal (0.1–120 Hz);
h(n)—low-pass filter (LPF);
g (n)—high-pass filter (HPF);
d (n)—the signal of the detail produced by HPF, e.g., d1, 1, d2, 1, d3, 1, d4, 1;
a (n)—the signal produced by LPF, is a rough approximation, e.g., a1, 1, a2, 1, a3, 1, a4, 1;
↓2—down sampling by two.

The wavelet transform is a way to implement a particular type of signal representation called multi-resolution analysis [57,58]. The analyzed signal is described by a succession of details and approximations that contain more information. Each level of approximation (Figures 1 and 2) contains information available at the previous level, which is an added component of detail. In Figure 3, the signal processed by discrete wavelet transform and Daubechies method using four decomposition levels for a patient before and after a short seizure is presented. In Figure 3, detail d1 represents gamma waves, detail d2 represents beta waves, detail d3 represents alpha waves, detail d4 represents theta waves, and the approximation a4 represents delta waves.

In Figure 4, the signal processed by discrete wavelet transform and Daubechies method using four decomposition levels for a patient with epileptic seizures is presented. In Figure 4, the detail d1 represents gamma waves, detail d2 represents beta waves, detail d3 represents alpha waves, detail d4 represents theta waves, and the approximation a4 represents delta waves. From Figure 4, it is evident that the presence of the gamma waves with values equal to or greater than 120 shows that a seizure phase is present. Moreover, the epileptic spikes are very evident in Figure 4.

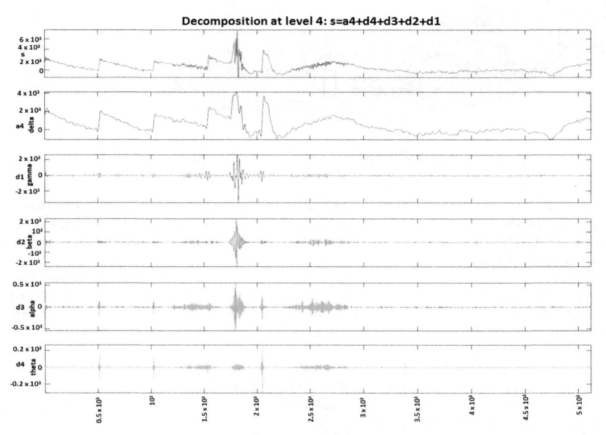

Figure 3. Patient before and after the seizure, signal decomposition on four levels using DWT.

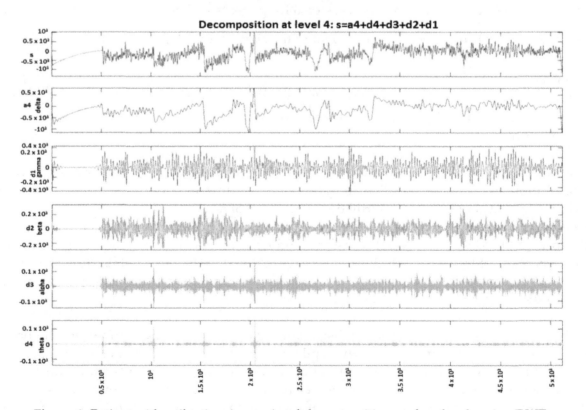

Figure 4. Patient with epileptic seizure, signal decomposition on four levels using DWT.

In Figure 5, the 3D spectrogram of the signals from all 13 channels of electro-cap used for monitoring a patient with an epileptic seizure is presented. The epileptic gamma waves spikes (with the yellow-red color market on the graphic) that are over 200 or 400, indicating abnormal frequencies for gamma waves that occur on seizures, are also evident from Figure 5.

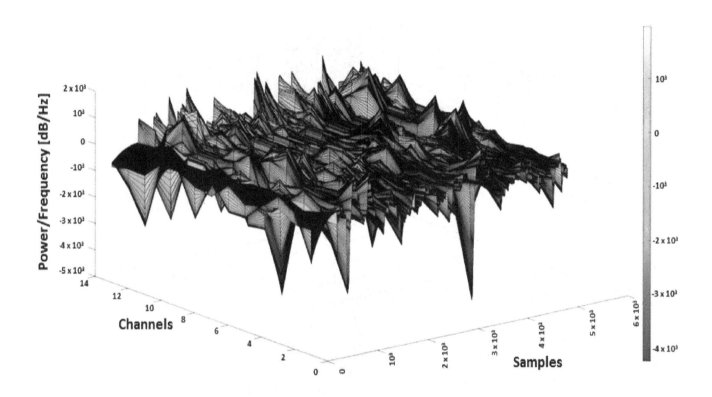

Figure 5. 3D spectrogram of EEG signals from 13 channels.

3. Biomedical Signal Selection

To analyze the correlation and covariance between signals, signals such as EEG (related to the frontal lobes FP1-F3, FP2-F4), EMG, and PPG from a patient n1 with no epileptic seizures and a patient n2 with epileptic seizures were selected.

The purpose of using PPG and EMG signals in correlation with EEG was to find a modification of the biomedical signals collected from wearable devices that could anticipate an epilepsy seizure and to use a software system to send medical alerts in advance [59–65]. From the CAP Sleep Database, the biomedical signals taken from 2 patients (n1 and n2) were used for the actual study. In Figures 6 and 7, the 3D spectrograms for the EEG signals (Fp2-F4, F4-C4, C4-P4, P4-O2, F8-T4, T4-T6, FP1-F3, F3-C3, C3-P3, P3-O1, F7-T3, T3-T5, C4-A1) taken from patients n1 and n2 are presented. In the case of patient n1, the epileptic spikes for gamma waves cannot be observed (Figure 6), but in the case of patient n2, these spikes are evident, marked with yellow-orange in the 3D spectrogram (Figure 7) and being above the 120 Hz threshold.

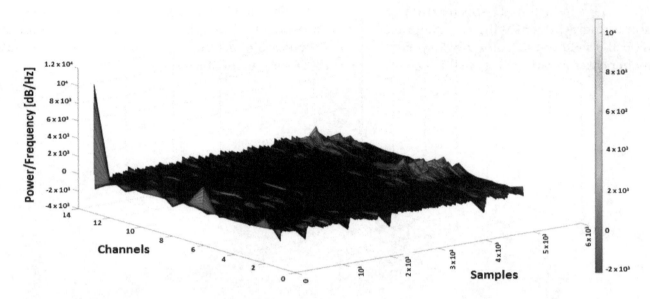

Figure 6. 3D spectrogram of signals EEG from 13 channels for patient n1 with no epileptic seizures.

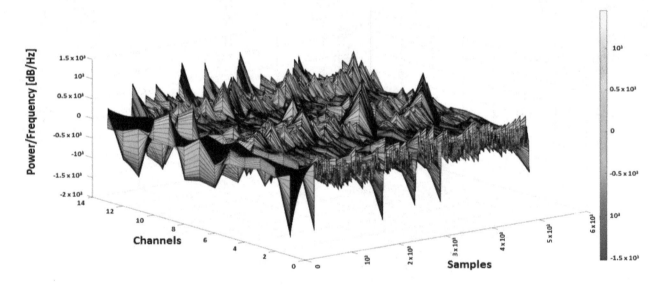

Figure 7. 3D spectrogram signals EEG from 13 channels for patient n2 with epileptic seizures.

4. Results Based on Predictive Analysis of the Signals Using Artificial Neural Networks

For predictive analysis of EEG signals, artificial feed-forward neural networks are used based on the Levenberg–Marquardt backpropagation optimization algorithm.

The functional units within the neural networks consisted of:

- Input units represented by the values of the EEG matrix for patients with epilepsy seizures.

    Hidden groups (data) given by the number of neurons (10, 50, 100, and 150 neurons, respectively).

- Outputs are represented by the values of the EEG matrix for patients who do not have seizures.

For optimization, the Levenberg–Marquardt algorithm was used, which approximates the Hessian matrix (H) as follows (1):

$$H = J^T J \tag{1}$$

where:

- J is the Jacobian matrix containing the derivatives of the error function concerning weights (w) and biases (b);
- J^T is the transposed Jacobian matrix;
- e is the vector of errors.

The Levenberg–Marquardt algorithm uses the following parameter updating rule (Equation (2)):

$$x_{k+1} = x_k - \left[J^T J + \mu I \right]^{-1} J^T e \qquad (2)$$

For this purpose, four neural networks were designed with n hidden neurons (Figure 8), where $n \in \{10, 50, 100, 150\}$, to estimate the occurrence of epilepsy seizures, compared with EEG signals taken from a healthy patient, respectively, with EEG signals received from the patient with no seizures. The artificial neural network (ANN) architecture models (with 10, 50, 100, and 150 respective hidden neurons) used for the prediction of the epileptic seizures have a two-layer feed-forward network with hidden sigmoid neurons and linear output neurons, and allow the training and evaluation of the performance using mean square error (MSE) and regression analysis (R). The proposed ANNs structures are based on the principal elements:

- input data (matrix 13 × 5120 samples);
- hidden layer with n neurons, $n \in \{10, 50, 100, 150\}$;
- output (target) data (matrix 13 × 5120 samples);
- train set (70% of samples) that is used to provide an independent measure of network performance during and after training;
- test set (15% of samples) that is used during training, and the network is adjusted according to its error;
- validation set (15% of samples) is used to measure network generalization, and to halt training when generalization stops improving.

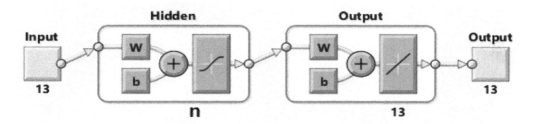

Figure 8. Artificial neural network (ANN) with n neurons, $n \in \{10, 50, 100, 150\}$.

In Table 1, the principal parameters for ANNs with 10, 50, 100, and 150 neurons are presented.

Table 1. ANN parameters.

Neurons No.	Input Data [Samples EEG3]	Output (Target) Data [Samples EEG1]	Train Set [Samples]	Test Set [Samples]	Validation Set [Samples]
10	Matrix 13 × 5120	Matrix 13 × 5120	3584	768	768
50	Matrix 13 × 5120	Matrix 13 × 5120	3584	768	768
100	Matrix 13 × 5120	Matrix 13 × 5120	3584	768	768
150	Matrix 13 × 5120	Matrix 13 × 5120	3584	768	768

Prediction and optimization were made with a feed-forward backpropagation multi-layer neural network.

The input data-independent variables (matrix input) X_1 = EEG signal (EEG3) taken when the patient does not have seizures.

The target data-dependent variables (matrix target) Y_1 = EEG signal (EEG1) taken from a patient with epilepsy. The target (Y_1) represents the desired output for the given input, X_1. We consider the real output matrix (D).

The continuous training of neural networks is based on extensive datasets; 70% (3584 samples) of the total data generated by the ANNs were used to train the model, while 15% (768 samples) of the data was used for testing and 15% (768 samples) for validation (Figures 9–12). Regression analysis of the ANN model showed the R^2 (regression) values for training between 0.57316 for the ANN with ten neurons, 0.65267 for the ANN with 50 neurons, 0.85089 for the ANN with 100 neurons, and 0.81819 for the ANN with 150 neurons, showing the higher accuracy and significance of the ANN model for the ANN with 100 neurons, respective to the ANN with 150 neurons.

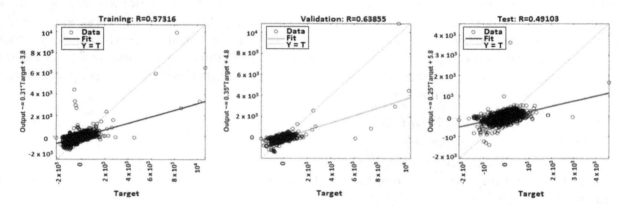

Figure 9. Regression (R^2) for validation, test, and training—ANN with ten neurons.

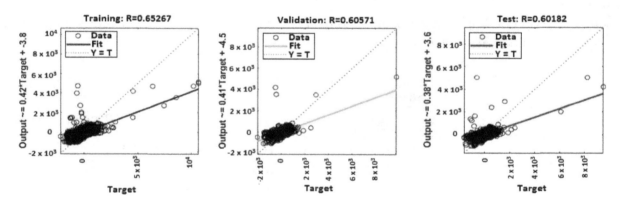

Figure 10. Regression (R^2) for validation, test, and training—ANN with 50 neurons.

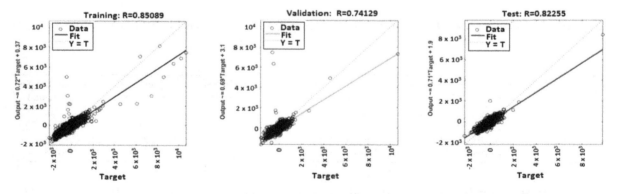

Figure 11. Regression (R^2) for validation, test, and training—ANN with 100 neurons.

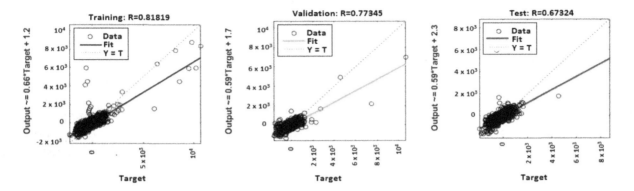

Figure 12. Regression (R^2) for validation, test, and training—ANN with 150 neurons.

MATLAB libraries were used to perform the functions and the code sequences within the neural networks. The regression plots (9–12) show a regression between network outputs and network targets. The parameterized linear regression model is given by mathematical relation (3). The R (Equation (3)) value indicates the relationship between the outputs (y) and targets. If $R = 1$, this indicates that there is an exact linear relationship between outputs and targets. If the R-value is close to zero, then there is no linear relationship between the outputs and targets.

$$R = D = \sum_{j=1}^{M} w_j x_j + \varepsilon \quad \Leftrightarrow \quad R = w^T x + \varepsilon \tag{3}$$

where:

- ε is the error;
- w_j is synaptic weight;
- x is the input matrix;
- M is the model order;
- T denotes matrix transposition (Equations (4) and (5)).

$$w = [w_1, w_2, \ldots, w_M]^T \tag{4}$$

$$x = [x_1, x_2, \ldots, x_M]^T \tag{5}$$

From the regression graphs for testing, training, and validation for neural networks with 10, 50, 100, and 150 neurons (Figures 9–12), and from values presented on Table 1, it is evident that the value of the R regression for training, validation, and testing is in a direct relationship with the number of neurons of the network. The regression value R close to zero indicates that is no linear relationship between outputs and targets. Moreover, if R is very close to 1, it shows a good match and an exact linear relationship between the outputs and targets. From the regression graphs, it is observed that the value of the regression for test, training, and validation is close to the value 1, which indicates a good match between inputs, outputs, and objectives. From Figure 9, it can be observed that, in the case of the neural network with ten hidden neurons, the values of the regression for test, validation, and training are in the inequality report $R_{Test} < R_{Training} < R_{Validation}$, the regression is lower than 1, and the higher one is the regression for validation ($R_{Validation} = 0.63855$). From Figure 10, we observed that, in the case of the neural network with 50 hidden neurons, the values of the regression for test, validation, and training are in the inequality report $R_{Test} < R_{Validation} < R_{Training}$, the regression is lower than 1, and the higher one is the regression for training ($R_{Training} = 0.65267$). In Figure 11, it can be observed that, in the case of the neural network with 100 hidden neurons, the values of the regression for test, validation, and training are in the inequality report $R_{Validation} < R_{Test} < R_{Training}$, the regression is lower than 1, and the higher one is the regression for training ($R_{Training}$ = 0.85089). From Figure 12, it is evident that, in the case of the neural network with 150 hidden neurons, the values of the regression for test, validation, and training are in the inequality report $R_{Test} < R_{Validation} < R_{Training}$, the regression is lower than 1, and the higher one is the regression for training ($R_{Training}$ = 0.81819).

From the histograms of errors (Figures 13 and 14), it can be observed that the increase in the number of neurons in the network leads to a decrease in the percentage of errors generated. The error histograms (Figures 13 and 14) show normal distributions with residuals (errors), indicating that many of the residuals fall on or near zero in the case of the ANN with 150 neurons. Analyzing Figures 13 and 14, we can conclude that the ANN model with 150 neurons used for the prediction can generate an excellent prediction of epileptic seizures.

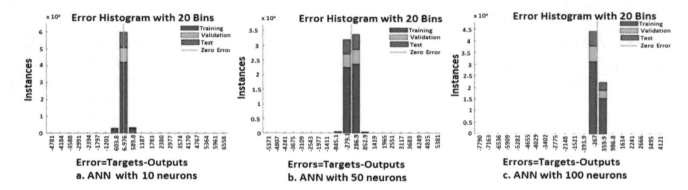

Figure 13. Error histograms—ANN with 10, 50, and 100 neurons.

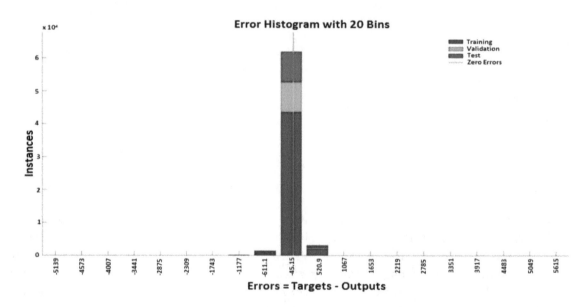

Figure 14. Error histogram—ANN with 150 neurons.

In Table 2 are presented for each neural network developed, the number of hidden neurons allocated, the processing time [seconds] of the neural network, and the values of the regression for training ($R_{Training}$), test (R_{Test}), and validation ($R_{Validation}$). In Table 2, the processing time represents the total time allocated for training, test, and validation.

In the proposed ANN with n (10, 50, 100, and 150) neurons, we defined the training set, test set, and validation set to check over-optimization. The validation set was used to measure network generalization, and to halt training when generalization stopped improving. The evaluation of the performance was done using mean square error (MSE) and regression analysis (R).

Table 2. Value $R = f$ (neural network neurons).

Neurons No.	R Training	R Validation	R Test	Processing Time [s]
10	0.57316	0.63855	0.49103	42
50	0.65267	0.60571	0.60182	745
100	0.85089	0.74129	0.82255	913
150	0.81819	0.77345	0.67324	2784

In Figures 15 and 16, the performances of the neural networks with 10 and 150 neurons, respectively, are presented. In Figures 15 and 16, error vs. epoch is plotted for the validation. The best validation is taken from the epoch with the lowest validation error. On the y axis of the charts, the mean squared error (MSE) (Equation (6)) is presented. The best validation is taken from the epoch with the lowest validation error. Mainly, the error reduces after more epochs of training.

$$\text{MSE}SE = \frac{1}{n}\sum_{i=1}^{n}(y_i - \hat{y}_i)^2 \tag{6}$$

where:

y_i is the vector of observed values;
$\hat{y}_i$ is the vector of predicted values.

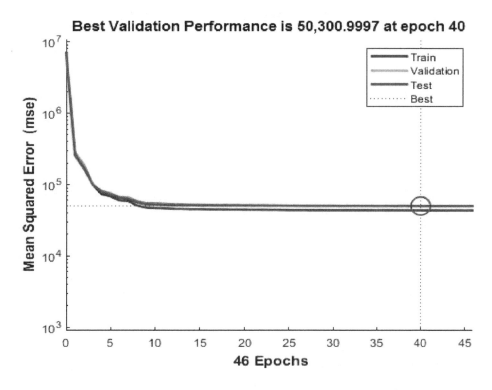

Figure 15. Neural network (10 neurons) best validation performance.

However, the best validation performance was generated in 40 epochs, whereas 47 epochs were run to confirm the model accuracy for the ANN with ten neurons (Figure 15). The best validation performance was generated in 9 epochs, whereas 15 epochs were run to confirm the model accuracy for the ANN with 150 neurons (Figure 16). In comparison with the ANN with ten neurons, the ANN with 150 neurons shows higher performance.

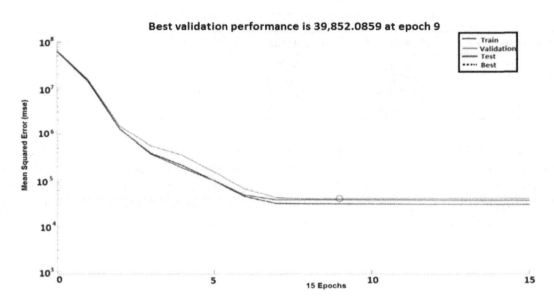

Figure 16. Neural network (150 neurons) best validation performance.

5. Discussion

5.1. Biomedical Signals Covariance Analysis

In order to evaluate if the previously presented biomedical signals (EMG, PPG, and EEG) can be used to predict epileptic seizures, it is necessary to investigate the covariance between all the analyzed signals. Mainly, for two discrete signals, $x(k)$ and $y(k)$, correlation is a discrete function in time (Equation (7)), defined by:

$$r_{xy}(k) = \sum_{n=-\infty}^{+\infty} x(n)y(n-k) \tag{7}$$

where $k = 0, 1, 2, \ldots$.

Using the correlation function of two signals, the similarity between the signals can be appreciated. The autocorrelation function has a maximum in origin when $k = 0$ and can be used to determine the periodicity of real signals. The autocorrelation function (Equation (8)) is defined by:

$$r_{xx}(k) = \sum_{n=-\infty}^{+\infty} x(n)y(n-k) \tag{8}$$

where: $k = 0, 1, 2, \ldots$.

The signals EEG1 (no seizure) and EEG3 (with seizure) collected from patient n1, respective to the signals EEG2 (with seizure) and EEG4 (no seizure) collected from patient n2, were sampled at a rate of 160 Hz and filtered using high-pass (0.1 Hz) and low-pass filters (60 Hz for EEG with no seizure activity, respective to 120 Hz for EEG with seizure).

By analyzing the covariance matrix for EEG_i, EEG_j (Equations (9), (11), (13), (15), (17) and (19)), and correlation coefficients (Equations (10), (12), (14), (16), (18) and (20)), we found that:

- between EEG1 and EEG3 is a negative covariance; this means that they are not in a linear dependence (Equation (9)). Because the correlation coefficient is negative (Equation (10)), it follows that EEG1 and EEG3 are in an inverse proportionality relationship.
- between EEG2 and EEG4 is a negative covariance, which means that EEG2 and EEG4 are not in a linear dependence (Equation (11)). Because the correlation coefficient is negative (Equation (12)), it follows that EEG1 and EEG3 are in an inverse proportionality relationship.

- between EEG1 and EEG4 is a positive covariance, which means that EEG1 and EEG4 are in a linear dependence (Equation (13)), and because the correlation coefficient is positive (Equation (14)), it follows that EEG1 and EEG4 are in a direct proportionality relationship.
- between EEG1 and EEG2 is a negative covariance (Equation (15)), which means that EEG1 and EEG2 are not in a linear dependence, and because the correlation coefficient is negative (Equation (16)), it follows that EEG1 and EEG2 are in an inverse proportionality relationship.
- between EEG2 and EEG3 is a positive covariance, which means that EEG2 and EEG3 are in a linear dependence (Equation (17)), and because the correlation coefficient is positive (Equation (18)), it follows that EEG1 and EEG4 are in a direct proportionality relationship.
- between EEG3 and EEG4 is a negative covariance (Equation (19)), which means that EEG3 and EEG4 are not in a linear dependence, and because the correlation coefficient is negative (Equation (20)), it follows that EEG3 and EEG4 are in an inverse proportionality relationship.

$$cov(EEG1,\ EEG3) = 1.0e+05 * \begin{vmatrix} 0.7206 & -0.0369 \\ -0.0369 & 0.7206 \end{vmatrix} \tag{9}$$

$$R_{EEG1,\ EEG3} = \begin{vmatrix} 1.0000 & -0.0272 \\ -0.0272 & 1.0000 \end{vmatrix} \Leftrightarrow r_{1,2} = r_{2,1} = -0.0272 \tag{10}$$

$$cov(EEG2,\ EEG4) = 1.0e+05 * \begin{vmatrix} 0.5555 & -0.0900 \\ -0.0900 & 5.7909 \end{vmatrix}, \tag{11}$$

$$R_{EEG2,EEG4} = \begin{vmatrix} 1.0000 & -0.0502 \\ -0.0502 & 1.0000 \end{vmatrix} \Leftrightarrow r_{1,2} = r_{2,1} = -0.0502, \tag{12}$$

$$cov(EEG1,\ EEG4) = 1.0e+05 * \begin{vmatrix} 0.7206 & 0.0196 \\ 0.0196 & 5.7909 \end{vmatrix}, \tag{13}$$

$$R_{EEG1,\ EEG4} = \begin{vmatrix} 1.0000 & 0.0096 \\ 0.0096 & 1.0000 \end{vmatrix} \Leftrightarrow r_{1,2} = r_{2,1} = 0.0096, \tag{14}$$

$$cov(EEG1,\ EEG2) = 1.0e+04 * \begin{vmatrix} 7.2061 & -0.5302 \\ -0.5302 & 5.5551 \end{vmatrix}, \tag{15}$$

$$R_{EEG1,\ EEG2} = \begin{vmatrix} 1.0000 & -0.0838 \\ -0.0838 & 1.0000 \end{vmatrix} \Leftrightarrow r_{1,2} = r_{2,1} = -0.0838, \tag{16}$$

$$cov(EEG2,\ EEG3) = 1.0e+05 * \begin{vmatrix} 0.5555 & 0.3163 \\ 0.3163 & 2.5545 \end{vmatrix}, \tag{17}$$

$$R_{EEG2,EEG3} = \begin{vmatrix} 1.0000 & 0.2655 \\ 0.2655 & 1.0000 \end{vmatrix} \Leftrightarrow r_{1,2} = r_{2,1} = 0.2655, \tag{18}$$

$$cov(EEG3,\ EEG4) = 1.0e+05 * \begin{vmatrix} 2.5545 & -0.2580 \\ -0.2580 & 5.7909 \end{vmatrix}, \tag{19}$$

$$R_{EEG3,\ EEG4} = \begin{vmatrix} 1.0000 & -0.0671 \\ -0.0671 & 1.0000 \end{vmatrix} \Leftrightarrow r_{1,2} = r_{2,1} = -0.0671 \tag{20}$$

Using the Shapiro–Wilk test (Figure 17) to evaluate the distribution of EEG1, EEG2, EEG3, and EEG4 signals in the Brainstorm application, it can be seen that the values for $W_{EEG1} = 0.9378$, $W_{EEG2} = 0.9236$, $W_{EEG3} = 0.9133$, and $W_{EEG4} = 0.8299$, are very close to 1, which means that the signals have a distribution close to the normal distribution.

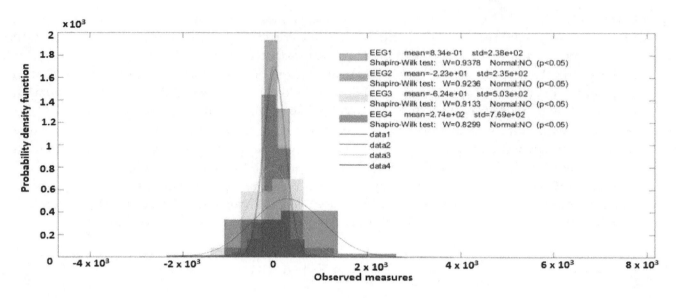

Figure 17. Distribution probabilities (Shapiro–Wilk test, Brainstorm).

The analysis of the covariances and correlations between EMG2 and EEG2 (Equations (21) and (22)) and PPG3 and EEG3 (Equations (23) and (24)), respective of those between EMG3 and EEG3 (Equations (25) and (26)), shows that there is a positive correlation and a direct covariance between signal pairs ((PPG3, EEG3) and (EMG3, EEG3)), respective of those between signal pairs (EMG2, EEG2), which could be exploited in anticipation of epilepsy seizures by predictive analysis using an ANN and a support decision system.

$$cov(EMG2, EEG2) = 1.0e + 04 * \begin{vmatrix} 0.6864 & 0.0422 \\ 0.0422 & 9.2137 \end{vmatrix}, \tag{21}$$

$$R_{EMG2,EEG2} = \begin{vmatrix} 1.0000 & 0.0168 \\ 0.0168 & 1.0000 \end{vmatrix} \Leftrightarrow r_{1,2} = r_{2,1} = 0.0168, \tag{22}$$

$$cov(PPG3, EEG3) = 1.0e + 05 * \begin{vmatrix} 0.2690 & 0.0909 \\ 0.0909 & 4.9304 \end{vmatrix}, \tag{23}$$

$$R_{PPG3, EEG3} = \begin{vmatrix} 1.0000 & 0.0789 \\ 0.0789 & 1.0000 \end{vmatrix} \Leftrightarrow r_{1,2} = r_{2,1} = 0.0789 \tag{24}$$

$$cov(EMG3, EEG3) = 1.0e + 05 * \begin{vmatrix} 2.1729 & 0.0122 \\ 0.0122 & 4.9304 \end{vmatrix}, \tag{25}$$

$$R_{EMG3,EEG3} = \begin{vmatrix} 1.0000 & 0.0037 \\ 0.0037 & 1.0000 \end{vmatrix} \Leftrightarrow r_{1,2} = r_{2,1} = 0.0037, \tag{26}$$

In conclusion, the correlations and covariances between the biomedical signals (EEG, PPG, and EMG) collected from sensors are significant because, in the case of the patients with epilepsy, the heart rate increases and may generate uncontrolled tremors of the muscles or their stiffening. Furthermore, to patients having epilepsy, the comorbidity phenomena are present [66–68] and consist of overlapping of several diseases (diabetes, cardiovascular diseases, etc.)

5.2. Comparative Analysis

To observe the performance of our proposed methodology, we compared our methods (DWT and ANN), validation, and accuracy of the results with the existing methods based on machine learning from the literature. Comparison is presented in Table 3, which contains the feature extraction methods, the machine learning methods, the validation methods, and also the classification accuracy.

Table 3. Methodology description of recent state-of-the-art compared with our results.

Literature	Features Extraction Method	Learning Machine Method	Validation	Classification Accuracy
Method 1	-	[69] Convolutional neural network (CNN) with 3 layers	6-fold cross validation	83.8–95%
Method 2	spectral and spatial features	[70] SVM	-	96%
Method 3	wavelet transform for decomposition	[71] ANN and genetic algorithm	-	-
Method 4	wavelet transform for decomposition	[72] negative correlation learning (NCL) and a mixture of experts (ME)	25% of the train set was randomly selected for the validation set	96.92%
Method 5	Multi-wavelet Transform	[73] ANN	-	90%
Method 6	-	[74] pyramidal one-dimensional CNN (P-1D-CNN)	10-fold cross validation	99.1%
Method 7	-	[75] 13-layer CNN	10-fold cross-validation	88.67%
Method 8	DWT	[76] SVM		96%
Method 9	Minimum redundancy maximum relevance (mRMR), Principal component analysis (PCA)	[77] SVM, k-nearest neighbors (k-NN), and discriminant analysis	Leave-one-out cross-validation	51% (SVM) 80% (k-nn with mRMR)
Method 10	-	[78] CNN	20-fold and 10-fold cross-validation	84.26%
Method 11	-	[79] U-Time—convolutional encoder-decoder network	5-fold cross-validation	-
Our work	DWT	ANN	15% of the samples were selected for the validation set	91.1%

5.3. Limitation and Future Scope

The proposed methods give significant results, but the ratio between best validation performance and processing time exhibits an inverse relationship and generates the limitation in real-time data processing because the neural network with 150 neurons has the best validation performance, but the increasing the number of neurons in the ANN generates an increase in the time required for data processing.

The other state-of-the-art methods do not analyze the problem of real-time processing through the perspective of the ratio between best performance validation and time.

However, an investigation for a new set of parameters and to learn algorithms to improve this is needed. Moreover, analyzing other physiological signals such as the heart's electrical activity (ECG) along with EMG, PPG, and EEG may improve the investigations to detect biomedical parameters changes before or during the seizures.

6. Conclusions

In this work, we used artificial neural networks (ANN) for automatic detection of epileptic seizures before onset. We used DWT with Daubechies function for decomposing the signals and analyzing EEG recordings before onset and during the seizure for patients with epileptic seizures and with no epileptic seizures. To design the model, we used the predictive analysis of EEG signals, artificial feed-forward neural networks based on the Levenberg–Marquardt backpropagation optimization algorithm. In addition, we analyzed the covariance between biomedical signals (EEG, PPG, and EMG) to select the signals that can be used on predicting epileptic seizures.

We can conclude that using the ANN with 150 neurons has an excellent performance in comparison with the ANN with ten neurons. However, this ANN analyzes requests an increased time in comparison with an ANN with a lower neuron number (e.g., ten neurons). Even if the use of an ANN with a large number of neurons gives more precision, it requires a very long time for data processing, and it is preferable to choose neural networks that provide an adequate solution about the issues regarding the accuracy of the outputs and the time allocated for processing [80].

The analysis of the covariance and correlation between signals allows the identification of biomedical signals that can be used in the predictive ANN applications for medical alert systems to send alerts if the regression at time t has a different value from the regression recorded in the analysis of signals taken from patients with no seizures activity [80].

The proposed methods showed promising results compared to other state-of-the-art methods. Our method opens new perspectives to the successful automatic detection of epileptic seizures before onset, enabling a real-time brain monitoring wearable system.

In the future, we plan to apply this method to epileptic signal detection on wearable devices. Our next research object is to develop a successful seizure forecasting model by analyzing, in addition, heart electrical activity (ECG).

Author Contributions: Conceptualization, R.M.A.; methodology, R.M.A.; software, R.M.A.; validation, R.M.A.; formal analysis, R.M.A., S.P., and A.F.; investigation, R.M.A.; writing—original draft preparation, R.M.A.; writing—review and editing, R.M.A. and A.F.; visualization, R.M.A.; supervision, S.P. and A.F.; project administration, R.M.A., A.F., and S.P.; and funding acquisition, A.F. All authors have read and agreed to the published version of the manuscript.

References

1. Hammad, M.; Pławiak, P.; Wang, K.; Acharya, U.R. ResNet-Attention model for human authentication using ECG signals. *Expert Syst.* **2020**, e12547. [CrossRef]
2. Tuncer, T.; Ertam, F.; Dogan, S.; Aydemir, E.; Pławiak, P. Ensemble residual network-based gender and activity recognition method with signals. *J. Supercomput.* **2020**, *76*, 2119–2138. [CrossRef]
3. Pławiak, P.; Acharya, U.R. Novel deep genetic ensemble of classifiers for arrhythmia detection using ECG signals. *Neural Comput. Appl.* **2019**, 1–25. [CrossRef]
4. Tuncer, T.; Dogan, S.; Pławiak, P.; Acharya, U.R. Automated arrhythmia detection using novel hexadecimal local pattern and multilevel wavelet transform with ECG signals. *Knowl. Based Syst.* **2019**, *186*, 104923. [CrossRef]
5. Plawiak, P.; Tadeusiewicz, R. Approximation of phenol concentration using novel hybrid computational intelligence methods. *Int. J. Appl. Math. Comput. Sci.* **2014**, *24*, 165–181. [CrossRef]
6. Kandala, R.N.; Dhuli, R.; Pławiak, P.; Naik, G.R.; Moeinzadeh, H.; Gargiulo, G.D.; Gunnam, S. Towards Real-Time Heartbeat Classification: Evaluation of Nonlinear Morphological Features and Voting Method. *Sensors* **2019**, *19*, 5079. [CrossRef] [PubMed]
7. Alqatawneh, A.; Alhalaseh, R.; Hassanat, A.; Abbadi, M. Statistical-Hypothesis-Aided Tests for Epilepsy Classification. *Computers* **2019**, *8*, 84. [CrossRef]
8. Chenane, K.; Touati, Y.; Boubchir, L.; Daachi, B. Neural Net-Based Approach to EEG Signal Acquisition and Classification. *BCI Appl. Comput.* **2019**, *8*, 87.
9. Borghini, G.; Aricò, P.; Di Flumeri, G.; Sciaraffa, N.; Babiloni, F. Correlation and similarity between cerebral and non-cerebral electrical activity for user's states assessment. *Sensors* **2019**, *19*, 704. [CrossRef] [PubMed]
10. Usami, K.; Matsumoto, R.; Sawamoto, N.; Murakami, H.; Inouchi, M.; Fumuro, T.; Shimotake, A.; Kato, T.; Mima, T.; Shirozu, H.; et al. Epileptic network of hypothalamic hamartoma: An EEG-fMRI study. *Epilepsy Res.* **2016**, *125*, 1–9. [CrossRef] [PubMed]

11. Übeyli, E.D.; Cvetkovic, D.; Cosic, I. AR spectral analysis technique for human PPG, ECG and EEG signals. *J. Med. Syst.* **2008**, *32*, 201–206. [CrossRef] [PubMed]

12. Bonita, J.D.; Ambolode, L.C.C.; Rosenberg, B.M.; Cellucci, C.J.; Watanabe, T.A.A.; Rapp, P.; Albano, A.M. Time domain measures of inter-channel EEG correlations: A comparison of linear, nonparametric and nonlinear measures. *Cogn. Neurodyn.* **2013**, *8*, 1–15. [CrossRef] [PubMed]

13. Mirowski, P.; Madhavan, D.; LeCun, Y.; Kuzniecky, R. Classification of patterns of EEG synchronization for seizure prediction. *Clin. Neurophysiol.* **2009**, *120*, 1927–1940. [CrossRef]

14. Kuhlmann, L.; Freestone, D.R.; Lai, A.; Burkitt, A.N.; Fuller, K.; Grayden, D.B.; Seiderer, L.; Vogrin, S.; Mareels, I.; Cook, M.J. Patient-specific bivariate-synchrony-based seizure prediction for short prediction horizons. *Epilepsy Res.* **2010**, *91*, 214–231. [CrossRef] [PubMed]

15. Shibasaki, H.; Rothwell, J.C.; Deuschl, G.; Eisen, A.; EMG-EEG Correlation. Recommendations for the practice of Clinical Neurophysiology: Guidelines of the International Federation of Clinical Neurophysiology. Electroenceph Clin Neurophysiol. Electroenceph. *Clin. Neurophysiol. Suppl.* **1999**, *52*, 269–274.

16. Williamson, J.R.; Bliss, D.W.; Browne, D.W.; Narayanan, J.T. Seizure prediction using EEG spatiotemporal correlation structure. *Epilepsy Behav.* **2012**, *25*, 230–238. [CrossRef]

17. Sharma, A.; Rai, J.K.; Tewari, R.P. Multivariate EEG signal analysis for early prediction of epileptic seizure. In Proceedings of the 2015 2nd International Conference on Recent Advances in Engineering & Computational Sciences (RAECS), Chandigarh, India, 21–22 December 2015.

18. Teixeira, C.; Direito, B.; Bandarabadi, M.; Le Van Quyen, M.; Valderrama, M.; Schelter, B.; Schulze-Bonhage, A.; Navarro, V.; Sales, F.; Dourado, A. Epileptic seizure predictors based on computational intelligence techniques: A comparative study with 278 patients. *Comput. Methods Programs Biomed.* **2014**, *114*, 324–336. [CrossRef] [PubMed]

19. Buchbinder, M. Neural imaginaries and clinical epistemology: Rhetorically mapping the adolescent brain in the clinical encounter. *Soc. Sci. Med.* **2014**, *143*, 304–310. [CrossRef] [PubMed]

20. Bandarabadi, M.; Teixeira, C.; Rasekhi, J.; Dourado, A. Epileptic seizure prediction using relative spectral power features. *Clin. Neurophysiol.* **2015**, *126*, 237–248. [CrossRef]

21. Smith, S.J.M. EEG in the diagnosis, classification, and management of patients with epilepsy. *J. Neurol. Neurosurg. Psychiatry* **2005**, *76*, ii2–ii7. [CrossRef]

22. Costa, R.P.; Oliveira, P.; Rodrigues, G.; Leitao, B.; Dourado, A. Epileptic seizure classification using neural networks with 14 features. In Proceedings of the International Conference on Knowledge-Based and Intelligent Information and Engineering Systems, Budapest, Hungary, 3–5 September 2008; Springer: Berlin, Germany.

23. Damayanti, A.; Pratiwi, A.B. Epilepsy detection on EEG data using backpropagation, firefly algorithm, and simulated annealing. In Proceedings of the 2nd International Conference on Science and Technology-Computer (ICST), Yogyakarta, Indonesia, 27–28 October 2016.

24. Aldabbagh, A.M.; Alshebeili, S.A.; Alotaiby, T.N.; Abd-Elsamie, F.E. Low computational complexity EEG epilepsy data classification algorithm for patients with intractable seizures. In Proceedings of the 2015 2nd International Conference on Biomedical Engineering (ICoBE), Penang, Malaysia, 30–31 March 2015.

25. Harikumar, R.; Shanmugam, A.; Rajan, P. VLSI Synthesis of Heterogeneous and SIRM Fuzzy System for Classification of Diabetic Epilepsy Risk Levels. In Proceedings of the 2008 Cairo International Biomedical Engineering Conference, Cairo, Egypt, 18–20 December 2008.

26. Quintero-Rincón, A.; Prendes, J.; Pereyra, M.; Batatia, H.; Risk, M. Multivariate Bayesian classification of epilepsy EEG signals. In Proceedings of the IEEE 12th Image, Video, and Multidimensional Signal Processing Workshop (IVMSP), Bordeaux, France, 11–12 July 2016.

27. Despre Electroencefalografie. Ce Diagnostice Poate Descoperi? Available online: http://www.unicare.ro/blog/despre-electroencefalografie-ce-diagnostice-poate-descoperi.htm (accessed on 15 December 2017).

28. Kreuzer, M. EEG based monitoring of general anesthesia: Taking the next steps. *Front. Comput. Neurosci.* **2017**, *11*, 56. [CrossRef]

29. Jameson, L.C.; Sloan, T.B. Using EEG to monitor anesthesia drug effects during surgery. *J. Clin. Monit.* **2006**, *20*, 445–472. [CrossRef]

30. Takeda, Y.; Inoue, Y.; Tottori, T.; Mihara, T. Acute psychosis during intracranial EEG monitoring: Close relationship between psychotic symptoms and discharges in amygdala. *Epilepsia* **2001**, *42*, 719–724. [CrossRef]

31. Gandelman-Marton, R.; Kimiagar, I.; Itzhaki, A.; Klein, C.; Theitler, J.; Rabey, J.M. Electroencephalography findings in adult patients with West Nile virus—associated meningitis and meningoencephalitis. *Clin. Infect. Dis.* **2003**, *37*, 1573–1578. [CrossRef]

32. Yi, G.-S.; Jiang, W.; Bin, D.; Xi-Le, W. Complexity of resting-state EEG activity in the patients with early-stage Parkinson's disease. *Cogn. Neurodyn.* **2017**, *2*, 147–160. [CrossRef] [PubMed]

33. Dauwels, J.; Francois, V.; Andrzej, C. Diagnosis of Alzheimer's disease from EEG signals: Where are we standing? *Curr. Alzheimer Res.* **2010**, *7*, 487–505. [CrossRef]

34. Melissant, C.; Alexander, Y.; Edward, E.F.; Cornelis, J.S. A method for detection of Alzheimer's disease using ICA-enhanced EEG measurements. *Artif. Intell. Med.* **2005**, *33*, 209–222. [CrossRef] [PubMed]

35. Jeong, J. EEG dynamics in patients with Alzheimer's disease. *Clin. Neurophysiol.* **2004**, *115*, 1490–1505. [CrossRef]

36. Deng, B.; Li, L.; Shunan, L.; Ruofan, W.; Haitao, Y.; Jiang, W.; Xile, W. Complexity extraction of electroencephalograms in Alzheimer's disease with weighted-permutation entropy. *Chaos Interdiscip. J. Nonlinear Sci.* **2015**, *25*, 043105. [CrossRef]

37. Bonanni, L.; Astrid, T.; Pietro, T.; Bernardo, P.; Sara, V.; Marco, O. EEG comparisons in early Alzheimer's disease, dementia with Lewy bodies and Parkinson's disease with dementia patients with a 2-year follow-up. *Brain* **2008**, *131*, 690–705. [CrossRef]

38. Kumar, S.S.P.; Ajitha, L. Early detection of epilepsy using EEG signals. In Proceedings of the International Conference on Control, Instrumentation, Communication, and Computational Technologies (ICCICCT), Kanyakumari, India, 10–11 July 2014; pp. 1509–1514.

39. Ahmad, M.Z.; Saeed, M.; Saleem, S.; Kamboh, A.M. Seizure detection using EEG: A survey of different techniques. In Proceedings of the International Conference on Emerging Technologies (ICET), Islamabad, Pakistan, 18–19 October 2016; pp. 1–6.

40. Al-Omar, S.; Kamali, W.; Khalil, M.; Daher, A. Classification of EEG signals to detect epilepsy problems. In Proceedings of the 2nd International Conference on Advances in Biomedical Engineering, Tripoli, Lebanon, 11–13 September 2013; pp. 5–8.

41. Sun, Z.; Wang, G.; Li, K.; Zhang, Z.; Bao, G. Cerebral functional connectivity analysis based on scalp EEG in epilepsy patients. In Proceedings of the 7th International Conference on Biomedical Engineering and Informatics, Dalian, China, 14–16 October 2014; pp. 283–287.

42. David, A.S.; Ruth, A.G. Neuropsychological study of motor neuron disease. *Psychosomatics* **1986**, *27*, 441–445. [CrossRef]

43. Lesný, I. Study in Different Forms of Cerebral Palsy. *Dev. Med. Child Neurol.* **2008**, *5*, 593–602. [CrossRef]

44. Screens, Tests and Evaluations. Available online: http://www.cerebralpalsy.org/about-cerebral-palsy/diagnosis/evaluations (accessed on 15 December 2017).

45. Şenbil, N.; Birkan, S.; Ömer, F.A.; Yahya, K.Y.G. Epileptic and non-epileptic cerebral palsy: EEG and cranial imaging findings. *Brain Dev.* **2002**, *24*, 166–169. [CrossRef]

46. Anderson, J.L.; Stewart, I.H.; Rae, C.; Morley, J.W. Brain function in Duchenne muscular dystrophy. *Brain* **2002**, *125*, 4–13. [CrossRef]

47. Electroencephalogram (EEG). Available online: https://www.nhs.uk/conditions/electroencephalogram (accessed on 12 February 2020).

48. Chen, D.; Wan, S.; Xiang, J.; Bao, F.S. A high-performance seizure detection algorithm based on Discrete Wavelet Transform (DWT) and EEG. *PLoS ONE* **2017**, *12*, e0173138. [CrossRef]

49. Terzano, M.G.; Parrino, L.; Smerieri, A.; Chervin, R.; Chokroverty, S.; Guilleminault, C.; Hirshkowitz, M.; Mahowald, M.; Moldofsky, H.; Rosa, A.; et al. Atlas, rules, and recording techniques for the scoring of cyclic alternating pattern (CAP) in human sleep. *Sleep Med.* **2002**, *3*, 187–199. [CrossRef]

50. Goldberger, A.L.; Amaral, L.; Glass, L.; Hausdorff, J.M.; Ivanov, P.C.; Mark, R.G.; Mietus, J.; Moody, G.B.; Peng, C.K.; Stanley, H. PhysioBank, PhysioToolkit, and PhysioNet: Components of a new research resource for complex physiologic signals. *Circulations* **2000**, *101*, e215–e220. [CrossRef]

51. Mingai, L.; Shuoda, G.; Guoyu, Z.; Yanjun, S.; Jinfu, Y. Removing ocular artifacts from mixed EEG signals with FastKICA and DWT. *J. Intell. Fuzzy Syst.* **2015**, *28*, 2851–2861. [CrossRef]

52. Real-Time Meditation Feedback. Available online: http://www.choosemuse.com (accessed on 20 April 2018).

53. Faust, O.; Acharya, R.U.; Adeli, H.; Adeli, A. Wavelet-based EEG processing for computer-aided seizure detection and epilepsy diagnosis. *Seizure* **2015**, *26*, 56–64. [CrossRef]

54. Ren, L.; Kucewicz, M.T.; Cimbalnik, J.; Matsumoto, J.Y.; Brinkmann, B.H.; Hu, W.; Worrell, G.A. Gamma oscillations precede interictal epileptiform spikes in the seizure onset zone. *Neurology* **2015**, *84*, 602–608. [CrossRef]

55. Al-Qazzaz, N.K.; Hamid Bin Mohd Ali, S.; Ahmad, S.A.; Islam, M.S.; Escudero, J. Selection of mother wavelet functions for multi-channel EEG signal analysis during a working memory task. *Sensors* **2015**, *15*, 29015–29035. [CrossRef] [PubMed]

56. Haddad, T.; Ben-Hamida, N.; Talbi, L.; Lakhssassi, A.; Aouini, S. Temporal epilepsy seizures monitoring and prediction using cross-correlation and chaos theory. *Healthc. Technol. Lett.* **2014**, *1*, 45–50. [CrossRef] [PubMed]

57. Orosco, L.; Correa, A.G.; Diez, P.F.; Laciar, E. Patient non-specific algorithm for seizures detection in scalp EEG. *Comput. Boil. Med.* **2016**, *71*, 128–134. [CrossRef]

58. Graps, A. An introduction to wavelets. *IEEE Comput. Sci. Eng.* **1995**, *2*, 50–61. [CrossRef]

59. Fergus, P.; Hussain, A.; Hignett, D.; Al-Jumeily, D.; Abdel-Aziz, K.; Hamdan, H. A machine learning system for automated whole-brain seizure detection. *Appl. Comput. Inform.* **2016**, *12*, 70–89. [CrossRef]

60. Subasi, A.; Ercelebi, E. Classification of EEG signals using neural network and logistic regression. *Comput. Methods Programs Biomed.* **2005**, *78*, 87–99. [CrossRef]

61. Ramgopal, S.; Thomé-Souza, S.; Jackson, M.; Kadish, N.E.; Fernández, I.S.; Klehm, J.; Bosl, W.; Reinsberger, C.; Schachter, S.; Loddenkemper, T. Seizure detection, seizure prediction, and closed-loop warning systems in epilepsy. *Epilepsy Behav.* **2014**, *37*, 291–307. [CrossRef]

62. Jeppesen, J.; Beniczky, S.; Johansen, P.; Sidenius, P.; Fuglsang-Frederiksen, A. Detection of epileptic seizures with a modified heart rate variability algorithm based on Lorenz plot. *Seizure* **2015**, *24*, 1–7. [CrossRef]

63. Osorio, I.; Manly, B.F.J. Probability of detection of clinical seizures using heart rate changes. *Seizure* **2015**, *30*, 120–123. [CrossRef]

64. Stefanidou, M.; Carlson, C.; Friedman, D. The relationship between seizure onset zone and ictal tachycardia: An intracranial EEG study. *Clin. Neurophysiol.* **2015**, *126*, 2255–2260. [CrossRef]

65. Vandecasteele, K.; De Cooman, T.; Gu, Y.; Cleeren, E.; Claes, K.; Van Paesschen, W.; Van Huffel, S.; Hunyadi, B. Automated Epileptic Seizure Detection Based on Wearable ECG and PPG in a Hospital Environment. *Sensors* **2017**, *17*, 2338. [CrossRef]

66. Seidenberg, M.; Pulsipher, D.; Hermann, B. Association of epilepsy and comorbid conditions. *Future Neurol.* **2009**, *4*, 663–668. [CrossRef]

67. Pellock, J.M. Understanding co-morbidities affecting children with epilepsy. *Neurology* **2004**, *62*, S17–S23. [CrossRef]

68. Zaccara, G. Neurological comorbidity and epilepsy: Implications for treatment. *Acta Neurol. Scand.* **2009**, *120*, 1–15. [CrossRef]

69. Zhou, M.; Tian, C.; Cao, R.; Wang, B.; Niu, Y.; Hu, T.; Guo, H.; Xiang, J. Epileptic Seizure Detection Based on EEG Signals and CNN. *Front. Aging Neurosci.* **2018**, *12*, 95. [CrossRef]

70. Shoeb, A.H.; Guttag, J.V. Application of machine learning to epileptic seizure detection. In Proceedings of the International Conference on Machine Learning (Haifa), Haifa, Israel, 21–24 June 2010; pp. 975–982.

71. Patnaik, L.; Manyam, O.K. Epileptic EEG detection using neural networks and post-classification. *Comput. Methods Programs Biomed.* **2008**, *91*, 100–109. [CrossRef]

72. Ebrahimpour, R.; Babakhan, K.; Arani, S.A.A.A.; Masoudnia, S. Epileptic seizure detection using a neural network ensemble method and wavelet transform. *Neural Netw. World* **2012**, *22*, 291. [CrossRef]

73. Akareddy, S.M.; Kulkarni, P. EEG signal classification for Epilepsy Seizure Detection using Improved Approximate Entropy. *Int. J. Public Health Sci. (IJPHS)* **2013**, *2*. [CrossRef]

74. Ullah, I.; Hussain, M.; Qazi, E.-U.-H.; Abualsamh, H.A. An automated system for epilepsy detection using EEG brain signals based on deep learning approach. *Expert Syst. Appl.* **2018**, *107*, 61–71. [CrossRef]

75. Acharya, U.R.; Oh, S.L.; Hagiwara, Y.; Tan, J.H.; Adeli, H. Deep convolutional neural network for the automated detection and diagnosis of seizure using EEG signals. *Comput. Boil. Med.* **2018**, *100*, 270–278. [CrossRef]

76. Acharya, U.R.; Yanti, R.; Swapna, G.; Sree, V.S.; Martis, R.J.; Suri, J.S. Automated diagnosis of epileptic electroencephalogram using independent component analysis and discrete wavelet transform for different electroencephalogram durations. *Proc. Inst. Mech. Eng. Part H J. Eng. Med.* **2012**, *227*, 234–244. [CrossRef]

77. Machado, F.; Sales, F.; Santos, C.; Dourado, A.; Teixeira, C. A knowledge discovery methodology from EEG data for cyclic alternating pattern detection. *Biomed. Eng. Online* **2018**, *17*, 185. [CrossRef] [PubMed]

78. Mousavi, S.; Afghah, F.; Acharya, U.R. SleepEEGNet: Automated sleep stage scoring with sequence to sequence deep learning approach. *PLoS ONE* **2019**, *14*, e0216456. [CrossRef] [PubMed]

79. Perslev, M.; Jensen, M.; Darkner, S.; Jennum, P.; Igel, C. U-time: A fully convolutional network for time series segmentation applied to sleep staging. In Proceedings of the Advances in Neural Information Processing Systems (NeurIPS 2019), Vancouve, BC, Canada, 8–14 December 2019.

80. Maria, A.R. Correlation Analysis of Biomedical Signals for Predictive Modeling. Master's Thesis, Politehnica University of Bucharest, București, Romania, 2019.

11

Automatic and Real-Time Computation of the 30-Seconds Chair-Stand Test without Professional Supervision for Community-Dwelling Older Adults

Antonio Cobo [1,2], Elena Villalba-Mora [1,2,*], Rodrigo Pérez-Rodríguez [3], Xavier Ferre [1], Walter Escalante [1], Cristian Moral [1] and Leocadio Rodriguez-Mañas [4,5]

[1] Centre for Biomedical Technology (CTB), Universidad Politécnica de Madrid (UPM), Pozuelo de Alarcón, 28223 Madrid, Spain; antonio.cobo@ctb.upm.es (A.C.); xavier.ferre@ctb.upm.es (X.F.); walter.escalante@ctb.upm.es (W.E.); cristian.moral@ctb.upm.es (C.M.)

[2] Centro de Investigación Biomédica en Red en Bioingeniería, Biomateriales y Nanomedicina (CIBER-BBN), 28029 Madrid, Spain

[3] Fundación para la Investigación Biomédica, Hospital de Getafe, Getafe, 28905 Madrid, Spain; rprodrigo@salud.madrid.org

[4] Servicio de Geriatría, Hospital de Getafe, Getafe, 28905 Madrid, Spain; leocadio.rodriguez@salud.madrid.org

[5] Centro de Investigación Biomédica en Red en Fragilidad y Envejecimiento Saludable (CIBER-FES), 28029 Madrid, Spain

* Correspondence: elena.villalba@ctb.upm.es

Abstract: The present paper describes a system for older people to self-administer the 30-s chair stand test (CST) at home without supervision. The system comprises a low-cost sensor to count sit-to-stand (SiSt) transitions, and an Android application to guide older people through the procedure. Two observational studies were conducted to test (i) the sensor in a supervised environment ($n = 7$; m = 83.29 years old, sd = 4.19; 5 female), and (ii) the complete system in an unsupervised one ($n = 7$; age 64–74 years old; 3 female). The participants in the supervised test were asked to perform a 30-s CST with the sensor, while a member of the research team manually counted valid transitions. Automatic and manual counts were perfectly correlated (Pearson's r = 1, $p = 0.00$). Even though the sample was small, none of the signals around the critical score were affected by harmful noise; p (harmless noise) = 1, 95% CI = (0.98, 1). The participants in the unsupervised test used the system in their homes for a month. None of them dropped out, and they reported it to be easy to use, comfortable, and easy to understand. Thus, the system is suitable to be used by older adults in their homes without professional supervision.

Keywords: frailty syndrome; sit-to-stand; 30-s chair stand test; wearable sensors; signal processing

1. Introduction

The present paper describes a system for older people to self-administer the 30-s chair stand test (CST) at home without supervision. The system comprises a low-cost sensor that automatically detects and counts sit-to-stand (SiSt) transitions in real-time, and a home care application that guides older people through the whole procedure. Since using novel technologies is not a trivial issue for older adults, we studied whether such a system would be able to match older people's abilities and expectations, so they can use it without supervision. The 30-s CST is a medical exam used to assess older adults' lower-limb strength [1]. It requires a subject to spend thirty seconds repeatedly standing up from, and sitting down on, a chair, with his arms folded on his chest, as fast as possible [1]. The number of times the said subject reached an upright position is then taken as a proxy to lower-limb strength [1]. It is used in combination with other medical exams to assess the functional status of older people.

Depending on the results of such a functional assessment, older people may be diagnosed as robust, pre-frail, or frail [2]. Frailty is a state of increased vulnerability to low power stressors, leading to difficulties in maintaining homeostasis that increases the risk of disability and other adverse outcomes, such as falls, hospitalization, permanent institutionalization, and death [3–6]. In fact, frailty is a major predictor of disability, with frail elders showing twice the risk of disability than non-frail older adults [7].

Disability is one of the major challenges for elderly care, because improvements in life expectancy are not coming together with similar improvements in impairment-free life expectancy (IFLE); on the contrary, a decline in the latter has even been observed in some countries [8]. Disability imposes a heavy psychological and economic burden on older people and their relatives over a long time; fortunately, frailty, which may precede the development of disability by several years [2], can be reversed [9–11]. Hence the paramount role of frailty detection in the prevention of disability. Several models have been proposed to explain frailty, with two of them prevailing as major approaches, namely, Rockwood's deficit accumulation model [12–14] and Fried's phenotypic model [2]. The latter is the most widespread, and identifies the following markers of frailty: (i) weight loss, (ii) exhaustion, (iii) weakness, (iv) slowness, and (v) low physical activity [2]. An older adult is classified as pre-frail if he tests positive to one or two of the frailty components in the phenotypic model, and as frail if he tests positive to three or more of them; otherwise he is classified as robust [2] (see Table 1).

Table 1. The phenotypic model for frailty involves the assessment of five different components (weight loss, exhaustion, weakness, slowness, and low physical activity); and then diagnosing the subject as robust, pre-frail, or frail, according to the number of components that resulted positive in the tests: robust (green rows) for zero components, pre-frail (yellow rows) for 1 or 2 components, or frail (red rows) for 3, 4, or 5 components.

If a Subject Tests Positive to:	He is Diagnosed as:
0 components	Robust.
1 component 2 components	Pre-frail.
3 components 4 components 5 components	Frail.

Frail older adults can reduce their levels of frailty, and even be restored back to robustness, with exercise-based interventions, especially if combined with early diagnosis and continuity of care [9,11,15]. Many different instruments are currently involved in the diagnosis and assessment of frailty. For instance, hand grip strength is used to assess weakness, in fact, the data in the original study of Fried et al. came from hand grip strength measurements [2], but it has also been explored as a measurement of overall frailty on its own; just as the stand up and go (TUG) test, which is a standard test for gait speed [6]. On the other hand, other sources of weakness measurements, such as those based on lower-limb strength, have been observed to be associated with either hand grip strength, gait speed, and even overall frailty [16]. In fact, instruments to assess lower-limb strength, such as the 30-s CST [1], and the STS5 (measuring how long it takes for an older person to repeatedly stand up from a chair five times) [17], are usually included as part of a comprehensive geriatric assessment (CGA). Both early diagnosis and continuity of care require frailty to be frequently assessed in search of early signs of functional decline. For instance, if two consecutive measurements of lower-limb strength taken two weeks apart with the 30-s CST show a decrease bigger that a given threshold, an alarm should be raised. However, it is not feasible to assess every older adult at risk of developing frailty every two weeks with the currently available means to conduct the functional assessment exams. Most of them require the involvement of a specifically trained professional in a geriatrics department to supervise their execution, and compute their corresponding scores. Obviously, a geriatrics department in specialized care cannot afford to undertake such a screening task. In fact, they should be focusing on taking care of the most severe cases. As a result, older people do not have their functional capacity assessed for early signs of frailty very often.

Automatic sensors that do not require the involvement of any specifically trained personnel could help to alleviate this problem. On the one hand, a single staff member in a geriatrics department could supervise several tests on multiple patients simultaneously. On the other hand, and probably involving a bigger potential impact, general practitioners or nurses in primary care could add functional assessment to routine follow-ups of their older adult patients. The potential benefits of such automatic sensors become even more remarkable within the current context of the COVID-19 pandemic. Olde people are at greater risk of developing severe complications and dying from COVID-19 [18]. Therefore, they have been advised to carefully comply with distancing measures to lower the risk of transmission. However, distancing measures favor social isolation and sedentary behaviors. Such sedentary behaviors increase the risk of developing frailty [19], and have been hypothesized to persist and become habits, based on observations from previous natural disasters, in particular, from the three years following the 2011 earthquake and tsunami in East Japan [20]. In such a scenario (i.e., fewer visits to the doctor and increased risk of frailty due to sedentary behavior) older adults would benefit from having automatic sensors to conduct functional assessment exams at home, on their own or helped by their care givers. In the particular case of the 30-s CST, the setup is rather simple; it just requires a regular rigid chair to repeatedly stand-up and sit-down, and a timer to control the duration of the test [1]. Nevertheless, a trained professional is required to judge which SiSt transitions are valid and must be added to the final score. Valid SiSt transitions occur when the subject reaches an upright position [1]. However, some older adults suffer from mobility constraints, and upright positions might differ from one subject to another.

A 30-s CST is not a transparent procedure embedded into people's daily lives. It requires older adults to interrupt their daily activities and go through a specific sequence of actions. Our approach involves a system that comprises an automatic sensor and a home care application to guide older adults through the procedure. One of the determinant factors of such a system is the specifics of the sensing device. According to Millor et al., the study of SiSt and stand-to-sit (StSi) transitions with inertial sensors can be traced back to the mid-1990s [21]; in particular to Kerr et al., in 1994 [22]. Over half of the works that Millor et al. reviewed were based on the assessment of daily life activities [21]. Only a few of them involved the assessment of repeated SiSt/StSi cycles in traditional tests for frailty assessment [21]. While some works relied on the use of multiple devices on different parts of the body, a low number of devices is recommendable to simplify the setup, lower the cost, and eventually improve acceptance and adoption. A very popular approach is to place a single inertial measurement unit (IMU) on the subject's lower back (L3–L5 region), close to the body center of mass, and take advantage of the quasi-periodic nature of the body movement [23,24]. This approach is exemplified in the works of van Lummel et al. (where the authors apply it to the STS5) [23] and Millor et al. (where the authors apply it to the 30-s CST) [24].

In particular, van Lummel et al. developed a fully automated method of processing repeated sit-to-stand-to-sit (STS) cycles [23]. They used triaxial acceleration and triaxial angular velocity signals from a single IMU device (dynaport) on the lower back to compute trunk pitch-angle and vertical velocity signals. They used the morphological properties of the trunk pitch-angle signal to identify and delimit the sub-phases and transitions in repeated STS cycles. They used the vertical velocity signal to spot and discard failed attempts. However, they do not explain which features of the vertical velocity and which criteria were used to classify an attempt as a failure.

On the other hand, Millor et al. developed a fully automated method to process repeated STS cycles in a 30-s CST [24]. They computed vertical velocity and vertical position from the vertical acceleration signal, from a single IMU device (MTx Orientation Tracker—Xsens Technologies B.V. Enschede, Netherlands) on the lower back. They applied double integration, combined with fourth-level polynomial curve adjustment and cubic splines interpolation. They used the morphological properties of the vertical position signal to identify and delimit complete STS cycles. A complete STS cycle can be found between two minima in the vertical position signal. They also used the MTx's onboard Kalman filter estimation for the X-orientation, and combined it with the vertical acceleration, the vertical velocity, and the vertical position signals to identify the sub-phases (i.e., impulse, stand up, and sit down) within each STS cycle. In a subsequent paper Millor, Lecumberri, Gómez, Martínez-Ramírez, and Izquierdo argued that they automatically detected failed attempts "... based on a threshold applied to both the time elapsed between a maximum and a minimum of the Z-position and to their difference." [25], (p. 4). However, they did not clarify what the values for these thresholds were nor how they were computed.

In both cases, the authors complemented their studies by computing multiple kinematic parameters, such as transition duration (TD), maximum and minimum values of the vertical acceleration (max., min., V-acc.), Area Under the Curve (AUC) of V-acc., and roll range, and processed them to obtain additional information beyond the test score [25]. van Lummel et al. were able to identify seat-off and seat-on instants [26], establish a relationship between the subjects' stand up strategies and their overall muscle strength [27], and compare the sensitivity of stair ascending (SA) and Leg-Extension Power (LEP) to detect age-related changes [28]. When they analyzed the associations between clinical outcomes (both health and functional outcomes) and the functional tests results, they observed stronger associations for their instrumented STS5 test than for manual records [29]. On the other hand, Millor et al. were able to detect differences in frailty status (robust, pre-frail, frail) across different subjects directly from their kinematic parameters [25]. They even identified the set of most informative parameters (i.e., anterior-posterior (AP) orientation range during the Imp phase, maximum vertical acceleration and vertical power peaks during SiSt phase, and total impulse during the StSi phase) [30]. In fact, they claimed that these parameters outperformed the number of completed cycles in the 30-s CST, as a criterion for frailty classification [30].

Other locations for the sensing devices, such as the chest, have also been explored [31]. Recently, in that line, Jovanov, Wrigth, and Ganegoda presented some preliminary results from their automated 30-s CST [32]. Instead of attaching a sensor directly to the subject's chest, they took advantage of the fact that the 30-s CST requires the subject to fold his arms over his chest, and used the inertial sensors onboard a smartwatch. They used 3D acceleration signals from two different models (Fossil Gen 4 and Polar M600). They obtained excellent reliability between automated and manual counts, with little processing load. However, their experimental subjects were not older adults (12 subjects, mean age: 39.1 y.o.). They did not provide any explanation of the STS cycle identification and delimitation criteria and algorithms, and they did not mention any mechanism to spot and dismiss failed attempts.

Lately, we have explored a different approach ourselves by using an ambient sensor instead of a body-worn sensor [33]. In our study we explored " ... the feasibility of using the quasi-periodic nature of the distance between a subject's back and the chair backrest during a 30-s CST to carry out unsupervised measurements based on readings from a low-cost ultrasound sensor" [33], (p. 3). Our sensor comprised an ultrasound sensing module, an Arduino controller board, and a wireless communications module. All three of them were integrated into our own design for a portable device that the end-users could attach to the backrest of any regular rigid chair. We observed older people to generate very noisy signals. We applied a moving minimum filter to cancel the effects of said noise and an adaptable threshold to tell the difference between sitting and standing regions in the signal. Even though intra-class correlation coefficients showed good levels of reliability between the sensor outcomes and the trained professional's manual counts, the differences between these outcomes resulted in the performance of some subjects not being correctly classified as average, better than average, or worse than average.

In the present paper we come back to the body-worn sensor approach. We propose to measure the thigh angle with respect to a horizontal plane perpendicular to the direction of gravity (i.e., tilt) with a single device on the subject's thigh itself, and to use the variation of the angle as the subject stands up and down over time to identify SiSt and StSi transitions. Measurements of the thigh angle from a single device have already been used in previous literature to study SiSt and StSi transitions, mostly to identify different postures and activities (sitting, standing, walking, ramp or stair ascending, etc.) while performing activities of daily living (either in controlled lab settings or in free-living conditions) [34–37]. However, we have not found any descriptions of an instrumented version of the 30-s CST based on this approach. The accurate estimation of tilt based on IMU readings relies on the fusion of accelerometer and gyroscope data [38]. Smartphones come equipped with IMUs and relatively high computing power. However, smartphone adoption among the geriatric population (i.e., people over 70 years old) is low, especially among low-income and low-education elders, because they use much simpler and cheaper mobile phones. Smartphones would be too expensive, and oversize, for the single purpose of being used as a sensor; since a home kit for frailty monitoring usually comprises multiple sensors, devices of a much lower cost are required. Kalman and complementary filters are the most widespread data fusion methods for IMU-based applications [38]. Kalman filters are computationally expensive and, as stated by Abhayasinghe, Murray, and Sharif Bidabadi, 32-bit microcontrollers with a digital signal processor (DSP) are necessary to run them in real time [39]. Conversely, the algorithm for the complementary filter is much simpler and, even though it involves the computation of an arc tangent, can be run on much cheaper 8-bit microcontrollers in real time [39]. According to Tognetti et al., making use of a simple accelerometer instead of a complete IMU may contribute to further decreasing the complexity and cost of the sensing device [40]; however, the complementary filter still relies on fusing accelerometer and gyroscope data. Fortunately, tilt can be estimated solely from accelerometry if the main contributor to the accelerometer readings is gravity. During a 30-s CST, however, an accelerometer will be exposed to sudden acceleration and deceleration forces when reaching the upright and sitting positions. Thus, the question remains whether the resulting noise will harm the correct identification of valid transitions.

On the other hand, using novel technologies is not a trivial issue for older adults. Moreover, the sensors described above have been tested in controlled settings, under the supervision of their corresponding research teams. We have found no works reporting older adult's performance when using this kind of automatic sensors on their own. Our approach involves a system that comprises an automatic sensor and a home care application to guide older adults through the procedure. Thus, the question remains whether such a system will match older people's abilities and expectations so they can use it without supervision. We implemented our own design for a low-cost sensor for counting SiSt transitions, which estimates the thigh angle solely form the readings of a single accelerometer. In addition, we implemented a home care app for Android that guides the older adults throughout the whole procedure. We first tested the sensor in a supervised environment, and then we tested the complete system in an unsupervised one. To test the sensor, we studied the impact of noise by analyzing the statistical significance of the estimated probability of finding harmless noise in a valid SiSt transition. We observed the noise in all the valid transitions in the critical scenario (i.e., test scores around the value used to spot patients not fit enough to remain independent) to be harmless. We then delivered the complete system to seven older adults' homes for a month, and conducted an acceptability study. The participants reported finding it easy to use, feeling comfortable using it, understanding the features and functionalities of the app, and feeling able to use it on their own.

2. Materials and Methods

The sensor was tested in an observational study, described in Section 2.1, where the participants used it while taking a 30-s CST, under the supervision of a trained member of the research team. The home care system was tested in another observational study, described in Section 2.2, where the participants used it to take several 30-s CSTs over the course of a month, at their own homes and without any kind of supervision.

2.1. Supervised Validation of the Sensor

2.1.1. Participants

Seven older subjects (age: m = 83.29 years old, sd = 4.19; gender: 5 female and 2 male) were recruited from a pool of participants that expressed a general interest in participating in research studies from the University Hospital of Getafe.

All subjects gave their informed consent for inclusion before they participated in the study. The study was conducted in accordance with the Declaration of Helsinki, and the protocol was approved by the Ethics Committee of the Universidad Politécnica de Madrid on 9 May 2019 (POSITIVE: Maintaining and improving the intrinsic capacity involving primary care and caregivers). The following inclusion and exclusion criteria were applied:

- A subject COULD ENTER the study if ALL the following INCLUSION CRITERIA applied:

  o   The subject is willing and able to give written informed consent for participation in the study.
  o   The subject is 70 years old or older.
  o   The subject is able to perform the 30-s CST in a safe way.
  o   The subject has not been diagnosed with cognitive impairment.

- A subject COULD NOT ENTER the study if ANY of the following EXCLUSION CRITERIA applied:

  o   Subjects suffering from any major disability.
  o   Subjects suffering from cognitive impairment.

2.1.2. Apparatus

The overall setup is depicted in Figure 1, and consisted of a regular rigid chair with a backrest, an instance of the wearable device under study, and a tablet device. The chair played the same role as usual in any regular 30-s CST. The subjects wore the sensing device on one of their thighs. The sensor is longitudinally aligned with the subject's femur and tightly attached to her thigh with a Velcro strap as shown in Figure 2. Since the sensor is sensitive to orientation, a green sticker was attached to one of its ends to signal which one has to remain closer to the knee. However, it is not visible in Figure 2, because once the sensor is put in place and secured, the Velcro strap covers it. The tablet hosts an app to control the sensor, and it is paired to the latter via Bluetooth. A member of the research team used the app to switch the sensor into either calibration or measurement mode, and to visualize the sensor automatic count at the end of each 30-s CST. In calibration mode, the readings from the accelerometer in the device are used to compute the thigh angle in both a sitting and an upright static posture, as a measurement of the subject's mobility constraints; then, the parameters in the automatic count algorithm are set accordingly to a personalized value. In measurement mode, the subject takes the 30-s CST itself, and the accelerometer readings are processed by the automatic count algorithm (aka STS analysis algorithm). Finally, the sensor sends the automatic count to the tablet via Bluetooth once the test is over. Further details about the sensor hardware, the automatic count algorithm, and the tablet app can be found in Sections 2.1.2.1 to 2.1.2.3, respectively.

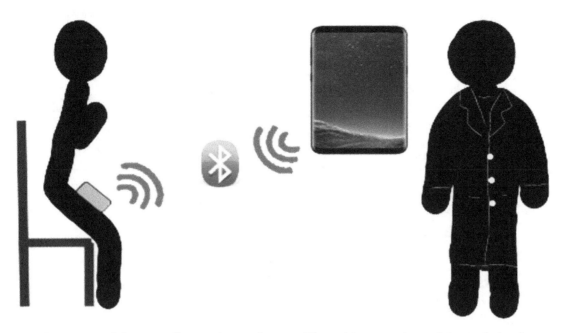

Figure 1. Depiction of the overall experimental setup: The subject stands up from and sits down on a regular rigid chair with the sensing device on one of his thighs; the sensing device is paired with a tablet via Bluetooth; a member of the research team uses the app on board the tablet device to switch the sensor into either calibration or measurement modes, and to visualize the sensor automatic count once the 30-s chair stand test (CST) is over.

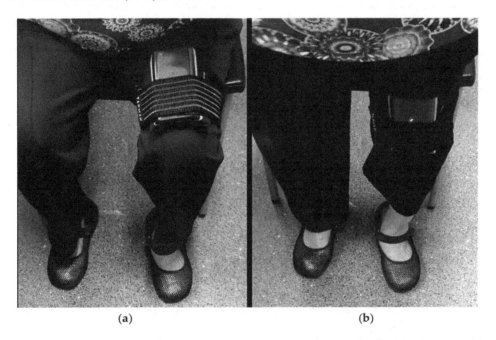

| (a) | (b) |

Figure 2. Position and alignment of the sensing device on a subject's thigh. (**a**) The wearable sensor is placed on the subject's thigh longitudinally aligned with her femur. The sensor is tightly attached to the subject's thigh with a Velcro strap to prevent it from sliding. The LED in the sensor is turned off when the subject is sitting; (**b**) and it is turned on every time a valid SiSt transition is detected.

2.1.2.1. The Wearable Sensor Device

The device consists of three main building blocks, as shown in Scheme 1. These blocks are, from left to right:

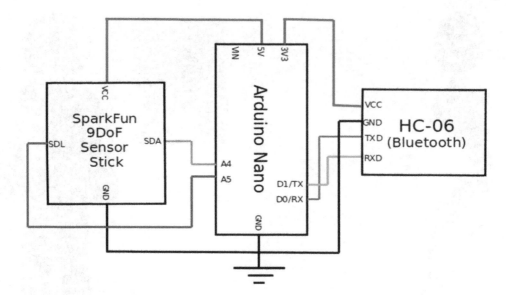

Scheme 1. Schematic block diagram of the interconnection between the device components. The Arduino Nano board (center) acts as the control and processing unit, collecting readings from the accelerometer (SparkFun block on the left), computing the estimations of the thigh angle over time, and analyzing the resulting signal. The Arduino Nano board also makes use of the Bluetooth module (HC-06 block on the right) to exchange messages with the external mobile device over a wireless communication channel. The whole device was powered by a 9V 6LP3146 battery. While the Arduino Nano board was directly powered by the battery, the accelerometer and the Bluetooth boards were indirectly powered by connecting them to the Arduino's 5V and 3.3V DC outputs, respectively. The battery was omitted in this scheme for the sake of clarity.

- An accelerometer (a SparkFun 9DoF Sensor Stick board with an LSM9DS1 IMU chip). This SparkFun board comes with a nine degrees of freedom IMU (i.e., it comprises a triaxial accelerometer, a triaxial gyroscope, and a triaxial magnetometer). However, we did not use the gyroscope and the magnetometer because, as explained in Section 2.1.2.2, acceleration readings are enough to compute an estimation of the thigh angle.

- A control and processing unit (an Arduino Nano board with an ATmega328P microcontroller). The Arduino board acts as the processing unit in the device thanks to its onboard micro-controller. Our processing algorithm runs on board the Arduino, and is responsible for collecting the accelerometer readings, computing the estimations of the thigh angle over time, and analyzing the resulting signal to automatically detect and count SiSt and StSi transitions in real time, without storing or transmitting the individual samples.

- A communications unit: (HC-06 Bluetooth 2.0 + EDR module). End users (in this case, the researcher conducting the experiment) control the behavior of the sensing device by interacting with a mobile app in an external tablet device. This communication unit enables wireless communication between the two devices via Bluetooth. The researcher can issue calibration and measurements commands to the sensing device, and the latter automatically sends the results to the tablet once a 30s-CST is over.

The device is powered by a 9 V battery (6LP3146). However, only the Arduino Nano board was directly powered by this battery. The accelerometer board was powered by connecting it to the Arduino's 5 V DC output, and the Bluetooth board was indirectly powered via the Arduino as well, by connecting the Bluetooth board to the Arduino's 3.3V DC output. The device also has an on/off switch, a LED, and a vibrator. The color of the LED helps to tell the difference between calibration mode and measurement mode. Once the device enters into measurement mode, the vibrator tells the subject when to start and stop the test. All these additional elements (the battery and its corresponding case, the on/off switch, the LED, and the vibrator) were omitted in Scheme 1 for the sake of clarity.

2.1.2.2. The STS Analysis Algorithm

The STS analysis algorithm itself involves two steps. First, the thigh angle is estimated in real-time as the acceleration samples arrive. The thigh angle in the 30-s CST was defined as the angle between the subject's thigh and a horizontal plane perpendicular to gravity (e.g., the seat of the chair), as shown in Figure 3b. During a 30-s CST, this angle is expected to vary over time between 0° in the sitting position (Figure 3a) and 90° in the upright position (Figure 3c).

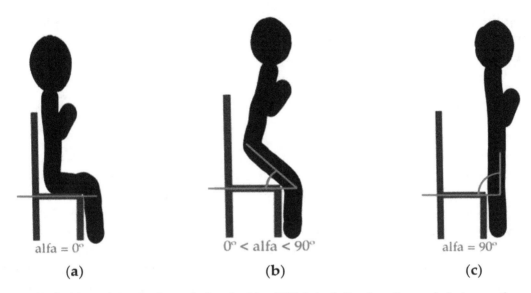

| (a) | (b) | (c) |

Figure 3. Definition of the thigh angle for the 30-s CST. It is defined as the angle between the subject's thigh and a horizontal plane perpendicular to gravity (e.g., the seat of the chair). It is depicted as the angle (alfa) between the red line along the longitudinal direction of the subject's thigh and the red line on the seat of the chair; therefore, (**a**) the expected value of the thigh angle in the sitting position is 0; (**b**) the value of the thigh angle at any time during SiSt and StSi transitions is bigger than 0 and lower than 90°; and (**c**) the expected value of the thigh angle in the upright position is 90°.

The thigh angle can then be computed from the gravity readings of the accelerometer on the subject's thigh, as demonstrated in Figure 4. The thigh angle (red angle, dubbed as alfa) is equal to the angle between gravity itself and the Z-gravity component of the accelerometer readings (green angle, dubbed as beta) because the gravity is always perpendicular to the horizontal plane (the seat of the chair), and the Z-gravity component is always perpendicular to the thigh.

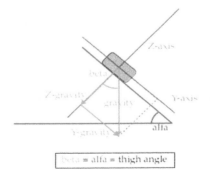

Figure 4. Computation of the thigh angle from the decomposition of gravity into orthogonal components along the axis of the reference system (blue lines) of an accelerometer on the subject's thigh. According to the convention applied in the preceding figure the thigh angle is represented by the red angle (alfa). Gravity and its components are depicted in green. The green angle (beta) between gravity itself and its Z-component is equal to the thigh angle (alfa), because gravity is always perpendicular to the horizontal plane, and the Z-gravity component is always perpendicular to the thigh.

Thus, if the Y-axis of the accelerometer is aligned with the thigh itself, as it is in the case of our experimental setting, the angle value at any given moment can be computed from the accelerometer Z-gravity and Y-gravity readings according to the following expression:

$$\alpha = \arctan\left(-g_y / g_z\right) \tag{1}$$

Obtaining the gravity components from the accelerometer readings would require filtering the raw acceleration signals. However, in order to lower the computational complexity of our algorithm we estimated the thigh angle directly from raw acceleration samples as:

$$\hat{\alpha} = \arctan\left(-a_y / a_z\right) \tag{2}$$

where a_y (i.e., the Y-acceleration component) and a_z (i.e., the Z-acceleration component) include the contribution of both gravity and the forces exerted by the subject to execute the SiSt and StSi transitions. The outcome of the expression above is limited by the fact that the tangent function is a periodic function, and the arc tangent function only returns values for the first period of the angle values, i.e., values between $-p/2$ and $p/2$. Theoretically, this should not be a problem because, as stated before, the value of the thigh angle is expected to oscillate within that range (between 0 and $p/2$ radians, i.e., between 0° and 90°). However, when the subject is close to the upright position, there are some non-ideal behaviors that should result in an angle estimation bigger than 90°, but will not if we applied Equation (2). For instance, the value of the Z-acceleration component is expected to always have a negative sign, except at the upright position where it is expected to be zero. Nevertheless, nearby the upright position, the noise from the acceleration and deceleration forces exerted by the older adult could alter the Z-acceleration sign, and turn it into a positive value. In that case, Equation (2) does not return a value bigger than $p/2$ but a negative value between $-p/2$ and zero. In order to make a correct estimation of the angle, the sign of the accelerometer readings must be taken into account according to the following expression:

$$\hat{\alpha} = \left\{ \begin{array}{l} -\arctan\left(a_y / a_z\right), \text{if} a_z \leqslant 0 \\ \pi - \arctan\left(a_y / a_z\right), \text{if} a_z > 0 \end{array} \right\} \tag{3}$$

Please note that the sign of the Y-acceleration component cannot be negative while the sign of the Z-acceleration component is positive, unless the device is upside down, because gravity always points downwards.

While the variation of the actual thigh angle over time, and even an estimation based on gravity components, are smooth quasi-periodic signals like the blue line in Figure 5, the values of the thigh angle estimated from raw acceleration readings, and their variation over time, result in a noisy signal like the green line in Figure 5. The said noise is particularly strong close to the maxima and minima of the actual angle, due to the abrupt deceleration forces applied to the sensor upon reaching the upright and sitting positions. Consequently, while the blue signal shows smoothly and clearly defined maxima that can be used to identify the end of a SiSt transition into the upright position, the local maxima and minima in the noisy green signal do not serve that purpose anymore. Which brings us to the second step in the STS analysis algorithm. In the second step, hysteresis thresholding was applied to the signal to remove the effect of the noise in the green signal. The output of such a filter was a binary signal (standing vs. sitting) like the red line in Figure 5. The threshold values and the computational algorithm described below were defined to filter the signal and spot valid SiSt transitions in real time.

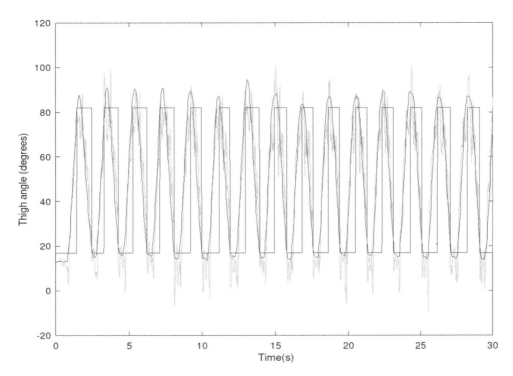

Figure 5. Graphical representation of the outcomes of a 30-s CST. The blue line represents the evolution of the thigh angle over time, computed from the estimation of the gravity components (it is not computed by the device). The green line represents the estimation of the thigh angle used in the device; it is directly computed from raw readings from the accelerometer. The red line represents the output of applying hysteresis thresholding to the green signal.

The output of the hysteresis thresholding algorithm switches between two different states (i.e., sitting and standing) as follows: The estimated value of the thigh angle is compared to two values configured in a previous stage (see the next paragraph). These two values are known as the sitting-threshold and the standing-threshold. If the previous sample was in a standing state and the current estimated thigh angle reaches a value greater than $0°$, and lower than the sitting-threshold, the subject is considered to have completed a StSi transition, the state changes to sitting, and the subsequent SiSt transition is an eligible candidate to count as a valid attempt; otherwise the subsequent SiSt transition will not count as a valid attempt no matter what. On the other hand, if the previous sample was in a sitting state and the extension angle reaches a value greater than the standing-threshold, and lower than $90°$ during an eligible SiSt transition, the state changes to standing, and the transition counts as a valid attempt; otherwise it is dismissed as a failure.

The rationale behind using the sitting-threshold and the standing-threshold comes from the fact that even though the expected angle values theoretically range from $0°$ (sitting) to $90°$ (standing), there are two sources of non-ideal behavior that require the definition of more flexible threshold values. First, mobility constraints may narrow this range for some older subjects. A subject's readings whose default standing position does not exceed $80°$, will never reach the theoretical $90°$ standing-angle. Thus, valid standing attempts would be dismissed and the automatic count of valid SiSt transitions would result in a wrong score. Analogously, a subject's readings whose default sitting position does not fall down below $10°$, will never reach the theoretical $0°$ sitting-angle. Thus, subsequent valid standing attempts would be dismissed and the automatic count of valid SiSt transitions would result in a wrong score as well.

The other source of non-ideal behavior is the non-ideal nature of the sensor readings themselves. Even if a subject reaches his default standing position, the sensor might provide a reading slightly lower than the subject's default standing angle. In such a case a valid attempt would be dismissed as a failure, and the automatic count of SiSt transitions would result in a wrong score. The analogous situation applies to the sitting position and the subject's default sitting angle.

To avoid the negative impact of these situations on the sensor performance, the sensor is calibrated before initiating a 30-s CST. The subject's thigh angle in a static sitting position is measured and recorded. In particular, the sitting angle is computed as the mean value of the angle readings collected while the subject is sitting in a static position for four seconds. Then, a correction is applied to allow for some error tolerance. The sitting-threshold is set to its final value by adding 10° to the subject's default sitting angle. Analogously, the subject's thigh angle in a static upright position is measured and recorded, and then the standing-threshold is set to its final value by subtracting 10° from the subject's default standing angle.

2.1.2.3. The Tablet App

The application was developed in Java for Android. The tablet device was a Huawei M2-A01L with Android 5.1.1. The application is used to configure the personalized parameters in the sensor algorithm (i.e., the sitting-threshold and the standing-threshold), to issue a command to the sensor for it to begin the measurement process, and to visualize the test results after completion. The application home screen shows a list of all the sensor devices paired with the tablet so the end-user gets to pick which one to configure. In the case of the data collection stage in the present study, only one device was paired with the tablet. The application has two operation modes, namely, calibration mode and measurement mode. In calibration mode, the values for the sitting-threshold and the standing-threshold are computed and set according to the following process:

1. The researcher puts the sensor into calibration mode by issuing the corresponding command with the app.
2. The researcher asks the sensor to compute sitting angle readings for four seconds and send them back to the app by issuing the corresponding command with the app.
3. The app computes the mean value of these sitting-angle readings and stores them as the subject's default sitting-angle.
4. The researcher asks the sensor to compute standing-angle readings for four seconds and send them back to the app by issuing the corresponding command with the app.
5. The app computes the mean value of these standing-angle readings and stores them as the subject's default standing-angle.
6. The researcher enters an error tolerance value for each default angle.
7. The researcher asks the sensor to set the value of the sitting-threshold and the standing-threshold by issuing the corresponding command with the app. The sitting-threshold is computed as the sum of the subject's default sitting-angle and the error tolerance value for the sitting position. On the other hand, the standing-threshold is computed as the subtraction of the error tolerance value for the standing position from the subject's default standing-angle.

In measurement mode the application waits for the sensor to send the results of the 30-s CST according to the following process:

1. The researcher puts the sensor into measurement mode by issuing the corresponding command with the app.
2. The researcher asks the sensor to start the 30-s CST measurement sequence by issuing the corresponding command with the app.
3. The application waits idle for the results of the 30-s CST.
4. The application shows the results of the 30-s CST on screen.

2.1.3. Procedure

Seven older subjects were administered a 30-s CST each, in accordance with the following procedure. A member of the research team gave instructions to the subjects to guide them through the process. First, a member of the research team paired the wearable sensor with the tablet device via Bluetooth, and asked the subject to put on the wearable device. The subject was then asked to sit down on the chair to calibrate the sensor sitting-threshold. Next, the subject was asked to stand up to calibrate the sensor standing-threshold. After the calibration stage, the subject was asked to repeatedly stand up from, and sit down on, the chair as fast as possible for 30 s. The subject was asked to do so with his arms folded over his chest, and starting from a sitting position. The sensor emitted a short vibration to indicate to the subject when to start. A trained member of the research team manually counted SiSt transitions. Once the 30 s were over, the sensor emitted another short vibration to signal the subject to stop. Then, the sensor sent the outcomes of the automatic count algorithm to the mobile app, which showed them on screen. A member of the research team took note of the values for the manual and automatic counts.

2.1.4. Analysis

The correlation between the manual and the automatic counts were studied. These two variables are of the interval type, therefore we decided to compute their correlation with Pearson's moment-product correlation coefficient. Before applying Pearson's r to the data, the normality of the two data sets (manual vs. automatic counts) was tested. Due to the size of the sample, normality was studied with a Shapiro–Wilk test that resulted not statistically significant in both cases. Therefore, both data sets could be considered to be normally distributed, and we proceeded with Pearson's r. The Shapiro–Wilk test was calculated using the shapiro.test function, and Pearson's r was calculated using the cor.test function; in both cases R statistical software, version 3.6.3, was used. The 95% CI for the Pearson's r estimate was computed by applying Fisher's transformation.

To further characterize the impact of noise on the sensor performance we studied the statistical significance of our estimation for the probability of finding harmless noise levels in a valid SiSt transition. This situation was modeled as a binomial experiment, where each SiSt transition in the data set corresponds to a binomial event, a correct SiSt identification means harmless noise and, therefore, success, and an incorrect SiSt identification means harmful noise and, therefore, failure. The probability of harmless noise was estimated as the number of correct identifications in the data set divided by the total number of SiSt transitions in the data set. The 95% CI for the probability of success was calculated by applying a binomial test with the binom.test function in the R statistical software, version 3.6.3.

2.2. Unsupervised Validation of the Home Care System

2.2.1. Participants

Seven older subjects (3 female and 4 male), between 64 and 74 years old, participated in the unsupervised validation of the home care system. All subjects gave their informed consent for inclusion before they participated in the study. The study was conducted in accordance with the Declaration of Helsinki, and the protocol was approved by the Ethics Committee of the Universidad Politécnica de Madrid on 9 May 2019 (POSITIVE: Maintaining and improving the intrinsic capacity involving primary care and caregivers).

The following inclusion and exclusion criteria were applied:

- A subject COULD ENTER the study if ALL the following INCLUSION CRITERIA applied:

  - The subject is willing and able to give written informed consent for participation in the study.
  - The subject is 64 years old or older.
  - The subject is able to perform the 30-s CST in a safe way.

    o   The subject has not been diagnosed with cognitive impairment.

• A subject COULD NOT ENTER the study if ANY of the following EXCLUSION CRITERIA applied:

    o   Subjects suffering from any major disability.
    o   Subjects suffering from cognitive impairment.

2.2.2. Apparatus

2.2.2.1. The Sensor

The sensor hardware was ported to a more ergonomic case which included a sticker with clear instructions about the proper orientation of the ends of the device, with the help of two tags, namely, "Rodilla", which is the Spanish word for knee, and "Cabeza", which is the Spanish word for head (see Figure 6).

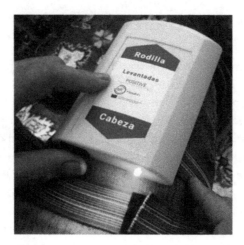

Figure 6. Second version of the sensor casing. The sticker on the sensor reports the correct orientation of the sensor with the help of two tags: "Rodilla", which is the Spanish word for knee, and "Cabeza", which is the Spanish word for head.

2.2.2.2. The Home Care Application

The home care application was developed in Java for Android and was a user friendly evolution of the application in Section 2.1.2.3. The application included a user-friendly interface specifically designed for older adults. Once the default and the threshold values of the participants sitting and standing angles were calibrated for the first time, the application recorded the outcomes so it was not necessary to re-calibrate every time the participant took a test. The app provided explanatory pictures, audio, and video to help the participant in preparing for taking a test, and audio instructions were also available to guide him through the whole procedure.

2.2.2.3. The Acceptability and General Impressions Questionnaires

In order to assess the system acceptability, a semi-structured interview comprising the questions in the second column in Table 2 was conducted. Furthermore, the participants' general impressions were also collected by conducting another semi-structured interview, comprising the questions in the third column in Table 2. The first three questions in each questionnaire are related to the participant's opinions on the sensor. The remaining ones are related to the participant's opinions on the application in the tablet.

Table 2. List of questions in the acceptability and general impressions questionnaires. The first three questions in each questionnaire ask about the participant's experience while using the sensor. Whereas, the remaining ones ask about the participant's experience while using the home care application on the tablet.

Type of Question	Acceptability Questionnaire	General Impressions Questionnaire
Related to the sensor	1. What difficulties did you find while using the sensor? 2. What is your opinion on the sensor? 3. How did you feel while using the sensor?	1. Was the device easy to put on? 2. Do you find the device comfortable? 3. Do you think you would be able to use the device at home on your own?
Related to the application	4. What difficulties did you find while using the tablet? 5. What is your opinion on the tablet? 6. How did you feel while using the tablet?	4. Which activities did you find the most difficult to achieve while using the tablet? 5. Which features did you find the hardest to understand in the tablet? 6. What are your general impressions on the tablet? 7. Do you think you would be able to use the app at home on your own?

2.2.3. Procedure

A trained technician went to the participants' homes to set up the system and explain to them how to use it (only one user per home was configured). The technician delivered a tablet device with the home care application pre-installed. Once in the participant's dwelling, the technician paired the sensor and the tablet via Bluetooth and proceeded to calibrate the participant's default sitting and standing angles as described in Section 2.1.2.3. The application recorded the values so the participant did not have to repeat this step every time he took a 30-s CST. The participants could contact the technician to get help to fix any technical issues that could arise over the course of the study.

The participants used the system for a month. The participant initiates a test by entering into the "My medical tests" in the app. The participants had to follow the instructions of the home care application to complete a 30-s CST, without any supervision or further assistance, and according to the following procedure. The participant put the tablet on a nearby surface. The participant then had to put the device on over his knee, secure it with the strap, and click next on the tablet. Then the participant had to switch on the device and click next on the tablet. After that, the participant had to fold his arms over his chest and wait for the start signal. Then he had to stand up and sit down repeatedly until the stop signal. After that, the participant could switch the device off and take it off Once the 30-days period of study was over, a member of the research team went to the participants' homes to pick up the equipment and to conduct an interview to evaluate acceptability and general impressions by administering the corresponding questionnaires.

2.2.4. Analysis

The results of the acceptability and general impressions questionnaires were qualitatively assessed.

3. Results

3.1. Supervised Validation of the Sensor

Table 3 summarizes the outcomes from the data collection process. Most of the people in older populations are female, and this pattern was also reflected in the composition of the sample of volunteers recruited for the present study (5 female and 2 male).

Table 3. Data collected during the experimental procedure. Each row in the table holds the data for one of the seven older adults in the experiment (age: m = 83.29 years old, sd = 4.19; gender: 5 female and 2 male). Each participant took a single 30-s CST. The outcomes from the sensor automatic count match the outcomes from the trained professional's manual count for all the seven participants. All the 67 SiSt transitions that took place were correctly identified, and the mean absolute error was equal to zero.

Participant ID	Gender	Age	Default Sitting-Angle	Default Standing-Angle	30 s CST Result (Manual Count)	30 s CST Result (Automatic Count)
1	male	88	25°	55°	5	5
2	female	87	25°	70°	6	6
3	male	81	27°	87°	13	13
4	female	79	25.5°	84°	8	8
5	female	79	18.7°	85°	8	8
6	female	81	44°	81°	9	9
7	female	88	19°	82°	18	18

The mean absolute error for the automatic count of SiSt transitions was computed, as usual, according to the following expression:

$$\text{error} = \frac{1}{7} \cdot \sum_{i=1}^{7} |\text{manualCount}_i - \text{autoCount}_i|. \tag{4}$$

The mean absolute error was equal to zero because the sensor output was error-free in all the seven 30-s CSTs, i.e., all the 67 SiSt transitions were correctly identified. This means the high frequency noise in the estimated angle signal was not larger than the gap between the sitting and the standing thresholds for any of the SiSt transitions in the data set. Therefore, the hysteresis thresholding mechanism had not been affected by said noise and no spurious transitions between states had taken place.

Additionally, the correlation between the manual and the automatic counts was studied to test the statistical significance of the perfect match in our observations. Being two variables of the interval type, we chose Pearson's r to study their correlation. Before computing Pearson's r, the normality of the two variables (manual count vs. automatic count) was studied with a Shapiro–Wilk test, as shown in Table 4.

Table 4. Results of the normality test for the manual count data set (left) and the automatic count data set (right). None of the tests were statistically significant. Thus, we did not find statistical significance to state that any of the data sets were not normally distributed. Therefore, we considered that they complied with the bivariate normality assumption, and proceeded to study their correlation with Pearson's r.

Manual Count	Automatic Count
W = 0.88227, p-value = 0.2367	W = 0.88227, p-value = 0.2367

The data set complies with the bivariate normality assumption because the Shapiro–Wilk test resulted not statistically significant for both variables. Therefore, we proceeded to study their correlation with Pearson's moment–product correlation ($r = 1$, $p = 0.00$). This correlation estimate showed full correlation between the sensor automatic count and the manual count. The 95% CI was computed as a means to measure the accuracy of our estimation. The cor.test function in R computes the CI by applying Fisher's transformation, and returned a 95% CI = (1, 1). This result suggests that our observation was indistinguishable from a perfect correlation. However, the Fisher transformation defines the lower and upper limits of the 95% CI as:

$$\tanh\left(\text{artanh}(\rho) \pm 1.96 / \sqrt{(n-3)}\right), \tag{5}$$

where r is the Pearson correlation coefficient and n is the sample size, which in this case equals the number of participants recruited for the study. The hyperbolic arc tangent function is defined only within the open interval $(-1, 1)$, but not for the case when r equals one. Since the hyperbolic arc tangent function tends to infinity as r tends to one, the contribution of the sample size to the value of the upper and lower values in Fisher's expression becomes irrelevant. Therefore, we think we are not getting much information about the impact of our sample size on the accuracy of our estimation.

In order to tackle this issue and study the accuracy of our sensor, we studied the probability of finding a SiSt transition with harmless levels of noise; because the higher the number of transitions with harmless levels of noise, the more accurate the sensor outcomes will be. The situation was modeled as a binomial experiment (as described in Section 2.1.4), which resulted in an estimated probability of success $p = 1$ with a 95% CI = (0.96, 1). Therefore, the older adults in our sample are expected to produce SiSt transitions with harmless levels of noise at least 96% of the time. Therefore, our sensor would need to observe 25 SiSt transitions in order to make a mistake due to a high level of noise. Since the mean number of SiSt transitions per 30-s CST in our sample is 9.57, the sensor would make a mistake once every 2.61 tests; thus, in order to observe one wrong score, you need to conduct three tests. In other words, according to our estimated 95% CI, in the worst case scenario, our sensor would provide an error free score for at least 67% of the tests conducted, while the remaining 33% would miss the correct score by one SiSt transition. These results show our sensor to be very accurate, however, it could be argued that a sample of seven older adults is too small to be representative of the many interpersonal differences in the general older population and, therefore, the results might have been poorer if the device had been tested on a wider variety of cases.

A larger sample might have shown cases with higher levels of noise; so we analyzed under which conditions angle signals would be noisier, and tested our algorithm behavior in those conditions. The noise in the angle signal is the result of the acceleration and deceleration forces applied to the sensor, especially upon reaching the upright and sitting positions. The faster, and the more sudden, the stand up and sit down moves are, the stronger these forces will be. On the one hand, subjects would have moved faster if they have completed a higher number of SiSt transitions within the 30 s in the test. On the other hand, given a fixed number of transitions, subjects need a larger momentum for those transitions with a wider range. Therefore, the angle signal is expected to be noisier for 30-s CSTs with a higher number of SiSt transitions and a wider range for the thigh angle. Rikli and Jones identified the normative standard values to use the 30-s CST outcomes to compare an older adult's performance with the average population [41]. According to these standards, a subject's performance might be considered to be (i) within, (ii) below, or (iii) over the reference range of the average population [41]. However, the reference ranges have different values depending on gender and age [41]. Thus, two people of the same gender with the same test score but belonging to different age groups need not be considered to have the same level of physical decline; and the same applies to two people of different gender but belonging to the same age group. According to these standards 90% of the men in the younger age group (between 60 and 64 years old) score below 22 [41]. The analogous scores for the remaining age groups in the case of men are lower than 22; as they are in the case of women of all age groups. On the other hand, Rikli and Jones also identified the critical values that predict physical independence until late in life [42]. An older adult scoring above the critical value is considered to be fit enough to remain independent until late in life; conversely an older adult scoring below the critical value is considered to be at risk of becoming dependent and requires taking action. These critical values depend on gender and age as well [42]. The critical value for men in the younger group (between 60 and 64 years old) is 17 [42]. The critical values for the remaining age groups in the case of men are lower than 17; as they are in the case of women for all age groups. Thus, we took 22 SiSt transitions as a reference value for an extreme and highly demanding scenario, and 17 SiSt transitions for a critical and likely scenario. Then, we conducted an exploratory study to inquire about the performance of our approach under those two scenarios.

A member of the research team took ten 30-s CSTs scoring 22 or above (highly demanding scenario) and another ten 30-s CSTs scoring around 17 (critical scenario). The data for this exploratory study were collected with a smartphone (Nokia 6 TA-1021 with Android 9) on the subject's thigh and were processed with GNU Octave 5.2.0; this was because the researchers were locked down at their homes, due to the COVID-19 pandemic, and did not have access to the prototypes of the sensor devices. The experiment in the highly demanding scenario resulted in a total of 230 SiSt transitions. Of which, 15 showed harmful noise. All 15 behaved like the transitions depicted around Time = 20 and Time = 25 s in Figure 7. Both transitions show a strong and narrow inverse peak of noise (green line in Figure 7) that tricks the algorithm into detecting a spurious StSi transition, and another spurious SiSt transition (red line in Figure 7). Thus, an extra SiSt transition was detected for each valid transition affected by this kind of noise; in the case of Figure 7, the final score was overestimated by two points, i.e., 25 SiSt transitions were reported instead of 23. All the signals collected, and the code to process and visualize them, are available as Supplementary Materials.

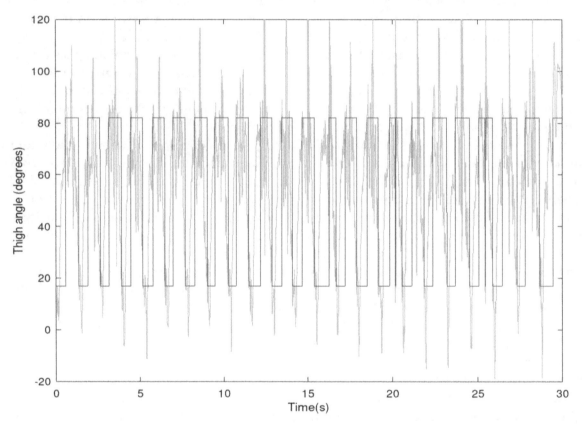

Figure 7. Graphical representation of the outcomes of a 30-s CST in the presence of some transitions with harmful levels of noise. The green line represents the estimation of the thigh angle over time, while the red line represents the transitions detected by the hysteresis algorithm. The transitions around Time = 20 and Time = 25 show a strong and narrow inverse peak of noise that tricks the algorithm into detecting a spurious StSi transition, and then another spurious SiSt transition. Thus, an extra SiSt transition was detected for each of them, and the final score was overestimated by two points; 25 SiSt transitions were reported instead of 23.

Like in the case of the older adults' data set, we studied the probability of finding a SiSt transition with harmless levels of noise. Again, it was modeled as a binomial experiment (as described in Section 2.1.4) and the experiment resulted in an estimated probability of success $p = 0.93$, with a 95% CI = (0.89, 0.96). According to the lower limit of this CI, it would be necessary to observe 10 SiSt transitions in order to observe one of them with a high level of noise. The mean number of SiSt transitions per 30-s CST in our sample is 23; thus, between two and three high level noise transitions would be observed per test. On the other hand, according to the upper limit of the 95% CI, i.e., p (harmless noise) = 0.96, only one in two tests would miss the correct score, and would do so by a single point.

Finally, the experiment in the critical scenario resulted in a total of 173 SiSt transitions. The algorithm successfully identified all of them. In this case, the estimated probability of success is $p = 1$ with a 95% CI = (0.98, 1). Therefore in the worst case (lower limit of the CI), it is necessary to observe 50 SiSt transitions in order to observe one error. Since the mean number of SiSt transitions in our sample is 17.3, an error would be observed every 2.89 tests. Thus, in order to observe one wrong score, you need to conduct three tests. Therefore, according to the 95% CI, the noise pattern around the critical value would result in a single wrong transition in only one in three tests. Under such a noise pattern our sensor would remain very accurate around the target critical value.

3.2. Unsupervised Validation of the Home Care System

3.2.1. The Acceptability Questionnaire

3.2.1.1. Question #1: What Difficulties Did You Find While Using the Sensor?

All but one of the participants declared they did not find any major problems while using the device. One participant declared having experienced some pain in his knee due to osteoarthritis. The same participant also declared being worried about the possibility of the device falling out during the course of the 30-s CST.

3.2.1.2. Question #2: What is Your Opinion on the Sensor?

All the participants provided favorable answers to this question. They highlighted that the sensor is comfortable and easy to use. They also remarked that the labels on the sensor sticker were easy to follow and helped them to know how to correctly put the device on the leg.

3.2.1.3. Question #3: How Did You Feel While Using the Sensor?

The participants declared that they felt comfortable using the device, and that they felt motivated to improve their performance over time. In line with the answers to Question #1, one participant declared to be worried about the possibility of the device falling out during the course of the tests.

3.2.1.4. Question #4: What Difficulties Did You Find While Using the Tablet?

Some participants struggled to understand the video instructions, and some participants faced a few technical issues, however, they declared not to have experienced any major problems once those issues were fixed.

3.2.1.5. Question #5: What is Your Opinion on the Tablet?

Most users reported satisfactory experiences and good opinions on the tablet.

3.2.1.6. Question #6: How Did You Feel While Using the Tablet?

Some participants experienced some technical issues that made them feel uncomfortable. However, their experience and feelings became more satisfactory once these issues were solved.

3.2.2. The General Impressions Questionnaire

3.2.2.1. Question #1: Was the Device Easy to Put on?

Six participants reported they found the device easy to put on. None of the participants reported that they did not find it easy, however, one of them reported the strap did not fit very well around his leg.

3.2.2.2. Question #2: Do You Find the Device Comfortable?

Six participants reported they found the device comfortable. In line with the answers to Question #1, one of them reported some issues regarding the length of the strap.

3.2.2.3. Question #3: Do You Think You Would Be Able to Use the Device at Home on Your Own?

All the participants felt able to use the device at home on their own.

3.2.2.4. Question #4: What Activities Did You Find the Most Difficult to Achieve While Using the Tablet?

Some participants detected some discrepancies between the explanatory videos and the textual description of the exercise, which made them have some doubts. The rest of the application features were reported to be easy to understand.

3.2.2.5. Question #5: Which Features Did You Find the Hardest to Understand in the Tablet?

In line with the answers to Question #4, all of the application functionality was reported to be easy to understand.

3.2.2.6. Question #6: What are Your General Impressions on the Tablet?

All the participants reported favorable opinions about the tablet. They highlighted the motivating potential of such an app and the subsequent health benefits.

3.2.2.7. Question #7: Do You Think You Would Be Able to Use the App at Home on Your Own?

All the participants felt able to use the app at home on their own. However, one of them highlighted that he would be able to do so as long as the application did not become more complex, and another one highlighted that technical support would be required.

4. Discussion

Our sensor took advantage of the quasiperiodic variation of the thigh angle over time (i.e., the angle between the longitudinal axis of the subject's thigh and a horizontal plane perpendicular to gravity, e.g., the seat of the chair). The thigh angle was computed from acceleration readings from an accelerometer on the subject's thigh. Previous works found in the literature have taken advantage of the quasiperiodic variation of some other variables such as the trunk pitch-angle [23], vertical velocity [23,24], and vertical position [24] to study repetitive STS cycles in STS5 and 30-s CST tests. They estimated the values of these variables from the readings of an IMU on the L3 region of the subject's lumbar spine. We think the thigh angle is a more convenient approach for two reasons. On the one hand, we think that older people might find it easier to correctly place the sensor on their thighs than on their lower backs, especially if they do not have any help to put them on. However, none of the papers studied their algorithm's sensitivity to misplacing of the sensor. The procedure for the estimation of the thigh angle described in the present paper (i.e., estimating the angle from the Y-acceleration and Z-acceleration components) requires the sensor X-axis to be aligned with the knee rotation axis. However, this constraint is easy to overcome by extending the angle estimation expression to its three-dimensional form. On the other hand, computing trunk pitch-angle, vertical velocity, and vertical position require integration and even double integration of the IMU readings. Due to the noisy nature of the latter, the result is distorted by drift and requires a lot of effort to estimate the original signal with computationally complex algorithms. Millor et al., for instance, applied double integration, combined with fourth-level polynomial curve adjustment and cubic splines interpolation [24]. Conversely, it is not necessary to integrate the acceleration readings to make an estimation of the thigh angle. Such an estimation can be computed from the values of the different components of gravity in the accelerometer reference system; and these values can be estimated by filtering raw acceleration readings.

We did not include any Kalman or complementary filters in our design to avoid the extra hardware and computational load. Instead, we estimated the thigh angle directly from raw acceleration readings; which resulted in noisy but drift-free angle estimations. In spite of the noisy nature of the angle estimations, the device showed an excellent performance. All the SiSt transitions were correctly identified in real time, and the device provided error-free outcomes for all the seven 30-s CST conducted with older adults. The narrow CI returned by the cor.test function in R suggests this observation is indeed statistically indistinguishable from a perfect correlation. However, the limitations described for the Fisher transformation in Section 3, to accommodate such an extreme value for Pearson's r, make us think we are not getting much information about the impact of our sample size on the accuracy of our estimated correlation.

Looking at the results of our study from a different perspective, we studied the accuracy of our device based on the probability of observing noise levels high enough to exceed the gap between their personalized upper and lower thresholds in the hysteresis stage. Since all the transitions were correctly identified in real time, we concluded that the participants in the study did not generate any transitions with such high levels of noise. According to the narrow 95% CI in our estimation, low levels of noise are expected to happen at least 96% of the time. Which would result in very accurate sensor outcomes. This result can be generalized to the SiSt transitions generated by any population represented by our sample. However, our sample is limited because it could be argued that seven older adults are too few to be representative of the many interpersonal differences in the general older population and, therefore, signals with a higher level of noise might have been observed if the device had been tested on a wider variety of cases. Nevertheless, we did not find any SiSt transitions with harmful levels of noise in our exploratory study for the critical scenario (around 17 transitions with high momentum). According to the narrow 95% CI obtained for that critical scenario (0.98, 1), even if any high noise transitions were to be observed, a single wrong transition would be observed in only one in three tests. Since the 30-s CST is expected to be scheduled to be taken once or twice a week in a home care scenario, we did not observe any risks of missing anyone not fit enough due to sustained overestimated scores over time. We observed that a frequent overestimation of the scores is likely to happen in the highly demanding scenario (over 22 transitions with high speed and high momentum). However, we think that this result does not have a strong impact on the utility of our approach for two reasons. First, less than 10% of the older population are able to reach such high scores, and second, even in case of overestimation, people scoring over 22 are far away from the critical threshold, and therefore are undoubtedly fit enough not to require any immediate intervention. Anyway, further experiments may be useful to characterize the noise profile between the scores of 17 and 22.

We integrated the sensor into a home care app that guides the user throughout the process of taking a 30-s CST, and conducted an acceptability study with older adults in free-living conditions (i.e., using a home care app at home for several weeks to interact with the device without any assistance). All the participants kept using the system throughout the course of the study and none of them dropped out. This observation is in line with their favorable opinions about both the sensor and the application; and, in particular, corroborates the participants' positive answers to whether they feel able to use the system at home on their own. Despite the excellent results of this acceptability study, further studies will be necessary to test, on the one hand, the long-term acceptability and adoption by older adults and their caregivers, and, on the other hand, to test the feasibility of this novel home care model for frailty in accommodating end-users' needs and expectations, not just on the older adults' side, but also on the health care professionals' side.

5. Conclusions

We developed a system for older people to self-administer the 30-s chair stand test (CST) at home without supervision. The system comprises a low-cost sensor that automatically detects and counts sit-to-stand (SiSt) transitions in real time, and a home care application that guides older people through the whole procedure. We studied whether such a system was able to match older people's abilities and expectations so they can use it at home on their own without any supervision. The sensor automatic counts were perfectly correlated to the researcher's manual count, so we concluded that the signals generated by the participants did not push the device to its operational limits. This observation is supported by a very narrow 95% CI for the probability of finding a SiSt transition with a low level of noise. The small size of our sample limits our ability to generalize this result to the general older population because more demanding signals might have been observed if the device had been tested on a larger sample. However, we did not find harmful levels of noise in any of the signals in our exploratory study around the critical score. Thus, we did not observe any risks of missing anyone not fit enough due to sustained overestimated scores over time. None of the participants in the unsupervised study of the complete system dropped out, and at the end of the study none of them reported any major problems in understanding the system and interacting with it. They declared they felt comfortable using it, and felt able to use it on their own. Thus, the system is suitable to be used by older adults in their homes without professional supervision.

Author Contributions: Conceptualization, E.V.-M., R.P.-R., X.F., and L.R.-M.; methodology, E.V.-M., R.P.-R., X.F., and L.R.-M.; software, W.E. and A.C.; validation, C.M.; formal analysis, A.C. and W.E.; investigation, W.E., A.C., and C.M.; resources, E.V.-M., X.F., R.P.-R., L.R.-M., W.E., and A.C.; data curation, W.E., and A.C.; writing—Original draft preparation, A.C.; writing—Review and editing, E.V., A.C., X.F., R.P.-R., and L.R.-M.; visualization, A.C.; supervision, E.V.-M., X.F., R.P.-R., and L.R.-M.; project administration, E.V., X.F., R.P.-R., and L.R.-M.; funding acquisition, L.R.-M., E.V., R.P.-R., and X.F. All authors have read and agreed to the published version of the manuscript.

Acknowledgments: We would like to thank FEDER funds for co-financing our home institutions. The authors would like to specially thank the volunteers in the study for their unselfish collaboration, enthusiasm, and dedication.

References

1.   Jones, C.J.; Rikli, R.E.; Beam, W.C. A 30-s Chair-Stand Test as a Measure of Lower Body Strength in Community-Residing Older Adults. *Res. Q. Exerc. Sport* **1999**, *70*, 113–119. [CrossRef]
2.   Fried, L.P.; Tangen, C.M.; Walston, J.; Newman, A.B.; Hirsch, C.; Gottdiener, J.; Seeman, T.; Tracy, R.; Kop, W.J.; Burke, G.; et al. Frailty in Older Adults: Evidence for a Phenotype. *J. Gerontol. Ser. A Biol. Sci. Med. Sci.* **2001**, *56*, M146–M157. [CrossRef]
3.   Campbell, A.J.; Buchner, D.M. Unstable disability and the fluctuations of frailty. *Age Ageing* **1997**, *26*, 315–318. [CrossRef]
4.   Rockwood, K.; Ehogan, D.B.; Macknight, C.; Rockwood, P.K. Conceptualisation and Measurement of Frailty in Elderly People. *Drugs Aging* **2000**, *17*, 295–302. [CrossRef]
5.   Walston, J.; Fried, L.P. Frailty and the Older MAN. *Med. Clin. N. Am.* **1999**, *83*, 1173–1194. [CrossRef]
6.   Clegg, A.P.; Young, J.; Iliffe, S.; Rikkert, M.O.; Rockwood, K. Frailty in elderly people. *Lancet* **2013**, *381*, 752–762. [CrossRef]
7.   Kojima, G. Frailty as a predictor of disabilities among community-dwelling older people: A systematic review and meta-analysis. *Disabil. Rehabil.* **2016**, *39*, 1897–1908. [CrossRef]
8.   Zheng, Y.; Cheung, K.S.L.; Yip, P.S. Are We Living Longer and Healthier? *J. Aging Health* **2020**, 0898264320950067. [CrossRef]

9.　Cesari, M.; Vellas, B.; Hsu, F.-C.; Newman, A.B.; Doss, H.; King, A.C.; Manini, T.M.; Church, T.; Gill, T.M.; Miller, M.E.; et al. A Physical Activity Intervention to Treat the Frailty Syndrome in Older Persons–Results From the LIFE-P Study. *J. Gerontol. Ser. A Biol. Sci. Med. Sci.* **2014**, *70*, 216–222. [CrossRef]

10.　Rodríguez-Mañas, L.; Fried, L.P. Frailty in the clinical scenario. *Lancet* **2015**, *385*, e7–e9. [CrossRef]

11.　Fairhall, N.; Langron, C.; Sherrington, C.; Lord, S.R.; Kurrle, S.E.; Lockwood, K.A.; Monaghan, N.; Aggar, C.; Gill, L.; Cameron, I.D. Treating frailty-a practical guide. *BMC Med.* **2011**, *9*, 83. [CrossRef]

12.　Mitnitski, A.B.; Mogilner, A.J.; Rockwood, K. Accumulation of Deficits as a Proxy Measure of Aging. *Sci. World J.* **2001**, *1*, 323–336. [CrossRef]

13.　Rockwood, K.; Mitnitski, A. Frailty in Relation to the Accumulation of Deficits. *J. Gerontol. Ser. A Biol. Sci. Med. Sci.* **2007**, *62*, 722–727. [CrossRef]

14.　Rockwood, K.; Mitnitski, A. Frailty Defined by Deficit Accumulation and Geriatric Medicine Defined by Frailty. *Clin. Geriatr. Med.* **2011**, *27*, 17–26. [CrossRef]

15.　Ko, F. The Clinical Care of Frail, Older Adults. *Clin. Geriatr. Med.* **2011**, *27*, 89–100. [CrossRef]

16.　Batista, F.S.; Gomes, G.A.D.O.; Neri, A.L.; Guariento, M.E.; Cintra, F.A.; Sousa, M.D.L.R.D.; D'Elboux, M.J. Relationship between lower-limb muscle strength and frailty among elderly people. *Sao Paulo Med. J.* **2012**, *130*, 102–108. [CrossRef]

17.　Guralnik, J.M.; Simonsick, E.M.; Ferrucci, L.; Glynn, R.J.; Berkman, L.F.; Blazer, D.G.; Scherr, P.A.; Wallace, R.B. A Short Physical Performance Battery Assessing Lower Extremity Function: Association with Self-Reported Disability and Prediction of Mortality and Nursing Home Admission. *J. Gerontol.* **1994**, *49*, M85–M94. [CrossRef]

18.　Zhou, F.; Yu, T.; Du, R.; Fan, G.; Liu, Y.; Liu, Z.; Xiang, J.; Wang, Y.; Song, B.; Gu, X.; et al. Clinical course and risk factors for mortality of adult inpatients with COVID-19 in Wuhan, China: A retrospective cohort study. *Lancet* **2020**, *395*, 1054–1062. [CrossRef]

19.　Song, J.; Lindquist, L.A.; Chang, R.W.; Semanik, P.A.; Ehrlich-Jones, L.S.; Lee, J.; Sohn, M.-W.; Dunlop, D.D. Sedentary Behavior as a Risk Factor for Physical Frailty Independent of Moderate Activity: Results from the Osteoarthritis Initiative. *Am. J. Public Heal.* **2015**, *105*, 1439–1445. [CrossRef]

20.　Hall, G.; Laddu, D.R.; Phillips, S.A.; Lavie, C.J.; Arena, R. A tale of two pandemics: How will COVID-19 and global trends in physical inactivity and sedentary behavior affect one another? *Prog. Cardiovasc. Dis.* **2020**. [CrossRef]

21.　Millor, N.; Lecumberri, P.; Gomez, M.; Martinez-Ramirez, A.; Izquierdo, M. Kinematic Parameters to Evaluate Functional Performance of Sit-to-Stand and Stand-to-Sit Transitions Using Motion Sensor Devices: A Systematic Review. *IEEE Trans. Neural Syst. Rehabil. Eng.* **2014**, *22*, 926–936. [CrossRef]

22.　Kerr, K.; White, J.; Barr, D.; Mollan, R. Standardization and definitions of the sit-stand-sit movement cycle. *Gait Posture* **1994**, *2*, 182–190. [CrossRef]

23.　Van Lummel, R.C.; Ainsworth, E.; Lindemann, U.; Zijlstra, W.; Chiari, L.; Van Campen, P.; Hausdorff, J.M. Automated approach for quantifying the repeated sit-to-stand using one body fixed sensor in young and older adults. *Gait Posture* **2013**, *38*, 153–156. [CrossRef]

24.　Millor, N.; Lecumberri, P.; Gómez, M.; Martínez-Ramírez, A.; Rodríguez-Mañas, L.; García-García, F.J.; Izquierdo, M. Automatic Evaluation of the 30-s Chair Stand Test Using Inertial/Magnetic-Based Technology in an Older Prefrail Population. *IEEE J. Biomed. Heal. Inform.* **2013**, *17*, 820–827. [CrossRef]

25.　Millor, N.; Lecumberri, P.; Gómez, M.; Martínez-Ramírez, A.; Izquierdo, M. An evaluation of the 30-s chair stand test in older adults: Frailty detection based on kinematic parameters from a single inertial unit. *J. Neuroeng. Rehabil.* **2013**, *10*, 86. [CrossRef]

26.　Van Lummel, R.C.; Ainsworth, E.; Hausdorff, J.M.; Lindemann, U.; Beek, P.J.; Van Dieën, J.H. Validation of seat-off and seat-on in repeated sit-to-stand movements using a single-body-fixed sensor. *Physiol. Meas.* **2012**, *33*, 1855–1867. [CrossRef]

27.　Van Lummel, R.C.; Evers, J.; Niessen, M.; Beek, P.J.; Van Dieën, J.H. Older Adults with Weaker Muscle Strength Stand up from a Sitting Position with More Dynamic Trunk Use. *Sensors* **2018**, *18*, 1235. [CrossRef]

28.　Van Roie, E.; Van Driessche, S.; Huijben, B.; Baggen, R.; Van Lummel, R.C.; Delecluse, C. A body-fixed-sensor-based analysis of stair ascent and sit-to-stand to detect age-related differences in leg-extensor power. *PLoS ONE* **2019**, *14*, e0210653. [CrossRef]

29. Van Lummel, R.C.; Walgaard, S.; Maier, A.B.; Ainsworth, E.; Beek, P.J.; Van Dieën, J.H. The Instrumented Sit-to-Stand Test (iSTS) Has Greater Clinical Relevance than the Manually Recorded Sit-to-Stand Test in Older Adults. *PLoS ONE* **2016**, *11*, e0157968. [CrossRef]

30. Millor, N.; Lecumberri, P.; Gomez, M.; Martinez, A.; Martinikorena, J.; Rodríguez-Mañas, L.; García-García, F.J.; Izquierdo, M. Gait Velocity and Chair Sit-Stand-Sit Performance Improves Current Frailty-Status Identification. *IEEE Trans. Neural Syst. Rehabil. Eng.* **2017**, *25*, 2018–2025. [CrossRef]

31. Regterschot, G.R.H.; Zhang, W.; Baldus, H.; Stevens, M.; Zijlstra, W. Sensor-based monitoring of sit-to-stand performance is indicative of objective and self-reported aspects of functional status in older adults. *Gait Posture* **2015**, *41*, 935–940. [CrossRef]

32. Jovanov, E.; Wright, S.; Ganegoda, H. Development of an Automated 30 Second Chair Stand Test Using Smartwatch Application. In Proceedings of the 2019 41st Annual International Conference of the IEEE Engineering in Medicine and Biology Society (EMBC), Berlin, Germany, 23–27 July 2019; Volume 2019, pp. 2474–2477.

33. Cobo, A.; Villalba-Mora, E.; Hayn, D.; Ferre, X.; Pérez-Rodríguez, R.; Sánchez-Sánchez, A.; Bernabé-Espiga, R.; Sánchez-Sánchez, J.-L.; López-Diez-Picazo, A.; Moral, C.; et al. Portable Ultrasound-Based Device for Detecting Older Adults' Sit-to-Stand Transitions in Unsupervised 30-Second Chair–Stand Tests. *Sensors* **2020**, *20*, 1975. [CrossRef]

34. Abhayasinghe, N.; Murray, I. Human activity recognition using thigh angle derived from single thigh mounted IMU data. In Proceedings of the 2014 International Conference on Indoor Positioning and Indoor Navigation (IPIN), Busan, Korea, 27–30 October 2014; pp. 111–115.

35. Steeves, J.A.; Bowles, H.R.; McClain, J.J.; Dodd, K.W.; Brychta, R.J.; Wang, J.; Chen, K.Y. Ability of Thigh-Worn ActiGraph and activPAL Monitors to Classify Posture and Motion. *Med. Sci. Sports Exerc.* **2015**, *47*, 952–959. [CrossRef]

36. Martinez-Hernandez, U.; Dehghani-Sanij, A.A. Probabilistic identification of sit-to-stand and stand-to-sit with a wearable sensor. *Pattern Recognit. Lett.* **2019**, *118*, 32–41. [CrossRef]

37. Pickford, C.G.; Findlow, A.H.; Kerr, A.; Banger, M.; Clarke-Cornwell, A.M.; Hollands, K.L.; Quinn, T.; Granat, M.H. Quantifying sit-to-stand and stand-to-sit transitions in free-living environments using the activPAL thigh-worn activity monitor. *Gait Posture* **2019**, *73*, 140–146. [CrossRef]

38. Gui, P.; Tang, L.; Mukhopadhyay, S. MEMS based IMU for tilting measurement: Comparison of complementary and kalman filter based data fusion. In Proceedings of the 2015 IEEE 10th Conference on Industrial Electronics and Applications (ICIEA), Auckland, New Zealand, 15–17 June 2015; pp. 2004–2009.

39. Abhayasinghe, N.; Murray, I.; Bidabadi, S.S. Validation of Thigh Angle Estimation Using Inertial Measurement Unit Data against Optical Motion Capture Systems. *Sensors* **2019**, *19*, 596. [CrossRef]

40. Tognetti, A.; Lorussi, F.; Carbonaro, N.; De Rossi, D. Wearable Goniometer and Accelerometer Sensory Fusion for Knee Joint Angle Measurement in Daily Life. *Sensors* **2015**, *15*, 28435–28455. [CrossRef]

41. Rikli, R.E.; Jones, C.J. Functional Fitness Normative Scores for Community-Residing Older Adults, Ages 60–94. *J. Aging Phys. Act.* **1999**, *7*, 162–181. [CrossRef]

42. Rikli, R.E.; Jones, C.J. Development and Validation of Criterion-Referenced Clinically Relevant Fitness Standards for Maintaining Physical Independence in Later Years. *Gerontologist* **2012**, *53*, 255–267. [CrossRef]

12

Two Potential Clinical Applications of Origami-Based Paper Devices

Zong-Keng Kuo [1], Tsui-Hsuan Chang [2], Yu-Shin Chen [1], Chao-Min Cheng [2,*] and Chia-Ying Tsai [3,4,*]

[1] Institute of Nanoengineering and Microsystems, National Tsing Hua University, Hsinchu 30013, Taiwan; ayudivac@gmail.com (Z.-K.K.); ericys2004@gmail.com (Y.-S.C.)
[2] Institute of Biomedical Engineering, National Tsing Hua University, Hsinchu 30013, Taiwan; allmyown74@gmail.com
[3] Department of Ophthalmology, Fu Jen Catholic University Hostpital, Fu Jen Catholic University, New Taipei City 24352, Taiwan
[4] School of Medicine, College of Medicine, Fu Jen Catholic University, New Taipei City 24205, Taiwan
* Correspondence: chaomin@mx.nthu.edu.tw (C.-M.C.); chiaying131@gmail.com (C.-Y.T.)

Abstract: Detecting small amounts of analyte in clinical practice is challenging because of deficiencies in specimen sample availability and unsuitable sampling environments that prevent reliable sampling. Paper-based analytical devices (PADs) have successfully been used to detect ultralow amounts of analyte, and origami-based PADs (O-PADs) offer advantages that may boost the overall potential of PADs in general. In this study, we investigated two potential clinical applications for O-PADs. The first O-PAD we investigated was an origami-based enzyme-linked immunosorbent assay (ELISA) system designed to detect different concentrations of rabbit IgG. This device was designed with four wing structures, each of which acted as a reagent loading zone for pre-loading ELISA reagents, and a central test sample loading zone. Because this device has a low limit of detection (LOD), it may be suitable for detecting IgG levels in tears from patients with a suspected viral infection (such as herpes simplex virus (HSV)). The second O-PAD we investigated was designed to detect paraquat levels to determine potential poisoning. To use this device, we sequentially folded each of two separate reagent zones, one preloaded with NaOH and one preloaded with ascorbic acid (AA), over the central test zone, and added 8 μL of sample that then flowed through each reagent zone and onto the central test zone. The device was then unfolded to read the results on the test zone. The three folded layers of paper provided a moist environment not achievable with conventional paper-based ELISA. Both O-PADs were convenient to use because reagents were preloaded, and results could be observed and analyzed with image analysis software. O-PADs expand the testing capacity of simpler PADs while leveraging their characteristic advantages of convenience, cost, and ease of use, particularly for point-of-care diagnosis.

Keywords: origami-based paper analytic device; origami ELISA; IgG; paraquat

1. Introduction

To improve the operation and expand the testing capacity and scope of paper-based analytical devices, we borrowed from the art of origami and folded papers into functional forms that facilitated the application of multiple reagents for conducting more complex and potentially more impactful paper-based, point-of-care biochemical analyses, including multiple, simultaneous chemical reaction-based assays and enzyme-linked immunosorbent assays (ELISAs). In recent years, paper-based analytical devices have demonstrated a variety of advantages for point-of-care diagnostics. Such devices are inexpensive, easily obtained, ecofriendly, naturally wicking, highly compatible with bioassays, and require only small sample amounts [1,2]. Accordingly, a wide array of bioassays have been developed using paper-based analytical devices, including ELISA, and commercialized rapid tests for influenza, bacterial infection, and pregnancy. For example, paper-based ELISA (P-ELISA) devices have been applied to diagnose biological sample protein targets, such as HIV [3], VEGF in aqueous humor [4–6], lactoferrin in tears [7], autoimmune antibodies in serum and blister fluid [8], human chorionic gonadotropin (hCG) in urine samples [9], a cancer marker (prostate-specific antigen, PSA) in serum [10], and *Escherichia coli* in water [11]. The list of analytes identifiable in urine or serum samples using paper-based analytical devices and biochemical analysis includes proteins, glucose, lactate, uric acid, pesticides, and others [4,12,13]. Although paper-based analytical devices are very competitive in terms of cost and sample requirements, they may yet be improved upon. Some P-ELISA procedures, for example, require a number of different reagents and complicated procedures that can be disadvantageous for point-of-care (POC) testing. Further, a more critical environment for biochemical reactions may be required for colorimetric detection of several analytes such as paraquat, a poisonous organophosphate [4,13], and accuracy may suffer when using small sample amounts in paper-based analytic devices. Here, we investigate the possibilities of a user-friendly origami-based paper device to ameliorate P-ELISA complexity and provide a more suitable environment for biochemical analysis.

Keratitis is a leading cause of ocular blindness globally. Gram-positive and gram-negative bacteria, viruses such as herpes simplex virus (HSV), and parasites such as *Acanthamoeba* are known to cause keratitis. Diagnosing keratitis from nonbacterial pathogens, i.e., from HSV or *Acanthamoeba*, is difficult, relies on clinical symptoms and signs, and requires specific treatment such as antiviral agents or chlorhexidine [14,15]. Early and specific diagnosis of keratitis and its cause is important for prognosis [16]. This may be more easily achieved with new methodology. Tears provide the first line of immunological defense for the ocular surface, and tears contain many proteins and cytokines that might be measured as markers of the local immunological state. Secretory immunoglobulins in tears, e.g., IgA, IgG, and IgM, are thought to be specific antimicrobial substances that may increase following ocular surface infection [17]. Secretory IgA, in particular, has been shown to protect the ocular surface from viral and bacterial infection, as well as from parasite infestation, and may operate by coating pathogenic microorganisms to prevent them from adhering to the corneal epithelium [18,19]. IgG and IgM are present in very low concentrations in tears, and IgG concentration is known to increase in inflammation [17–20]. In HSV infection, IgG could sensitize HSV, and lead to increased viral load [21,22] and secretory IgA may neutralize HSV [23]. The effect of neutralization of HSV in ocular tissue may depend on the concentration ratios of IgA and IgG [23]. One study showed similar total serum IgG level but significantly higher anti-*Acanthamoeba* IgG antibody levels in patients with *Acanthamoeba* keratitis compared to those in normal subjects [24]. Patients with *Acanthamoeba* keratitis also displayed lower levels of IgA in tears compared to normal subjects [24]. Efficient methods to detect levels and ratios of each of these compounds would be useful for diagnosis and treatment.

Paraquat is a commonly used herbicide around the world due to its low cost and ready accessibility, especially in developing countries [25]. It has been prohibited in many countries due to its lethal toxicity, but in many developing countries, paraquat is still widely used. Lethally exposed patients often die from multiple organ failure, and without adequate antidote, the mortality rate from exposure is as high as 60–80% [26–28]. In one study, repeat pulse therapy within 5 h of paraquat ingestion decreased the mortality rate to less than 42.9% [29]. To achieve treatment within 5 h, rapid diagnosis of paraquat is invaluable. A paper-based device has been developed to detect paraquat in human serum and could be used in developing countries [6,13]. In the process of detecting paraquat, it is very important to keep the samples wet to ensure accuracy, but this is difficult to do with the existing paper-based device. A folded device that protects the testing zone from drying out may be more useful for maintaining a moist environment that would be more conducive to accurate testing.

Origami is the ancient art of folding flat paper to fabricate three-dimensional sculptures or structures [13,30]. This ancient art form has recently been used with new, scientific intent, as several origami-influenced, paper-based analytical devices (O-PADs) have been developed by folding a single sheet of flat paper into elegantly functional designs using a single patterning step. This method eliminated the need for complicated, sequential, layer-by-layer stacking of individual layers of paper using double-sided tape [31]. In addition, these microfluidic O-PADs can be unfolded to reveal each layer for easy test result analysis [31]. The main purpose for leveraging origami in these studies was to simplify the fabrication of three-dimensional (3D) microfluidic channels or multiple working zones within paper microfluidic devices. Despite some design advances, these devices could not ameliorate the need for multiple reagent preloading or provide the optimal environment for detection [32,33]. Several studies have been undertaken to investigate the possibilities of using origami to fabricate PADs for performing bioassays [31–35], but each did require the use of multiple reagents. In this manuscript we describe our research into possible approaches for optimizing O-PADs that could be useful for continued research efforts.

We explored two particular potential clinical opportunities for POC O-PADS to demonstrate their advantages: (1) The development of an O-PAD ELISA for IgG level testing that reduced test complexity and the number of required reagents; (2) the development of an O-PAD for biochemical analysis that used paraquat as the proof-of-concept assay target. We believe our work could lay some groundwork for the use of O-PADs as an improvement to PADs for POC testing.

2. Materials and Methods

2.1. Design of Origami-Based PAD for ELISA

The O-PAD for ELISA (O-ELISA) was designed on Whatman qualitative filter paper No. 1 and patterned using a wax printer (Xerox Phaser 8650N color printer, Norwalk, CT, USA). Four wings were fashioned to house ELISA reagent loading zones for pre-loading, and the central area was designed and reserved as a testing zone for sample loading. After heating at 105 °C for 3 min, the melted wax wicked through the paper to create hydrophobic barrier wells in the paper. Reagents were then pre-loaded into reagent zone barrier wells. These reagents included the following: (1) 2 μL of blocking buffer (5% (w/v) bovine serum albumin (BSA) (Sigma, SI-A7906, St. Louis, MO, USA) in PBS (Corning, 21-040-CM, Corning, NY, USA); (2) 2 μL solution of alkaline phosphatase (ALP)-conjugated detection antibody (Cell signaling, #7054, Danvers, MA, USA) (20 μg/mL, 0.01% (v/v) Tween-20 (Sigma, P9416, St. Louis, MO, USA); and (3) 2 μL BCIP/NBT substrate (13.4 mM BCIP (Sigma, B6274), 9 mM NBT (Sigma, N5514), 25 mM $MgCl_2$ (Sigma, M8266), 500 mM NaCl (Sigma, S7653) in 500 mM Tris buffer pH 9.5 (Sigma, T4661). After loading each reagent, the device was placed under ambient conditions for 5 to 10 min until the reagents dried.

2.2. Performing Origami-Based PAD for ELISA

The process for creating and using O-PADS is outlined in Figure 2. Briefly, we first loaded 2 μL of sample into the testing zone and allowed it to dry for 10 min under ambient conditions. Then, we folded the reagent zone to contact the testing zone, and loaded 3 μL of PBS into the reagent zone and allowed PBS to transfer reagents to the testing zone. The reaction time for BSA blocking was 5 min and the time for reaction with ALP-conjugated antibody was 10 min. Then, we folded the wash zone to the testing zone, placed the O-PAD on paper towels and washed with 3 μL of PBS. Finally, we folded the substrate zone to the testing zone and loaded 3 μL of PBS to transfer substrate to the testing zone and allowed the enzymatic reaction to proceed for 20 min under ambient conditions. The O-PAD was subsequently scanned using a photo scanner (EPSON 3490 PHOTO). Gray-scale color intensity following the enzymatic reaction was quantified using ImageJ software (ImageJ 1.80, National Institutes of Health, Bethesda, MD, USA). In order to diminish both background noise and analytical variation, we subtracted the original background value of each test zone for each detection result. The experimental data were further analyzed using Sigmaplot (version 13.0, Systat Software, Inc., San Jose, CA, USA).

2.3. Fabrication of the Origami-Based PAD for Paraquat Detection

An O-PAD for paraquat detection is shown in Figure 3. The pattern created on the device was fabricated as described above. We preloaded 5 µL of 5N NaOH and 6 µL of 5% (*w/v*) ascorbic acid onto the left and right parts of the PAD, respectively. After loading each reagent, the device was placed under ambient conditions for 20 min until the reagents dried.

2.4. Performing Origami-Based Detection of Paraquat

To perform origami-based detection of paraquat, we sequentially folded the left and right parts of the structure over and onto the central portion. We then loaded 8 µL of sample onto the test zone and allowed it to rest for 10 min at 25 °C. Detection results were recorded using a digital camera and the signal was analyzed using ImageJ software. The RGB color value of each detection result was obtained, and the R value was used for further calculation [13,36]. We subtracted original test zone background values for each detection result.

3. Results and Discussion

3.1. O-PAD for ELISA

We designed and fabricated a P-ELISA device with multiple preloaded reagents and, borrowing from origami, folded it to make a multilayered, three-dimensional device that provided structural advantages. The design of this O-PAD device is provided in Figure 1a,b.

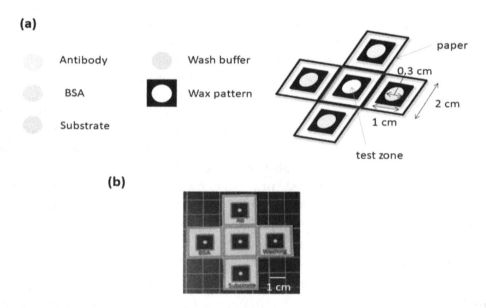

Figure 1. The design of an origami-influenced paper-based analytic device (O-PAD) for enzyme-linked immunosorbent assay (ELISA). (**a**) Reagents were pre-loaded into the four-wing fashioned zones, and the central area was reserved as testing zone for sample loading. (**b**) The picture of our O-PAD.

We used rabbit IgG as the analyte for demonstrating device performance (see schematic illustration in Figure 2. We used serial dilutions of IgG diluted in PBS (260 nM–2.6 pM) to investigate the limit of detection (LOD). The total time to complete testing with this novel device was approximately 46 min. Results from our test were scanned using a photo scanner and the mean gray-scale intensity of the color formed was measured using ImageJ (Figure 3). The LOD for this rabbit IgG system was calculated using the generated colorimetric results. We graphed colorimetric intensity versus rabbit IgG concentration (log scale) to produce the standard curve of this rabbit IgG system. We further employed nonlinear regression using the Hill equation, to generate a sigmoidal curve fit that has previously been used to describe the antibody–antigen reaction kinetics in paper [3]. Similar sigmoidal fits for both rabbit IgG [3] and human vascular endothelial growth factor [6] paper-based ELISA studies have been demonstrated. In the Hill equation (Equation (1)), è represents the fraction of occupied binding sites, [L] represents the ligand concentration (in mol), [L_{50}] describes the ligand concentration when half of the binding sites are occupied (in mol), and n is the Hill coefficient. The fraction of occupied binding sites can be described by the ratio of the observed intensity (I) of the colorimetrical signal to the maximum intensity (Equation (2)). The intensity is proportional to the amount of detected antigens (Equation (3)).

$$è = [L]^n/([L]^n + [L_{50}]^n) \tag{1}$$

$$è = I/I_{max} \tag{2}$$

$$I = I_{max}[L]^n/([L]^n + [L_{50}]^n) \tag{3}$$

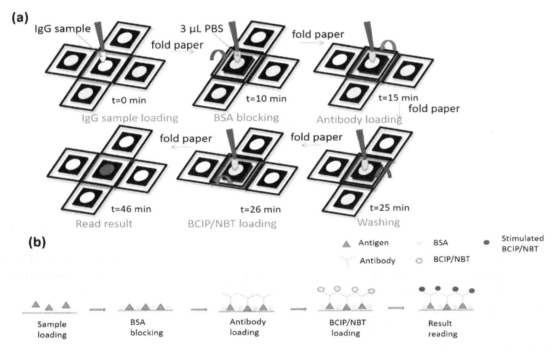

Figure 2. Schematic illustrations demonstrating use of O-PAD ELISA. (**a**) Reagents were pre-loaded into reagent zone barrier wells. These reagents included the following: (1) 2 µL of BSA blocking buffer (2) 2 µL solution of alkaline phosphatase (ALP)-conjugated detection antibody (3) 2 µL BCIP/NBT substrate. After loading each reagent, the device was placed under ambient conditions for 5 to 10 min until the reagents dried. (**b**) Schematic illustrations for BSA blocking, antibody loading, and BCIP/NBT loading.

Accordingly, we fitted the generated colorimetric results into the standard curve using Sigmaplot, and determined that the LOD of the IgG system using our device was about 201 pM, which was calculated by fitting the signal (25.4) that was three times the standard deviation of the blank control [3]. This low IgG LOD could be beneficial for analysis of low-volume specimens in clinical practice. Tear fluid for instance, an example of a low-volume sampling source, demonstrates increased inflammation caused by giant papillary conjunctivitis with an IgG concentration of 160 nM (i.e., IgG detection limit of 160 nM) [37] and viral infection, such as HSV [38], and could benefit from the availability of such a potential diagnostic tool.

Origami has previously been applied to fabricate a paper-based device for performing bioassays [32,33,39]. While the process requires the use of multiple reagents and complex steps, end-user time is saved by preloading with the necessary reagents for performing ELISA. With this ELISA O-PAD, users only need to load their sample to the test zone and apply a single, fixed volume of buffer to initiate testing. Results can be easily obtained via colorimetric readout. Moreover, the colorimetric signal can be scanned or photographed using a smartphone and the results more finely analyzed and compared. The mean color formation intensity can be quantified using versatile software applications including ImageJ or APPs, which can provide convenient POC diagnostic results.

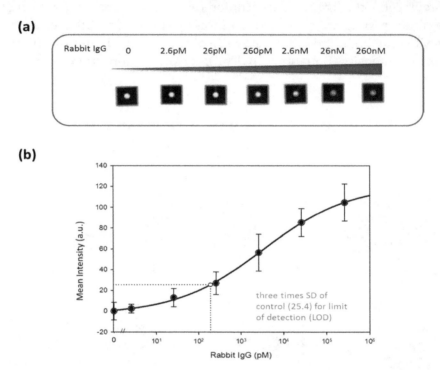

Figure 3. Results of rabbit IgG detection using the O-PAD. (**a**) Colorimetric response. (**b**) Calibration curve of rabbit IgG using mean gray-scale intensity versus several concentrations of rabbit IgG ($n = 6$).

Although an O-PAD with pre-loaded reagents is convenient for POC testing, the storage requirements of proteins, enzymes, substrates, and reagents may limit practicality. We used alkaline phosphatase-conjugated antibody as the detection antibody because commercialized alkaline phosphatase was provided to us as lyophilized powder shipped at ambient, room temperature. BCIP/NBT, the colorimetric substrate of alkaline phosphatase, was available in tablet form and could be crushed to a powder. For both of the above reasons, we felt that a preloaded alkaline phosphatase/BCIP/NBT system was suitable for our O-PAD. The horseradish peroxidase (HRP) and 3,3′,5,5′-tetramentylbenzidine (TMB) system commonly used for ELISA kits may be unsuitable for O-PAD development because the hydrogen peroxide involved in the colorimetric reaction is unstable [40], but we noted that Ramachandran et al. reported a method for long-term dry storage of HRP-conjugated antibody as well as its colorimetric substrate, diaminobenzidine (DAB) [41]. Indeed, some enzymes or proteins that have not undergone optimized drying procedures in suitable buffers may not be stable in a dried state for long-term storage. Our manuscript describes a process to leverage the known advantages of P-ELISA in a novel manner by folding it, origami-fashion, and pre-loading multiple reagents to create a multiplexed diagnostic tool. We believe that the versatility of this approach could lead to an exceptionally useful commercial product, especially if long-term dry-state storage solutions can be found for a broad array of test reagents.

A three-dimensional (3D) microfluidic paper-based analytical device (3D-μPAD) was reported by Liu et al. that used a sliding movable test strip that was dipped into reagent stored within the device [37]. After sliding the test strip to a different location under spots preloaded with stored reagent, buffer was loaded and the integrated, stored reagent was transferred to the test zone. ELISA could be completed by repeating this test-strip sliding action and loading additional buffer [37]. Using rabbit IgG as a model analyte, Liu et al. performed an ELISA in 43 min, with a detection limit of 330 pM. Although this device provides an alternative solution to previous P-ELISA methods, it was difficult to control the contact between test zones and stored, preloaded reagents. Moreover, mass fabrication of this particular 3D-μPAD was problematic.

3.2. O-PAD for Paraquat Detection

Our previous results showed that a folded, origami-inspired structure could facilitate efficient PAD procedures. However, successful detection of multiple analytes using a single PAD relied on maintaining particular, sometimes critical, conditions such as moisture level. In a previous study, we showed that paraquat detection in a PAD required a wet environment [13,36]. Traditional ELISA, however, requires application of multiple reagents, and the time to complete such a process using paper increases the likelihood of any moisture-sensitive components drying out. To remedy this we created an O-PAD for paraquat detection that used its protective folds to maintain moisture during the sample testing phase. This O-PAD for paraquat detection, with a printed wax pattern created as described above, is shown in Figure 4. We preloaded 5 µL of 5 N NaOH and 6 µL of 5% (*w/v*) ascorbic acid (AA) onto the left and right parts of our PAD, respectively. After preloading each reagent, we placed the device under ambient conditions for 20 min to allow the reagents to dry. We then folded the reagent zones containing NaOH and AA onto the test zone sequentially and loaded 8 µL of test sample onto the test zone before letting the device sit for 10 min at 25 °C. Paraquat, in contact with NaOH and AA, changed to paraquat radical ion (blue color) [13,36]. The resulting colorimetric response for each reagent was recorded using a digital camera and analyzed using ImageJ software. The RGB color value of each detection result was obtained. Because previous studies indicated that R value provided the best colorimetric reaction for evaluative and diagnostic purposes [13,36], we employed the same protocol here. In order to diminish background noise and analytical variation, we subtracted any original background values for each test zone result. We used five different concentrations of paraquat standard solution (i.e., 0, 10, 25, 50, and 100 ppm) to establish our standard curve (Figure 5). The LOD for paraquat detection using our O-PAD was 5.82 ppm, which was calculated by using the signal results of our 0 ppm groups plus three-fold standard deviations in the regression model of the standard curve (Figure 5).

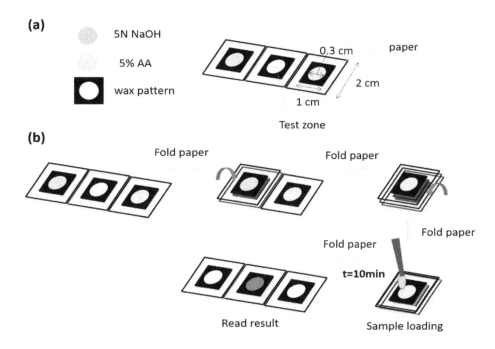

Figure 4. Schematic illustrations of O-PAD for paraquat detection. (**a**) 5 µL of 5 N NaOH and 6 µL of 5% (*w/v*) ascorbic acid (AA) were preloaded onto the left and right parts of our PAD, respectively. (**b**) The reagent zones containing NaOH and AA were folded onto the test zone sequentially. 8 µL of test sample was loaded onto the test zone, and the device stood for 10 min at 25 °C. Paraquat, in contact with NaOH and AA, changed to paraquat radical ion (blue color).

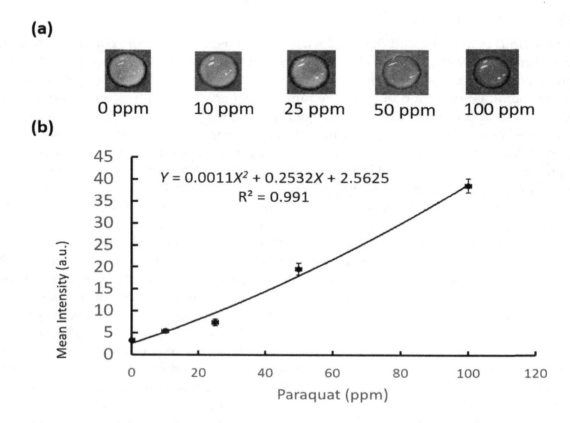

Figure 5. Result of paraquat detection using the O-PAD. (**a**) Colorimetric response. (**b**) The calibration curve of paraquat using mean RGB intensity versus several concentrations of paraquat ($n = 3$).

The LOD (5.82 ppm) using our O-PAD was comparable to the LOD (3.86 ppm) of a previous 96-well format PAD we developed [13]. The O-PAD was more convenient for users because the relevant reagents were preloaded and the results could be easily obtained following a single test sample loading step. Further, the O-PAD comprising three folded paper layers provided a moist environment for paraquat testing that was more suitable than the 96-well format testing device, which consisted of a single layer of paper. These advantages could provide useful point-of-care device development strategies for other analyte detection models. It is worth noting that the lack of long-term storage stability for preloaded reagents may limit the use of our O-PAD for paraquat detection, i.e., ascorbic acid oxidizes in the presence of oxygen. We believe that methods aimed at improving long-term, dry-state reagent storage could help to optimize and broaden the range of potential applications for O-PADs.

Recently, PADs have demonstrated advantages for POC diagnostics. Paper-based ELISA, for instance, require less sample volume and less time to complete than conventional ELISA because of the high surface-to-volume ratio of paper fibers within the test zones [3]. However, PADs are still plagued by some shortcomings that remain to be resolved (Table 1). For example, multiple reagents and more consumables are required to conduct assays, which increase process complexity. Moreover, single-layer PADs may suffer from dry conditions that are less ideal, even insufficient, for testing particular analytes. To ameliorate these disadvantages, we sought to leverage the folded structure of origami to fabricate user-friendly, sensitive, and accurate PADs. Reagents required for conducting assays on such a device could be preloaded and integrated among the device's protective folds. Use of one of these devices requires relatively straightforward folding and unfolding manipulations. Together, these advantages could increase ease, convenience, and acceptability of such devices especially for POC applications in resource-limited areas. We believe that reliance on an ancient art form, origami, could expand the future potential for the development of PADs for clinical diagnostics that could reap real benefits for human health.

Table 1. Comparisons of conventional ELISA and paper-based ELISA (P-ELISA) to origami-based paper devices (some information adapted from reference [3]).

	Conventional	P-ELISA	Origami
Pre-loaded reagents for assay	No	No	Yes
Reagents needed for conducting assay	Multiple reagents	Multiple reagents	One reagent or sample only
Equipment	Multiple tips	Multiple tips	Single tip
Convenience	Low	Low	High
Environment for reactions of detection	Less stable	Less stable	More stable
Required antigen volume	70 μL	3 μL	2 μL
Total complete time	213 min	51 min	46 min
LOD	5.7 pM	18 nM	201 pM

LOD—limit of detection.

4. Conclusions

O-PADs provide a more convenient, reliable, and easy-to-use approach for target sample detection. In this study, we successfully used an O-PAD to detect rabbit IgG level with a low LOD. Due to the limited information regarding the IgG LOD for ophthalmic viral infection or inflammation, we could not compare our results to the references. Overall, this study demonstrated two potential areas for clinical application of OPADs that could provide significant scientific and health benefits. Our device provides two advantages: (1) to reduce test complexity and the number of required reagents through pre-loaded reagents; and, (2) to provide a wet environment for moisture-sensitive analysis, e.g., paraquat detection. However, there are still several limitations associated with our device. First, while providing advantages over paper-based ELISA, our device still could not reach the sensitivity of conventional ELISA; this limitation may be improved by optimizing the assay to suppress the background signal. Second, the long-term storage stability of preloaded reagents such as ascorbic acid, which oxidizes if exposed to oxygen, may limit usage. We believe that additional developments, especially those aimed at improving long-term dry-state storage, would improve our device and broaden its applicability.

Author Contributions: Conceptualization, Z.-K.K. and C.-M.C.; methodology, C.-M.C.; software, T.-H.C.; validation, Y.-S.C.; formal analysis, T.-H.C.; investigation, Z.-K.K.; resources, C.-M.C.; data curation, Y.-S.C.; writing—original draft preparation, Z.-K.K., C.-Y.T.; writing—review and editing, C.-Y.T., C.-M.C.; visualization, Z.-K.K.; supervision, C.-M.C.; project administration, C.-M.C.; funding acquisition, C.-M.C., C.-Y.T.

Acknowledgments: This study was supported by grants (107-2628-E-007-001-MY3 and 108-2622-E-007-020-CC3) from the Ministry of Science and Technology, Taiwan, and a grant (PL-201809004-V) from the Fu Jen Catholic University Hospital, Taiwan.

References

1. Chen, Y.H.; Kuo, Z.K.; Cheng, C.M. Paper—A potential platform in pharmaceutical development. *Trends Biotechnol.* **2015**, *33*, 4–9. [CrossRef]

2. Sher, M.; Zhuang, R.; Demirci, U.; Asghar, W. Paper-based analytical devices for clinical diagnosis: Recent advances in the fabrication techniques and sensing mechanisms. *Expert Rev. Mol. Diagn.* **2017**, *17*, 351–366. [CrossRef]

3. Cheng, C.M.; Martinez, A.W.; Gong, J.; Mace, C.R.; Phillips, S.T.; Carrilho, E.; Mirica, K.A.; Whitesides, G.M. Paper-based ELISA. *Angew. Chem. Int. Ed. Engl.* **2010**, *49*, 4771–4774. [CrossRef] [PubMed]

4. Yen, T.H.; Chen, K.H.; Hsu, M.Y.; Fan, S.T.; Huang, Y.F.; Chang, C.L.; Wang, Y.P.; Cheng, C.M. Evaluating organophosphate poisoning in human serum with paper. *Talanta* **2015**, *144*, 189–195. [CrossRef] [PubMed]

5.   Hsu, M.Y.; Hung, Y.C.; Hwang, D.K.; Lin, S.C.; Lin, K.H.; Wang, C.Y.; Choi, H.Y.; Wang, Y.P.; Cheng, C.M. Detection of aqueous VEGF concentrations before and after intravitreal injection of anti-VEGF antibody using low-volume sampling paper-based ELISA. *Sci. Rep.* **2016**, *6*, 34631. [CrossRef] [PubMed]

6.   Hsu, M.Y.; Yang, C.Y.; Hsu, W.H.; Lin, K.H.; Wang, C.Y.; Shen, Y.C.; Chen, S.F.; Chau, S.F.; Tsai, H.Y.; Cheng, C.M. Monitoring the VEGF level in aqueous humor of patients with ophthalmologically relevant diseases via ultrahigh sensitive paper-based ELISA. *Biomaterials* **2014**, *35*, 3729–3735. [CrossRef]

7.   Yamada, K.; Takaki, S.; Komuro, N.; Suzuki, K.; Citterio, D. An antibody-free microfluidic paper-based analytical device for the determination of tear fluid lactoferrin by fluorescence sensitization of Tb3+. *Analyst* **2014**, *139*, 1637–1643. [CrossRef]

8.   Hsu, C.K.; Huang, H.Y.; Chen, W.R.; Nishie, W.; Ujiie, H.; Natzuga, K.; Fan, S.T.; Wang, H.K.; Lee, J.Y.Y.; Tsai, W.L.; et al. Paper-based ELISA for the detection of autoimmune antibodies in body fluid-the case of bullous pemphigoid. *Anal. Chem.* **2014**, *86*, 4605–4610. [CrossRef]

9.   Apilux, A.; Ukita, Y.; Chikae, M.; Chailapakul, O.; Takamura, Y. Development of automated paper-based devices for sequential multistep sandwich enzyme-linked immunosorbent assays using inkjet printing. *Lab Chip* **2013**, *13*, 126–135. [CrossRef]

10. Wang, S.; Ge, L.; Song, X.; Yu, J.; Ge, S.; Huang, J.; Zeng, F. Paper-based chemiluminescence ELISA: Lab-on-paper based on chitosan modified paper device and wax-screen-printing. *Biosens. Bioelectron.* **2012**, *31*, 212–218. [CrossRef]

11. Shih, C.M.; Chang, C.L.; Hsu, M.Y.; Lin, J.Y.; Kuan, C.M.; Wang, H.K.; Huang, C.T.; Chung, M.C.; Huang, K.C.; Hsu, C.E. Paper-based ELISA to rapidly detect *Escherichia coli*. *Talanta* **2015**, *145*, 2–5. [CrossRef] [PubMed]

12. Dungchai, W.; Chailapakul, O.; Henry, C.S. Use of multiple colorimetric indicators for paper-based microfluidic devices. *Anal. Chim Acta* **2010**, *674*, 227–233. [CrossRef] [PubMed]

13. Kuan, C.M.; Lin, S.T.; Yen, T.H.; Wang, Y.L.; Cheng, C.M. Paper-based diagnostic devices for clinical paraquat poisoning diagnosis. *Biomicrofluidics* **2016**, *10*, 034118. [CrossRef] [PubMed]

14. Barron, B.A.; Gee, L.; Hauck, W.W.; Kurinij, N.; Dawson, C.R.; Jones, D.B.; Wilhelmus, K.R.; Kaufman, H.E.; Sugar, J.; Hyndiuk, R.A. Herpetic Eye Disease Study: A controlled trial of oral acyclovir for herpes simplex stromal keratitis. *Ophthalmology* **1994**, *101*, 1871–1882. [CrossRef]

15. Schwab, I.R.J.O. Oral acyclovir in the management of herpes simplex ocular infections. *Ophthalmology* **1988**, *95*, 423–430. [CrossRef]

16. Bacon, A.S.; Dart, J.K.; Ficker, L.A.; Matheson, M.M.; Wright, P.J.O. Acanthamoeba keratitis: The value of early diagnosis. *Virology* **1993**, *100*, 1238–1243.

17. German, A.; Hall, E.; Day, M.J. Measurement of IgG, IgM and IgA concentrations in canine serum, saliva, tears and bile. *Vet. Immunol.* **1998**, *64*, 107–121. [CrossRef]

18. Bron, A.; Seal, D.J. The defences of the ocular surface. *Trans. Ophthalmol. Soc. UK* **1986**, *105*, 18–25.

19. McClellan, B.H.; Whitney, C.R.; Newman, L.P.; Allansmith, M.R. Immunoglobulins in tears. *Am. J. Ophthalmol.* **1973**, *76*, 89–101. [CrossRef]

20. Coyle, P.; Sibony, P.J. Tear immunoglobulins measured by ELISA. *Investig. Ophth. Vis. Sci.* **1986**, *27*, 622–625.

21. Ashe, W.K.; Mage, M.; Notkins, A.L. Kinetics of neutralization of sensitized herpes simplex virus with antibody fragments. *Short Commun.* **1969**, *37*, 290–293. [CrossRef]

22. Ashe, W.K.; Notkins, A.L. Kinetics of sensitization of herpes simplex virus and its relationship to the reduction in the neutralization rate constant. *Virology* **1967**, *33*, 613–617. [CrossRef]

23. Centifanto, Y.; Kaufman, H.E. Secretory immunoglobulin A and herpes keratitis. *Infect. Immun.* **1970**, *2*, 778–782.

24. Alizadeh, H.; Apte, S.; El-Agha, M.-S.H.; Li, L.; Hurt, M.; Howard, K.; Cavanagh, H.D.; McCulley, J.P.; Niederkorn, J.Y. Tear IgA and serum IgG antibodies against Acanthamoeba in patients with Acanthamoeba keratitis. *Cornea* **2001**, *20*, 622–627. [CrossRef]

25. Wesseling, C.; De Joode, B.V.W.; Ruepert, C.; León, C.; Monge, P.; Hermosillo, H.; Partanen, L.J. Paraquat in developing countries. *Int. J. Occup. Environ. Health* **2001**, *7*, 275–286. [CrossRef]

26. Pond, S.M.; Rivory, L.P.; Hampson, E.C.; Roberts, M.S. Kinetics of toxic doses of paraquat and the effects of hemoperfusion in the dog. *J. Toxicol. Clin. Toxicol.* **1993**, *31*, 229–246. [CrossRef]

27. Sittipunt, C. Paraquat poisoning. *Respir. Care.* **2005**, *50*, 383–385.

28. Weng, C.H.; Hu, C.C.; Lin, J.L.; Lin-Tan, D.T.; Hsu, C.W.; Yen, T.H. Predictors of acute respiratory distress syndrome in patients with paraquat intoxication. *PLoS ONE* **2013**, *8*, e82695. [CrossRef]

29. Hsu, C.W.; Lin, J.L.; Lin.Tan, D.T.; Chen, K.H.; Yen, T.H.; Wu, M.S.; Lin, S.C. Early hemoperfusion may improve survival of severely paraquat-poisoned patients. *PLoS ONE* **2012**, *7*, e48397. [CrossRef]

30. Johnson, M.; Chen, Y.; Hovet, S.; Xu, S.; Wood, B.; Ren, H.; Tokuda, J.; Tse, Z.T.H. Fabricating biomedical origami: A state-of-the-art review. *Int. J. Comput. Assist. Radiol. Surg.* **2017**, *12*, 2023–2032. [CrossRef]

31. Liu, H.; Crooks, R.M. Three-dimensional paper microfluidic devices assembled using the principles of origami. *J. Am. Chem Soc.* **2011**, *133*, 17564–17566. [CrossRef] [PubMed]

32. Ge, L.; Wang, S.; Song, X.; Ge, S.; Yu, J. 3D origami-based multifunction-integrated immunodevice: Low-cost and multiplexed sandwich chemiluminescence immunoassay on microfluidic paper-based analytical device. *Lab Chip* **2012**, *12*, 3150–3158. [CrossRef] [PubMed]

33. Govindarajan, A.V.; Ramachandran, S.; Vigil, G.D.; Yager, P.; Bohringer, K.F. A low cost point-of-care viscous sample preparation device for molecular diagnosis in the developing world; an example of microfluidic origami. *Lab Chip* **2012**, *12*, 174–181. [CrossRef] [PubMed]

34. Chen, C.-A.; Yeh, W.-S.; Tsai, T.-T.; Chen, C.-F. Three-dimensional origami paper-based device for portable immunoassay applications. *Lab Chip* **2019**, *19*, 598–607. [CrossRef] [PubMed]

35. Tian, T.; An, Y.; Wu, Y.; Song, Y.; Zhu, Z.; Yang, C. Integrated Distance-Based Origami Paper Analytical Device for One-Step Visualized Analysis. *ACS Appl. Mater. Interfaces* **2017**, *9*, 30480–30487. [CrossRef]

36. Chang, T.-H.; Tung, K.-H.; Gu, P.-W.; Yen, T.-H.; Cheng, C.-M. Rapid Simultaneous Determination of Paraquat and Creatinine in Human Serum Using a Piece of Paper. *Micromachines* **2018**, *9*, 586. [CrossRef]

37. Donshik, P.C.; Ballow, M. Tear immunoglobulins in giant papillary conjunctivitis induced by contact lenses. *Am. J. Ophthalmol.* **1983**, *96*, 460–466. [CrossRef]

38. Borderie, V.M.; Gineys, R.; Goldschmidt, P.; Batellier, L.; Laroche, L.; Chaumeil, C.J.C. Association of Anti–Herpes Simplex Virus IgG in Tears and Serum With Clinical Presentation in Patients With Presumed Herpetic Simplex Keratitis. *Cornea* **2012**, *31*, 1251–1256. [CrossRef]

39. Liu, X.; Cheng, C.; Martinez, A.; Mirica, K.; Li, X.; Phillips, S.; Mascarenas, M.; Whitesides, G. A portable microfluidic paper-based device for ELISA. In Proceedings of the 2011 IEEE 24th International Conference on Micro Electro. Mechanical Systems, Cancun, Mexico, 23–27 January 2011; pp. 75–78.

40. Verma, M.S.; Tsaloglou, M.-N.; Sisley, T.; Christodouleas, D.; Chen, A.; Milette, J.; Whitesides, G.M. Sliding-strip microfluidic device enables ELISA on paper. *Biosens Bioelectron.* **2018**, *99*, 77–84. [CrossRef]

41. Ramachandran, S.; Fu, E.; Lutz, B.; Yager, P.J.A. Long-term dry storage of an enzyme-based reagent system for ELISA in point-of-care devices. *Analyst* **2014**, *139*, 1456–1462. [CrossRef]

13

The Danger of Walking with Socks: Evidence from Kinematic Analysis in People with Progressive Multiple Sclerosis

Su-Chun Huang [1], Gloria Dalla Costa [1,2], Marco Pisa [1,2], Lorenzo Gregoris [2], Giulia Leccabue [2], Martina Congiu [1], Giancarlo Comi [1,2] and Letizia Leocani [1,2,*]

[1] Neurorehabilitation Department and Experimental Neurophysiology Unit, INSPE-Institute of Experimental Neurology, San Raffaele Hospital, 20132 Milan, Italy; huang.suchun@hsr.it (S.-C.H.); dallacosta.gloria@hsr.it (G.D.C.); pisa.marco@hsr.it (M.P.); congiu.martina@hsr.it (M.C.); comi.giancarlo@hsr.it (G.C.)

[2] Vita-Salute San Raffaele University, Via Olgettina, 58, 20132 Milan, Italy; gregorislorenzo96@gmail.com (L.G.); giulialeccabue95@gmail.com (G.L.)

* Correspondence: letizia.leocani@hsr.it

Abstract: Multiple sclerosis (MS) is characterized by gait impairments and severely impacts the quality of life. Technological advances in biomechanics offer objective assessments of gait disabilities in clinical settings. Here we employed wearable sensors to measure electromyography (EMG) and body acceleration during walking and to quantify the altered gait pattern between people with progressive MS (PwPMS) and healthy controls (HCs). Forty consecutive patients attending our department as in-patients were examined together with fifteen healthy controls. All subjects performed the timed 10 min walking test (T10MW) using a wearable accelerator and 8 electrodes attached to bilateral thighs and legs so that body acceleration and EMG activity were recorded. The T10MWs were recorded under three conditions: standard (wearing shoes), reduced grip (wearing socks) and increased cognitive load (backward-counting dual-task). PwPMS showed worse kinematics of gait and increased muscle coactivation than controls at both the thigh and leg levels. Both reduced grip and increased cognitive load caused a reduction in the cadence and velocity of the T10MW, which were correlated with one another. A higher coactivation index at the thigh level of the more affected side was positively correlated with the time of the T10MW (r = 0.5, $p < 0.01$), Expanded Disability Status Scale (EDSS) (r = 0.4, $p < 0.05$), and negatively correlated with the cadence (r = −0.6, $p < 0.001$). Our results suggest that excessive coactivation at the thigh level is the major determinant of the gait performance as the disease progresses. Moreover, demanding walking conditions do not influence gait in controls but deteriorate walking performances in PwPMS, thus those conditions should be prevented during hospital examinations as well as in homecare environments.

Keywords: multiple sclerosis; gait analysis; kinematics; surface EMG; accelerator; inertial sensor; T10MW

1. Introduction

Multiple sclerosis (MS) is a complex autoimmune disease characterized by multifocal and recurrent formation of demyelinating plaques possibly involving every area of the central nervous system (CNS) [1]. The disease usually affects multiple domains, but the motor pathway is constantly involved and usually it follows a disto-proximal gradient of severity with lower limbs being more precariously and severely impaired than the upper limbs [2]. Gait is one of the most disabling neurological symptoms in people with MS [3]. In the most advanced phases of the disease, gait dysfunction is typically due to pyramidal deficits, and sensory and cerebellar disturbances also coexist with variable extents [4].

Technological advances in biomechanics offer possibilities to objectively estimate gait disabilities such as joint kinematics, kinetics, and patterns of muscle activations during walking [5]. Non-invasive wireless wearable devices for the recording of surface electromyography and kinematics are commercially available [6]. These devices can be placed on different parts of the body based on clinical needs and they are capable of measuring gait quality in an everyday environment. For example, belt-mounted devices are used routinely in the clinical setting as they provide information on gait parameters such as cadence and velocity. The results of these simple techniques are highly consistent with more sophisticated laboratory equipment used in the research setting [7]. However, for people with MS the ideal conditions under which gait should be tested need to be better explored. Although for one of the most widely used walking tests, the 25 foot walk test, it is recommended to use comfortable shoes, in the clinical setting it can be useful to observe gait patterns without shoes in order to better appreciate subtle abnormalities in ankle or toe movements, and in order to reduce variability at longitudinal assessments due to changes of shoes. Even in research settings, gait parameters are collected during barefoot walking [8]. Sometimes, the barefoot condition is not fully reached and the patient is allowed to wear socks for better comfort. However, walking while wearing socks may be dangerous. Walking in socks without shoes or in slippers without a sole has been associated with falls in women [9]. Being barefoot or wearing socks without shoes may also increase the risk of falls from slipping or trauma from unexpected contact [10]. Older people going barefoot, wearing socks without shoes, or wearing slippers have an increased risk of serious injury at home due to a fall [11]. Falls are a common cause of harm in people with MS; it has been described that 50% of patients report falls in a 3-month period [12]. Walking under more demanding conditions, such as during cognitive loads, greatly influences motor performance [13]. Worsening of gait during a dual-task situation is also associated with an increased risk of falls in people with MS [8]. The aim of the current study was to explore whether walking with socks may be associated with a worsening in gait performance in people with progressive MS (PwPMS), similarly to what was already described for cognitive load.

2. Materials and Methods

2.1. Subjects

We examined gait performance in 40 consecutive patients attending the Department of Neurorehabilitation of San Raffaele Hospital (Milan, Italy), with a confirmed diagnosis of MS based on the 2017 McDonald criteria [14], age 18–65 years old, Expanded Disability Status Scale (EDSS) up to 6.5 (able to walk for at least 10 min safely with or without aids), absence of orthopedic pathologies that might influence walking performances, without depression nor cognitive involvements as per routine neurological and cognitive examinations at entry (token test, symbol digit modalities test, Beck Depression Inventory-II). All patients' data were collected as part of their clinical care according to the Guideline of Good Clinical Practice [15]; all patients provided written informed consent to the use of their data for research. Fifteen healthy subjects were enrolled as the control group with similar age and sex distribution; they first provided written informed consent to participate in the study, that was approved by our Institutional Ethics Committee (approval number: N13/2017) and all data were anonymized prior to analysis.

2.2. Gait Analysis

Gait analysis was assessed using a G-Walk (BTS bioengineering, Italy), an inertial sensor which measures tri-axial accelerations, while performing a timed 10 min walking test (T10MW). The subject was asked to walk straight for 10 min with the sensor attached to the waist with a belt, covering the lower lumbar area (L4–L5). Body accelerations along the anterior-posterior, medio-lateral, and vertical axes during the T10MW were recorded with a sampling frequency of 100 Hz. According to standard

T10MW procedure, patients were asked to complete the test at the maximum speed they could safely walk. A counting dual-task (DT) condition was also tested by adding a mental tracking cognitive task in which the subject was asked to count backward by 3 from 100 while performing the T10MW. As the dual task is routinely performed to test interference on gait by cognitive load, it was performed only in the more frequently used condition, while wearing shoes. Therefore, the T10MW was assessed in three different conditions: (1) walking with shoes on (2) walking with only socks on and (3) walking with shoes on while performing DT.

The acceleration data were analyzed with G-Studio (G-Studio software, BTS bioengineering, Milan, Italy) for the three conditions. Time, cadence, velocity, and step length were calculated for further analyses.

2.3. sEMG Recording

Surface EMG was used to record muscular activity simultaneously with the acceleration measurement. Eight wireless electrodes (FREEEMG-1000, BTS bioengineering, Milan, Italy) were attached directly to the skin overlying the Rectus Femoris (RF), long head of Biceps Femoris (BF), Tibialis Anterior (TA) and Medial Gastrocnemius (GM) bilaterally. EMG data were sampled at a rate of 1000 Hz and signals were remotely transferred to a USB receiver.

The sEMG data were processed with self-developed Matlab scripts (Matlab 2016b, MathWorks, Natickm, MA). The raw sEMG data were first band-pass filtered between 10 to 500 Hz, full-wave rectified, then smoothed with a low pass filter (3.5 Hz cut-off frequency). The averaged amplitude of the resting EMG (before the subject started walking) was subtracted from the smoothed EMG for each muscle. This subtracted data were then normalized to the largest recorded value of each muscle (max. EMG). Coactivation between each agonistic-antagonistic muscle pairs (RF-BF and TA-GM) were quantified as the coactivation index (CoI). The CoI was calculated as the overlap areas of the normalized EMG data divided by the duration of the overlapping, a higher CoI indicates more coactivation between the muscle pairs [16]. However, the length of the EMG data differs between subjects since it depends on the walking speed. In order to obtain a more stable CoI and enable the comparisons between subjects, CoI was calculated from five consecutive steps of the T10MW.

2.4. Clinical Assessment

The EDSS score was evaluated by the treating neurologist at hospital admissions. All patients also underwent a clinical evaluation of spasticity according to the Modified Ashworth Scale (MAS) on bilateral RF, BF, TA and GM. On the same muscular groups, strength was measured with Medical Research Council Scale (MRC) [17,18]. These scores were used to define the less affected (LA) and more affected (MA) side in each patient. Static balance performance was assessed with the Berg Balance Scale (BBS) [19].

Patient reported outcomes were also added to the clinical evaluation. The walking status of PwPMS was measured with a 12-Item MS Walking Scale (MSWS-12) [20]; fatigue was assessed with the Fatigue Severity Scale (FSS) [21]; the MS Spasticity Scale-88 (MSSS-88) and the Numeric Rating Scale of Spasticity (NRS) were used for estimating the impact of spasticity [22] on physical performances [23]. The risk of falls was evaluated with Conley scale [24]. The disability is evaluated using the Functional Independence Measure (FIM) [25] and the Barthel Index [26].

2.5. Statistics

For data demographics, the data are expressed in mean and standard deviations (SD). Independent t-test and chi-square tests were used to compare age, gender, and body mass index (BMI) distributions between PwPMS and healthy controls (HCs) respectively.

The spatiotemporal parameters and CoI from both PwPMS and HCs for all three conditions (shoes, socks, DT) were used for further statistics. Mixed two-way ANOVA (group x conditions) were employed to test significant differences between PwPMS and HCs under the three conditions.

The analyses of CoI were performed in less and more affected side (LA/MA), respectively. If the ANOVA model was significant, turkey post-hoc analysis with Bonferroni correction ($p < 0.01$) was used to search the difference between (1) shoes and socks condition and (2) shoes and the DT condition, while the difference between PwPMS and HCs were tested with the independent t-test.

Correlations were performed among the kinematic parameters, sEMG recording, and clinical assessments. The alpha-level was corrected with Bonferroni correction and set at 0.017 for two tails as the correlations were performed in three major categories. Spearman's correlation was used to explore the relationship between the quantitative data (spatiotemporal parameters and CoI) and the clinical assessment (EDSS, MSWS-12, FSS, MSSS-88, Conley, Barthel, FIM, BBS, and NRS). Pearson's correlation was used to examine the relationship between spatiotemporal parameters and CoI. All the statistical analyses were performed with Prism 5 (GraphPad Software, Inc., San Diego, CA).

3. Results

3.1. Subjects Demographics

Forty people with progressive MS (20 males; mean age: 51.0 ± 9.8 years; mean BMI = 24.0 ± 4.6) with a mean EDSS score of 5.5 ± 1 (ranging from 1.5 to 6.5) were examined and fifteen HCs (4 males; mean age: 52.7 ± 4.4 years; mean BMI = 24.0 ± 2.2) were enrolled. The characteristics and results of clinical assessments of the two groups are shown in Table 1. No significant difference was found in age ($p = 0.4971$), sex ($p = 0.3381$), nor BMI ($p = 0.9448$) distributions between the groups.

Table 1. Data demographics of the subjects and clinical assessments. No significant difference was found in gender ($p = 0.3381$), age ($p = 0.4971$) nor in body mass index (BMI, $p = 0.9448$) between groups. Data are shown in mean ± standard deviation format. PwPMS: patients with progressive multiple sclerosis; HCs: healthy controls. MAS: Modified Ashworth Scale; MRC Scale: Medical Research Council Scale; MSWS-12: 12-Item MS Walking Scale; FSS: Fatigue Severity Scale; MSSS-88: MS Spasticity Scale-88; FIM: Functional Independence Measure; BBS: Berg Balance Scale; NRS: Numeric Rating Scale of Spasticity.

Characteristics	PwPMS (n = 40)	HC (n = 15)
Gender (M/F)	20 / 20	4 / 9
Age (years)	50.9 ± 9.8	52.7 ± 4.4
BMI	24.0 ± 4.6	24.0 ± 2.2
EDSS	5.5 ± 1.1	-
More Affected Side (R/L)	23 / 17	-
MAS (more affected side)	2.4 ± 2.0	-
MRC scale (more affected side)	13.1 ± 3.2	-
MSWS-12	38.6 ± 9.7	-
FSS	39.5 ± 15.0	-
MSSS-88	188.6 ± 52.7	-
Conley scale	2.9 ± 1.8	-
Barthel scale	88.4 ± 10.3	-
FIM	112.5 ± 9.0	-
BBS	40.5 ± 7.7	-
NRS	3.9 ± 2.6	-

3.2. Comparisons of Spatiotemporal Parameters

Significant differences in both groups (PwPMS and HCs) and conditions (shoes, socks, and DT) were found in time (group: $p < 0.0001$; condition: $p = 0.0032$), cadence (group: $p < 0.0001$; condition: $p = 0.0032$), velocity (both $p < 0.0001$) and step length (both $p < 0.0001$). Interactions between group and conditions were only significant in time ($p = 0.0277$) and step length ($p = 0.0105$). Post-hoc analyses revealed that compared with the HCs, the PwPMS showed longer time, lower cadence, slower velocity, and shorter step length while performing T10MW in all three conditions ($p < 0.01$ for all post-hoc comparisons).

For intra-group comparisons, when wearing shoes, PwPMS showed shorter time ($p < 0.0001$), higher cadence ($p = 0.0005$), higher velocity ($p < 0.0001$), and longer step length ($p < 0.0001$) than walking with socks. On the other hand, HCs showed only smaller step size when wearing socks compared to shoes ($p = 0.0142$).

For the comparison between single and dual tasks, longer time ($p < 0.0001$), lower velocity ($p = 0.0002$), and shorter step length ($p = 0.0003$) was found in PwPMS while performing a counting DT, while cadence was not significantly different ($p = 0.09$). Interestingly, significantly reduced cadence during the DT compared to a single task was found in HCs ($p = 0.014$).

The results of spatiotemporal parameters are shown in Figure 1.

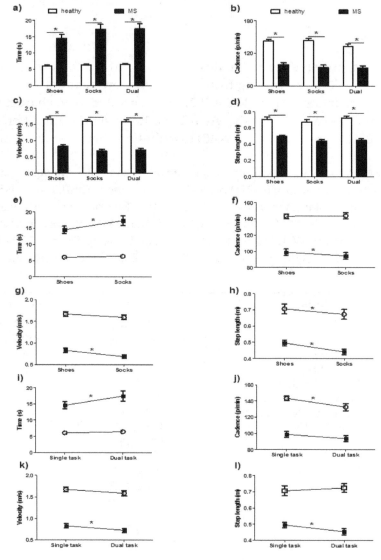

Figure 1. Inter- and intra group comparisons of spatiotemporal parameters. Significant group differences in time (**a**), cadence (**b**), velocity (**c**) and step size (**d**) were found in all three conditions. Intra-group comparison between shoes and socks conditions also showed significant differences in time (**e**), cadence (**f**), velocity (**g**), and step length (**h**) in PwPMS, while only step length in the HCs. For the comparison of single and dual tasks, longer time (**i**), lower velocity (**k**), and shorter step length (**l**) was found when PwPMS were performing a DT compared to performing a single task, while in the HCs only significantly reduced cadence (**j**) was found. *: $p < 0.01$ in post hoc analysis ((**a–d**): between-group comparison; (**j–l**): within-group comparisons).

3.3. Comparisons of Coactivation Index

Two-way ANOVA showed significant group differences of coactivation in both the MA and LA side in RF-BF ($p = 0.0007$ for both) and GM-TA (MA: $p = 0.0144$; LA: $p = 0.0047$) pairs, while no significant difference were found among conditions. Post-hoc analyses revealed that compared with HCs, PwPMS showed higher coactivation in the MA and LA sides for both antagonistic pairs among all three conditions ($p < 0.01$ for all).

For intra-group comparisons, in both PwPMS and the HC, no difference of the CoI was found when comparing between shoes and socks conditions, nor in shoes and with DT conditions. The results are shown in Figure 2.

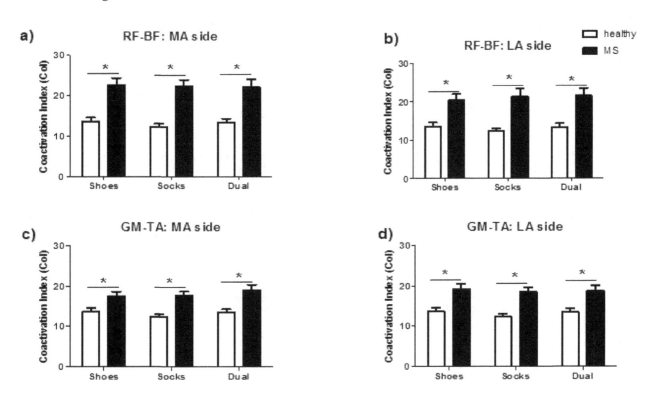

Figure 2. The inter-group difference of the coactivation index. Two-way ANOVA showed significant group difference of coactivation in both the MA and LA side in RF-BF (**a,b**) and GM-TA (**c,d**), while no significant difference was found among conditions. *: $p < 0.01$ in posthoc analyses.

3.4. Correlations among Measurements

For correlation between clinical assessments and spatiotemporal parameters, the EDSS score was correlated with time (shoes: r = 0.4785, $p = 0.0018$; socks: r = 0.4984, $p = 0.0011$; DT: r = 0.4006, $p = 0.0104$), cadence (shoes: r = −0.4932, $p = 0.0012$; socks: r = −0.4995, $p = 0.0010$; DT: r = −0.4270, $p = 0.0060$), and velocity (shoes: r = −0.4790, $p = 0.0018$; socks: r = −0.4967, $p = 0.0011$; DT: r = −0.4225, $p = 0.0066$) in all three conditions. On the other hand, with EMG results, the EDSS correlated with the CoI in the RF-BF pair of the MA side in socks (r = 0.4237, $p = 0.0169$) and with DT (r = 0.4761, $p = 0.0078$) conditions, also a trend correlation was found in the shoes condition (r = 0.3828, $p = 0.0368$). The FSS was correlated with the CoI in the RF-BF pair in both the MA and LA side in the socks condition (MA: r = −0.4953, $p = 0.0054$; LA: r = −0.5457, $p = 0.0105$). The FIM scores was correlated with time in shoes (r = −0.4026, $p = 0.0100$) and with the DT (r = −0.3875, $p = 0.0135$), and with velocity in all three conditions (shoes: r = 0.4080, $p = 0.0090$; socks: r = 0.4011, $p = 0.0103$; DT: r = 0.4235, $p = 0.0065$). The BBS correlated with time (r = −0.3961, $p = 0.0126$) and velocity (r = 0.3957, $p = 0.0127$) in shoes condition. The correlation results are summarized in Tables 2 and 3.

Table 2. Spearman's correlation coefficient between spatiotemporal parameters and clinical assessments in all the conditions. Spearman's correlation was performed to explore the relationship between kinematics and clinical measurements.

Variables	Conditions	EDSS	MSWS-12	FSS	MSSS-88	Conley	Barthel	FIM	BBS	NRS
Time (N = 40)	shoes	0.48 **	0.22	−0.23	−0.01	−0.07	−0.11	−0.40 *	−0.40 *	0.05
	socks	0.50 **	0.22	−0.27	−0.04	−0.08	−0.01	−0.35	−0.32	0.06
	DT	0.40 *	0.15	−0.16	0.03	−0.16	−0.00	−0.39 *	−0.29	−0.03
Cadence (N = 40)	shoes	−0.49 **	−0.20	0.31	0.08	0.11	0.08	0.33	0.36	0.07
	socks	−0.50 **	−0.21	0.32	0.06	0.13	0.02	0.33	0.35	0.07
	DT	−0.43 **	−0.13	0.15	−0.09	0.14	−0.07	0.29	0.27	0.16
Velocity (N = 40)	shoes	−0.48 **	−0.22	0.23	0.02	0.06	0.10	0.41 **	0.40 *	−0.05
	socks	−0.50 **	−0.20	0.27	0.03	0.11	0.03	0.40 *	0.36	−0.07
	DT	−0.42 **	−0.13	0.18	0.01	0.11	0.06	0.42 **	0.34	−0.08
Step Length (N = 40)	shoes	−0.27	−0.03	0.24	0.13	0.08	0.06	0.32	0.24	−0.13
	socks	−0.18	−0.06	0.14	0.03	−0.01	−0.04	0.11	0.04	−0.21
	DT	−0.15	−0.08	0.11	0.02	0.12	0.03	0.30	0.14	−0.13

The significance level was set to $p < 0.017$ *: $p < 0.017$; **: $p < 0.001$.

Table 3. Spearman's correlation coefficient between the coactivation index and clinical assessments in all the conditions. Spearman's correlation was performed to explore the relationship between sEMG recording and clinical exams.

Variables	Conditions	EDSS	MSWS-12	FSS	MSSS-88	Conley	Barthel	FIM	BBS	NRS
RF-BF MA (N = 31)	shoes	0.38	0.06	−0.27	−0.03	−0.10	−0.13	−0.30	−0.15	−0.41
	socks	0.42 *	−0.10	−0.50 **	−0.11	−0.18	−0.02	−0.14	−0.12	−0.30
	DT	0.48 **	−0.04	−0.38	−0.13	−0.05	0.05	−0.08	0.02	−0.35
RF-BF LA (N = 22)	shoes	0.12	−0.28	−0.46	−0.21	−0.09	−0.02	−0.13	0.02	−0.22
	socks	0.21	0.07	−0.55 *	−0.18	0.03	−0.05	−0.12	0.02	−0.02
	DT	0.26	−0.32	−0.41	−0.13	−0.08	−0.01	−0.00	0	−0.05
GM-TA MA (N = 40)	shoes	0.13	−0.04	0.02	0.16	−0.06	0.20	−0.03	0.10	0.17
	socks	0.07	0.02	−0.01	0.07	0.06	0.14	−0.08	0.01	0.13
	DT	0.17	−0.02	0.01	0.02	−0.05	0.22	−0.07	0.01	0.12
GM-TA LA (N = 40)	shoes	0.22	0.07	−0.09	0.07	0.11	0.12	−0.34	−0.39	0.18
	socks	0.16	0.10	0.13	0.18	0.33	0	−0.28	−0.30	0.22
	DT	0.02	−0.10	−0.11	−0.01	0.22	0.03	−0.14	−0.18	0.27

The significance level was set to $p < 0.017$. *: $p < 0.017$; **: $p < 0.001$.

Finally, when we compared the changes from the standard shoe condition to the two challenging conditions (i.e., socks or DT), we found significant positive correlations between the reduction in velocity (r = 0.3662, p = 0.0141) and cadence (r = 0.4158, p = 0.0076) when walking with socks versus shoes and when performing the dual versus simple task for PwPMS. A negative correlation was found between lower score of the BBS and the time increases from shoe condition to the socks condition (r = −0.3901, p = 0.0141) and a trend of negative correlation with the time increases from a single to a DT condition (r = −0.3247, p = 0.0437). The results are shown in Figure 3. No such correlations were found in HCs.

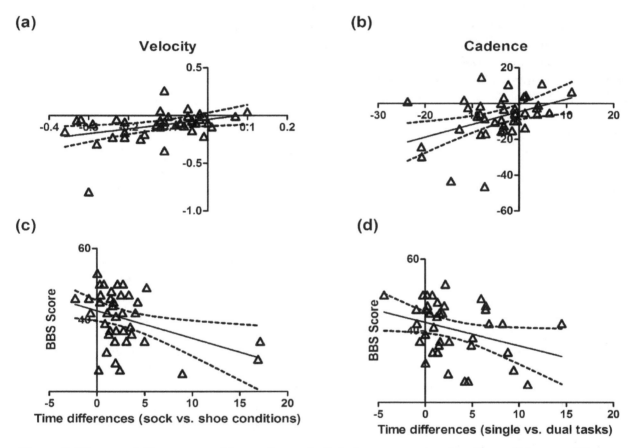

Figure 3. The correlations among kinematics and clinical assessments when the walking conditions changed for PwPMS. (**a,b**): x-axis: the difference between the shoes and the socks conditions (socks minus shoes); y-axis: the difference between the single task and DT conditions (single minus DT, both performed with shoes). Positive correlations were found in velocity (r = 0.3662, p = 0.0141) and cadence (r = 0.4158, p = 0.0076) between the differences of the shoes vs. socks condition and the single vs. DT conditions. (**c,d**): A significant negative correlation was found between the BBS scores and the time increases from shoe to sock conditions (r = −0.3901, p = 0.0141), and a trend correlation was found with time increases of single versus dual tasks (r = −0.3247, p = 0.0437).

4. Discussion

In the present study we employed wireless wearable devices to examine changes in gait control in demanding conditions. The T10MW was tested under three conditions (shoes, socks, and the counting DT) with the combined use of an accelerator and sEMG monitoring. As expected, PwPMS showed worse gait performance in kinematics and higher coactivation in antagonistic muscle pairs at thigh and leg levels than HCs. We found that only in the PwPMS, the kinematic measures changed when walking was performed under demanding conditions, while the pattern of coactivation remained the same. Further, the kinematic changes between the socks versus shoes conditions were positively correlated with those found between the single versus dual task condition. This result indicates that for PwPMS, the impact on gait performance when walking with socks without shoes, is correlated with that introduced by a cognitive load; similar findings were not present in the HC group. Both walking with socks and with a cognitive load were associated with increased risk of falls in women, elder people, or in people with MS [8–11].

A score of less than 45 in the Berg Balance Scale exposes one to a greater risk of falling [27]. We found that in the PwPMS group, lower scores of the Berg Balance Scale were related to worse gait control when walking in socks or performing a counting DT. No difference nor correlation was found regarding gender, age, nor BMI in different conditions. Therefore, for tests such as the T10MW or the timed 25 foot walk test, performing with socks should be avoided for all PwPMS.

The sEMG results showed increased coactivation in both the MA and LA side of the lower limbs during total stance in PwPMS compared with the HCs. However, due to the limitation of the devices used, the stance cannot be further separated into sub-phases. Boudarham et al. reported higher coactivation during the whole stance at the leg level, while at the thigh level only during the single support phase [28]. Compared with their group, our PwPMS group has a higher disability (mean EDSS: 5.5 vs. 3.8) and worse spasticity (MAS of MA side: 2.2 vs. 1), which could explain why we found excessive coactivation in the whole lower limbs. Also, in Budarham's study, no correlation between the EDSS and the CoI was found, while in our study the CoI of RF-BF at the MA side was correlated with the EDSS in more challenging walking conditions (i.e., with socks or the counting DT). Furthermore, the CoI of RF-BF at both the MA and LA side were correlated with worsening of most kinematic measurements. These results suggest that as the disease progresses, higher coactivation at the thigh level is the major source of the increasing walking impairment.

It is important to combine the information regarding muscle activation and joint kinematics to have a more comprehensive view of gait performance, which is fundamental for the clinicians to design more tailored rehabilitation protocols [29]. Thanks to the advance of technology, both sEMG and kinematics can be measured with wearable devices in the clinical setting. Additionally, wireless communication allows the remote transfer of data to laboratories and clinics for further analysis. This approach paves the way for remote assessment, as it is able to provide real-time information for both the patient and the clinician [6]. The costs for wearable devices used routinely in the clinical setting are usually lower compared with more sophisticated non-wearable equipment reserved to research laboratory environment [6]. These potential advantages make wearable devices a good candidate to be incorporated into home care and remote medicine, besides the hospital settings.

There are some limitations of the current study. First, the inertial sensor is not sensitive enough to reliably distinguish sub-phases of the stance cycle. All the data were reported as the performance of a whole gait cycle. However, for patients with a milder disability, the differences may only appear during the sub-phases. Second, as our cohort of patients was already characterized by moderate EDSS severity already indicating involvement of gait, we could not test whether kinematic parameters in the present study may be more sensitive than a clinical examination. Third, as the dual task has been performed with shoes, it is not possible to explore possible further worsening of gait measures under the combination of the two more difficult conditions (i.e., dual task with socks). Last, as the majority of our cohort included subjects with normal BMI, our results may not fully reflect the whole BMI variability.

5. Conclusions

Walking tests wearing socks should be discouraged to prevent falls for PwPMS. This concern should be embedded into guidelines for future remote medicine when these measurements can be performed during home care instead of hospital settings. The combined use of wearable accelerators and sEMG provide quantitative measurements of muscle activity and kinematics during walking, which can benefit future remote medicine programs, offering the opportunity to monitor disease progression and evaluate the efficiency of rehabilitation for PwPMS remotely.

Author Contributions: L.L.: Conceptualization, study design, method implementation, data collection supervision, analysis and interpretation, manuscript revision; L.G., G.L., M.C.: data collection; S.-C.H.: Data analysis; M.P.: data interpretation and manuscript revision; G.D.C.: statistical analysis and manuscript revision; S.C.H., L.G., G.L.: manuscript preparation; G.C.: manuscript revision for intellectual content. All authors have read and agreed to the published version of the manuscript.

References

1. Lassmann, H.; Bruck, W.; Lucchinetti, C.F. The immunopathology of multiple sclerosis: An overview. *Brain Pathol.* **2007**, *17*, 210–218. [CrossRef] [PubMed]

2. Institute of Medicine (US) Committee on Multiple Sclerosis. *Current Status and Strategies for the Future. Multiple Sclerosis: Current Status and Strategies for the Future*; Joy, J.E., Johnston, R.B., Jr., Eds.; National Academies Press: Washington, DC, USA, 2001.

3. Heesen, C.; Böhm, J.; Reich, C.; Kasper, J.; Goebel, M.; Gold, S.M. Patient perception of bodily functions in multiple sclerosis: Gait and visual function are the most valuable. *Mult. Scler. J.* **2008**, *14*, 988–991. [CrossRef] [PubMed]

4. Kalron, A.; Givon, U. Gait characteristics according to pyramidal, sensory and cerebellar EDSS subcategories in people with multiple sclerosis. *J. Neurol.* **2016**, *263*, 1796–1801. [CrossRef] [PubMed]

5. Lizama, L.E.C.; Khan, F.; Lee, P.V.; Galea, M.P. The use of laboratory gait analysis for understanding gait deterioration in people with multiple sclerosis. *Mult. Scler. J.* **2016**, *22*, 1768–1776. [CrossRef]

6. Shanahan, C.J.; Boonstra, F.M.C.; Lizama, L.E.C.; Strik, M.; Moffat, B.A.; Khan, F.; Kilpatrick, T.; Van Der Walt, A.; Galea, M.P.; Kolbe, S.C. Technologies for Advanced Gait and Balance Assessments in People with Multiple Sclerosis. *Front. Neurol.* **2018**, *8*, 708. [CrossRef] [PubMed]

7. Vítečková, S.; Horáková, H.; Poláková, K.; Krupička, R.; Růžička, E.; Brožová, H. Agreement between the GAITRite®System and the Wearable Sensor BTS G-Walk®for measurement of gait parameters in healthy adults and Parkinson's disease patients. *PeerJ* **2020**, *8*, e8835. [CrossRef]

8. Etemadi, Y. Dual task cost of cognition is related to fall risk in patients with multiple sclerosis: A prospective study. *Clin. Rehabil.* **2016**, *31*, 278–284. [CrossRef]

9. Larsen, E.R.; Mosekilde, L.; Foldspang, A. Correlates of falling during 24 h among elderly Danish community residents. *Prev. Med.* **2004**, *39*, 389–398. [CrossRef] [PubMed]

10. Menz, H.B.; Morris, M.E.; Lord, S.R. Footwear Characteristics and Risk of Indoor and Outdoor Falls in Older People. *Gerontology* **2006**, *52*, 174–180. [CrossRef]

11. Kelsey, J.L.; Procter-Gray, E.; Nguyen, U.-S.D.T.; Li, W.; Kiel, D.P.; Hannan, M.T. Footwear and falls in the home among older individuals in the MOBILIZE Boston Study. *Footwear Sci.* **2010**, *2*, 123–129. [CrossRef]

12. Coote, S.; Sosnoff, J.J.; Gunn, H. Fall Incidence as the Primary Outcome in Multiple Sclerosis Falls-Prevention Trials: Recommendation from the International MS Falls Prevention Research Network. *Int. J. MS Care* **2014**, *16*, 178–184. [CrossRef]

13. Leone, C.; Patti, F.; Feys, P. Measuring the cost of cognitive-motor dual tasking during walking in multiple sclerosis. *Mult. Scler. J.* **2014**, *21*, 123–131. [CrossRef] [PubMed]

14. Thompson, A.J.; Banwell, B.L.; Barkhof, F.; Carroll, W.M.; Coetzee, T.; Comi, G.; Correale, J.; Fazekas, F.; Filippi, M.; Freedman, M.S.; et al. Diagnosis of multiple sclerosis: 2017 revisions of the McDonald criteria. *Lancet Neurol.* **2018**, *17*, 162–173. [CrossRef]

15. ICH Harmonised Tripartite Guideline: Guideline for Good Clinical Practice. *J. Postgrad. Med.* **2001**, *47*, 199–203.

16. Unnithan, V.B.; Dowling, J.J.; Frost, G.; Ayub, B.V.; Bar-Or, O. Cocontraction and phasic activity during GAIT in children with cerebral palsy. *Electromyogr. Clin. Neurophysiol.* **1996**, *36*, 487–494. [PubMed]

17. Bohannon, R.W.; Smith, M.B. Interrater Reliability of a Modified Ashworth Scale of Muscle Spasticity. *Phys. Ther.* **1987**, *67*, 206–207. [CrossRef]

18. Hermans, G.; Clerckx, B.; Vanhullebusch, T.; Segers, J.; Vanpee, G.; Robbeets, C.; Casaer, M.P.; Wouters, P.; Gosselink, R.; Berghe, G.V.D. Interobserver agreement of medical research council sum-score and handgrip strength in the intensive care unit. *Muscle Nerve* **2011**, *45*, 18–25. [CrossRef]

19. Toomey, E.; Coote, S. Between-Rater Reliability of the 6-Minute Walk Test, Berg Balance Scale, and Handheld Dynamometry in People with Multiple Sclerosis. *Int. J. MS Care* **2013**, *15*, 1–6. [CrossRef]

20. Hobart, J.C.; Riazi, A.; Lamping, D.L.; Fitzpatrick, R.; Thompson, A.J. Measuring the impact of MS on walking ability: The 12-Item MS Walking Scale (MSWS-12). *Neurology* **2003**, *60*, 31–36. [CrossRef]

21. Krupp, L.B.; LaRocca, N.G.; Muir-Nash, J.; Steinberg, A.D. The fatigue severity scale. Application to patients with multiple sclerosis and systemic lupus erythematosus. *Arch. Neurol.* **1989**, *46*, 1121–1123. [CrossRef]

22. Hobart, J.C.; Riazi, A.; Thompson, A.J.; Styles, I.M.; Ingram, W.; Vickery, P.J.; Warner, M.; Fox, P.J.; Zajicek, J. Getting the measure of spasticity in multiple sclerosis: The Multiple Sclerosis Spasticity Scale (MSSS-88). *Brain* **2005**, *129*, 224–234. [CrossRef]

23. Farrar, J.T.; Troxel, A.B.; Stott, C.; Duncombe, P.; Jensen, M.P. Validity, reliability, and clinical importance of change in a 0–10 numeric rating scale measure of spasticity: A post hoc analysis of a randomized, double-blind, placebo-controlled trial. *Clin. Ther.* **2008**, *30*, 974–985. [CrossRef]

24. Guzzo, A.; Meggiolaro, A.; Mannocci, A.; Tecca, M.; Salomone, I.; La Torre, G. Conley Scale: Assessment of a fall risk prevention tool in a General Hospital. *J. Prev. Med. Hyg.* **2015**, *56*, E77–E87.

25. Ottenbacher, K.J.; Hsu, Y.; Granger, C.V.; Fiedler, R.C. The reliability of the functional independence measure: A quantitative review. *Arch. Phys. Med. Rehabil.* **1996**, *77*, 1226–1232. [CrossRef] [PubMed]

26. Mahoney, F.I.; Barthel, D.W. Functional Evaluation: The Barthel Index. *Md. State Med. J.* **1965**, *14*, 61–65. [PubMed]

27. Berg, K.O.; Wood-Dauphinee, S.L.; Williams, J.I.; Maki, B. Measuring balance in the elderly: Validation of an instrument. *Can. J. Public Health* **1992**, *83*, S7–S11.

28. Boudarham, J.; Hameau, S.; Zory, R.; Hardy, A.; Bensmail, D.; Roche, N. Coactivation of Lower Limb Muscles during Gait in Patients with Multiple Sclerosis. *PLoS ONE* **2016**, *11*, e0158267. [CrossRef]

29. Papagiannis, G.I.; Triantafyllou, A.I.; Roumpelakis, I.M.; Zampeli, F.; Eleni, P.G.; Koulouvaris, P.; Papadopoulos, E.C.; Papagelopoulos, P.J.; Babis, G.C. Methodology of surface electromyography in gait analysis: Review of the literature. *J. Med. Eng. Technol.* **2019**, *43*, 59–65. [CrossRef]

14

Preliminary Assessment of Burn Depth by Paper-Based ELISA for the Detection of Angiogenin in Burn Blister Fluid

Shin-Chen Pan [1,2]**, Yao-Hung Tsai** [3]**, Chin-Chuan Chuang** [3] **and Chao-Min Cheng** [3,*]

[1] Department of Surgery, Section of Plastic and Reconstructive Surgery, National Cheng Kung University Hospital, College of Medicine, National Cheng Kung University, Tainan 704, Taiwan; pansc@mail.ncku.edu.tw

[2] International Center for Wound Repair and Regeneration, National Cheng Kung University, Tainan 704, Taiwan

[3] Institute of Biomedical Engineering and Frontier Research Center on Fundamental and Applied Sciences of Matters, National Tsing Hua University, No. 101, Sec. 2, Kuang-Fu Rd., East Dist., Hsinchu 300, Taiwan; michaeltsai45@gmail.com (Y.-H.T.); jason20011122@gmail.com (C.-C.C.)

* Correspondence: chaomin@mx.nthu.edu.tw

Abstract: Rapid assessment of burn depth is important for burn wound management. Superficial partial-thickness burn (SPTB) wounds heal without scars, but deep partial-thickness burn (DPTB) wounds require a longer healing time and have a higher risk of scar formation. We previously found that DPTB blister fluid displayed a higher angiogenin level than SPTB blister fluid by conventional ELISA. In this study, we developed a paper-based ELISA (P-ELISA) technique for rapid assessment of angiogenin concentration in burn blister fluid. We collected six samples of SPTB blister fluid, six samples of DPTB blister fluid, and seven normal healthy serum samples for analysis. We again chose ELISA to measure and compare angiogenin levels across all of our samples, but we developed a P-ELISA tool and compared sample results from that tool to the results from conventional ELISA. As with conventional ELISA, DPTB blister fluid displayed higher angiogenin levels than SPTB in P-ELISA. Furthermore, our P-ELISA results showed a moderate correlation with conventional ELISA results. This new diagnostic technique facilitates rapid and convenient assessment of burn depth by evaluating a key molecule in burn blister fluid. It presents a novel and easy-to-learn approach that may be suitable for clinically determining burn depth with diagnostic precision.

Keywords: partial-thickness burn injury; burn blister fluid; P-ELISA; angiogenin; burn wound healing

1. Introduction

Burn wound prognosis depends on early and rapid diagnosis of burn depth. Superficial partial-thickness burn (SPTB) wounds heal spontaneously within two weeks of injury without scar formation. However, deep partial-thickness burn (DPTB) wounds take more than two weeks to heal and often result in hypertrophic scar formation if no aggressively surgical management. Optimal management of DPTB wounds can prevent skin scarring. Several methods were reported to assess the wound depth, including biopsy, thermography, laser Doppler techniques, and bedside clinical judgment [1]. Clinical observations are the gold standard for estimating clinical outcomes [2]. However, clinical assessment and prognosis of second-degree burn wounds with intact blisters become difficult in some cases, even for experienced surgeons. Measurements of tissue perfusion in injured wounds appear to be an option to assess tissue damage extent [3]. Although laser Doppler perfusion imaging was reported to be an efficient tool to evaluate blood flow of burn wounds [4–6], this machine is not readily available in all clinical settings.

Burn blisters, common to both SPTB and DPTB, are formed by an inflammatory response in early burn injury and exist between the epidermis and dermis [7]. The cytokines found in burn blister fluid can also be generated by activated or injured parenchymal cells after appropriate stimulation [8]. In our previous study, we observed that SPTB and DPTB blister fluids expressed different levels of angiogenin. When compared with SPTB, DPTB blister fluids displayed a higher angiogenin level [9]. In addition, angiogenin promoted in vitro angiogenesis such as endothelial cell proliferation and differentiation of circulating angiogenic cells as well as in vivo neovascularization [9]. Angiogenin, originally identified from a conditioned culture medium of colon cancer cells [10], is a potent angiogenic inducer and an independent prognostic factor in many cancers [11]. Because the angiogenin levels of SPTB and DPTB blister fluids were significantly different, the measurement of angiogenin in burn blister fluids can be used as a novel, noninvasive, or minimally invasive tool for surveying burn wound status.

ELISA is a well-established diagnostic tool for evaluating disease activity and assessing burn depth via analysis of fluid contents [9,12]. However, commercial ELISA kits are expensive, time-consuming, and are only available in clinical settings equipped with an ELISA reader. In order to simplify and expand clinical use of ELISA for early and efficient assessment of burn wounds, the development of a low-cost and rapid diagnostic tool for assessing burn depth is vital. Dot immunoassays on nitrocellular and filter papers is an established diagnostic tool [13–15]. Paper-based ELISA (P-ELISA), first developed by the Whitesides Research Group [16], has been an established diagnostic tool for decades. It is a useful procedure for performing immunoassays using a piece of filter paper for antibody–antigen recognition and has been applied for the diagnosis of infectious diseases (e.g., HIV and dengue fever), ophthalmological diseases (e.g., proliferative diabetic retinopathy, age-related macular degeneration), female genital diseases, and bullous pemphigoid [17–20]. The advantages of P-ELISA include speed, cost, small sample demands, and similar levels of sensitivity and specificity compared to conventional plate ELISA. Due to differential angiogenin levels between SPTB and DPTB blister fluids, the objective of this study is to develop a new application of the P-ELISA tool for the measurement of angiogenin expression in burn blister fluids in order to diagnose burn depth and facilitate improved burn wound care. Through conducting a small amount of clinical testing, we prove the clinical applicability of the device and guide the engineering process for further point-of-care and care-at-home devices with potential pre/clinical applications [21,22].

2. Material and Methods

2.1. Patient Samples

In order to study the differential expression of angiogenin in burn blisters from wounds of different depths, burn blister fluids were blindly aspirated with a needle from individually intact blisters within the first 3 days following injury and before identification of burn depth. Blister fluids were not classified into superficial or deep groups when fluids were harvested. Burn depth was confirmed by retrospective review of patient data according to healing status after the wound was healed. SPTB wounds were defined as those that healed within 14 days, and DPTB wounds were defined as those that required more than 14 days to heal or required burn wound debridement in the early assessment of wounds. Exclusion criteria included any potential bias such as fever, wound infection, or other severe medical problems including end-stage renal disease. Blood serum samples taken from healthy subjects were regarded as control samples. Informed consent was obtained from all patients, and study procedures were conducted in accordance with the Declaration of Helsinki and were approved by the Ethics Committee of National Cheng Kung University Hospital (No. A-ER-106-239, approval date 11 November 2017). All experiments were performed in accordance with relevant guidelines and regulations.

2.2. Preparation of Paper-Based 96-Well Plates Via Wax Printing

We designed a wax printing method for patterning Whatman No.1 filter papers (GE Healthcare, Buckinghamshire, UK) [20]. Briefly, a 96-well template was designed on a computer with Microsoft Office and then printed onto paper with wax. Complete, paper-depth hydrophobic barriers were created by melting the paper with printed-on wax at 105 °C for 5 min. Paper is highly permeable, which allows the wax to penetrate into the fiber matrix and then solidify to form defined hydrophobic barriers. This process is well-established and easy to complete.

2.3. Procedure of Paper-Based ELISA and Plate ELISA

Test zones were initially rinsed with 2 μL of Tris-buffered saline (TBS). Three microliters of burn fluid sample was then loaded onto the test zone and allowed to rest for 10 min. The test zone was then blocked with 3 μL 1% bovine serum albumin (BSA) for 10 min before adding 3 μL of rabbit anti-human angiogenin polyclonal primary antibody (Cat. No.: ab95389. Abcam, Cambridge, UK) and waiting another 10 min. Test zones were subsequently washed with 5 μL TBST (TBS+0.05% Tween 20), and then washed again with 10 μL TBST for a total of 2 washes. The washing process relied on a piece of blotting paper at the bottom to remove the washing buffer with capillary force. After washing, the test zone was incubated for 10 min with anti-rabbit IgG secondary antibody conjugated with horseradish peroxidase (HRP, Cat. No.: ab6721. Abcam, Cambridge, UK) before being washed again with 5 μL and 10 μL TBST (two washes). The color of the tested paper was developed after incubation with 3 μL of substrate solution (3,3′,5,5′-Tetramethylbenzidine (TMB): H_2O_2 = 1:1, Cat. No.: 555214. BD, Franklin Lakes, New Jersey, USA) for 10 min. The image signal was recorded using a camera at two time periods: (1) after 10 min of incubation with a secondary antibody; and (2) after 10 min of reaction time with the substrate solution. Both images were processed with Photocap software and analyzed with ImageJ software. To determine color intensity change, before and after images were first converted into 8-bit grayscale. Mean intensity was determined by comparing grayscale value differences from before and after images. Further normalization of the results was achieved by expressing values in terms of relative intensity, which was defined as (mean intensity of [experiment group]−mean intensity of [control group])/mean intensity of [control group]). Plate ELISA (Cat. No.: ab10600. Abcam, Cambridge, UK; Avastin® (bevacizumab), Roche, Basel, Switzerland) was used to measure the angiogenin and VEGF (Vascular endothelial growth factor) values in burn blister fluids. Each sample was applied in triplicate, and the average data from two plates were taken as final readouts. Values were expressed as mean ± SD. To also examine the role of pH on burn wound status, burn blister fluid pH values were collected with pH test strips (Cat. No.: 92111. Machery-Nagel, Düren, DE).

2.4. Data Analysis

Differences in angiogenin levels between SPTB and DPTB blister fluids was assessed using the Mann–Whitney U test. Analysis of variance was used to determine statistical differences among multiple groups. The relationship between the titer from the conventional plate ELISA and the relative intensity of P-ELISA was correlated using Pearson's correlation coefficient. Values of $p < 0.05$ were considered statistically significant. The results were expressed as mean ± SD.

3. Results

We have attempted to analyze the angiogenin levels in burn blister fluids to assess burn depth using P-ELISA. To determine optimal primary antibody concentration, we examined colorimetric responses to different dosages of recombinant angiogenin antibody on test paper impregnated with blister fluid. The results showed that 1 μg /mL of anti-angiogenin antibody provided the best signal. (Figure S1). To achieve the best staining with minimal background interference, we tested three different concentrations (0.05, 0.04, and 0.033 μg/mL) of secondary antibody. After testing serial dilutions of secondary antibody, we found that 0.033 μg/mL demonstrated the highest signal-to-background ratio for our primary antibody (Figure S2). We washed the test paper twice, first with 5 μL of TBST solution and then again with 10 μL of TBST solution, to remove unbound material. To determine optimal BSA concentration during the blocking step, we coated filter paper with different concentrations (1%, 0.5%, 0.1%) of blocking solution and compared reaction results to blister fluid harvested from DPTB patients and control blood serum. Mirroring the expected conventional plate ELISA results, our data showed that 1% of BSA displayed the best blocking effect for burn blister fluid when compared to our healthy human blood serum control (Figure S3). In addition to optimizing blocking, determining the best washing volume is essential for removing unbound reagents and reducing background signal. Unlike the conventional plate ELISA wash volume of 300 μL, P-ELISA requires only minute wash volumes. We tested the efficacy of three different wash solution amounts, 15 μL, 10 μL, and 5 μL, and found that three separate washes (the typical number of washes for conventional ELISA) with 5 μL removed all unbound nonspecific material (Figure S4). While the typical number of washes with conventional ELISA is three, we discovered that two cycles, one with 5 μL of wash buffer and one with 10 μL of wash buffer, provided the lowest background and strongest signal strength for P-ELISA (Figure S5).

Paper-based diagnostics provide a low-cost and easy-to-handle approach for studying a variety of target factors. Here, we demonstrated this approach by adding burn blister fluids and select reagents to test zones to detect angiogenin levels. As shown in Figure 1, burn fluid was added by hand, reagent was spotted onto each test zone, and the reaction was allowed to proceed for several minutes. Primary and secondary antibody were then added and optimized washing processes carried out to remove unbound antibody from the paper. Colorimetric responses were digitally recorded before and after color development. By analyzing the change in grayscale intensity of before and after images, we could determine the amount of angiogenin in burn blister fluids.

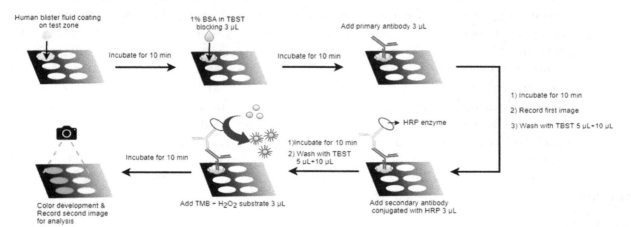

Figure 1. Procedure of paper-based ELISA (P-ELISA) for angiogenin analysis in burn blister fluid. Three microliters of burn fluid was loaded onto the test zone, and the test paper was incubated for 10 min. Three microliters of 1% BSA was then added for blocking, and the test paper was incubated for 10 min. The first image was recorded after loading 3 μL primary antibody, and the test paper was incubated for 10 min. The test paper was washed with 5 μL and then 10 μL TBST (Tris-buffered saline + 0.05% Tween 20) before adding 3 μL of horseradish peroxidase (HRP)-conjugated secondary antibody. The final procedure was to wash again with TBST and add 3 μL of substrate solution. After 10 min of incubation, we recorded the second image.

Relative mean intensity for angiogenin from SPTB burn blister fluids (Figure 2a) and DPTB burn blister fluids (Figure 2b) were tested and compared. In keeping with our previous study results, we found that angiogenin levels were significantly higher in DPTB fluids (4.2 ± 1.5, 95% confidence interval, 1.3–6.5, $n = 6$) than SPTB fluids (1.4 ± 0.3, 95% confidence interval, 0–4.0, $n = 6$) and healthy blood serum samples (0.9 ± 0.3, 95% confidence interval, 0.4–1.2, N = 7, $p < 0.01$) as measured by P-ELISA (Figure 2c). This demonstrates the reliability of P-ELISA to determine burn severity by evaluating angiogenin levels in burn blister fluids. Burn fluid samples have previously been tested via conventional ELISA plates for angiogenin and VEGF. Angiogenin is a downstream molecule of VEGF-regulated angiogenesis [23]. Observation of the role of VEGF in burn wound determination is interesting. Although no significant differences in VEGF were observed (SPTB: 31.5 ± 3.6 ng/mL, 95% confidence interval, 20.0–42.9 ng/mL, DPTB: 47.1 ± 10.9 ng/mL, 95% confidence interval, 16.8–77.5 ng/mL), there was a trend for higher angiogenin concentration in DPTB fluids compared with SPTB fluids as determined by conventional plate ELISA analysis (SPTB: 119.2 ± 28.4 ng/mL, 95% confidence interval, 28.8–209.6 ng/mL, DPTB: 331.5 ± 81.0 ng/mL, 95% confidence interval, 123.3–539.7 ng/mL, Figure 3, Table S1). No significant differences in VEGF level were observed between two different burn fluids, as shown in Figure 3, which was consistent with our previous study and another study indicating that VEGF was not responsible for differentiation of circulating angiogenic cells [9] or tumor growth and angiogenesis [23]. The consistent comparability of our P-ELISA results with conventional plate ELISA results was further supported by a correlation test using Pearson's correlation analysis. A moderate positive correlation (rho = 0.5906, p = 0.0722) between the titer of the plate ELISA and the relative intensity of P-ELISA was observed and is displayed in Figure 4.

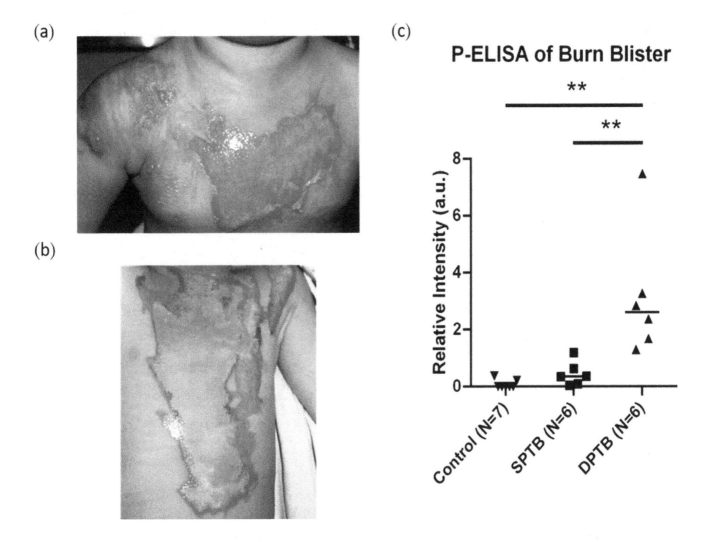

Figure 2. Analysis of angiogenin levels from superficial partial-thickness burn (SPTB) and deep partial-thickness burn (DPTB) blister fluids using P-ELISA. (**a,b**) Clinical pictures of superficial partial-thickness burn (SPTB, **a**) and deep partial-thickness burn (DPTB, **b**) wounds. (**c**) Comparison of angiogenin levels from two different burn fluids and healthy human blood serum as the control (n = 6 in SPTB and DPTB, n = 7 in control, mean ± S.D, ** p < 0.01).

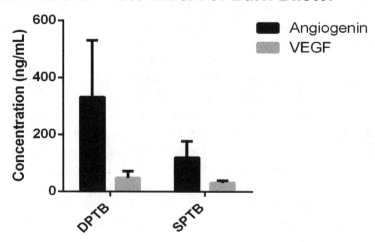

Figure 3. Analysis of angiogenin and VEGF (Vascular endothelial growth factor) concentrations in SPTB and DPTB blister fluids with conventional plate ELISA. A trend toward higher angiogenin concentration in DPTB fluids was detected, compared to SPTB ($n = 4$ in SPTB, $n = 6$ in DPTB, mean ± S.D.; $p = 0.07$). No significant difference in VEGF levels was observed between two different blister fluids ($n = 4$ in SPTB, $n = 5$ in DPTB, mean ± S.D.; $p = 0.26$).

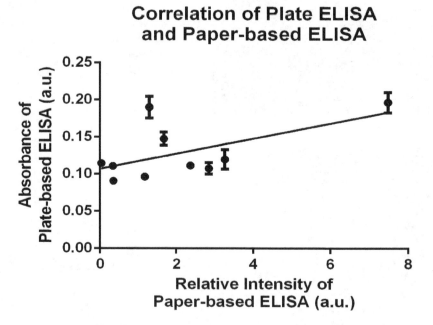

Figure 4. Correlation of the angiogenin detection between conventional plate ELISA and paper-based ELISA in burn blister fluids. The data show a moderate correlation between the results of P-ELISA and conventional plate ELISA ($r = 0.5906$, $p = 0.0722$).

In our laboratory, we have developed and explored the capacities for P-ELISA made of simple filter paper. To support the concept of P-ELISA material and process viability, we used patterned filter paper to collect directly absorbed blister fluid from human burn wounds (Supporting Movie) and had the test paper delivered to our laboratory on dry ice within 24 h, where we used it to successfully detect angiogenin levels via P-ELISA (Figure 5).

P-ELISA for Clinical Test

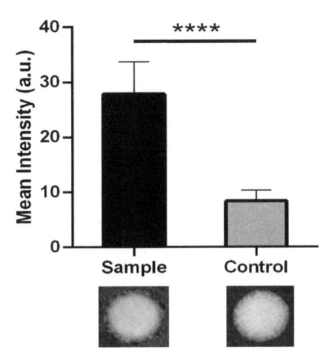

Figure 5. Clinical examination of angiogenin concentration by paper-based ELISA. Test paper was designed to absorb blister fluid from burn patients. Angiogenin signals were captured and analyzed. The mean intensity of detected angiogenin in burn blister fluid was significantly higher than that in normal serum control (mean ± S.D.; **** $p < 0.0001$, $n = 6$).

4. Discussion

Advances in diagnostic techniques have allowed clinicians to monitor disease severity in a rapid and noninvasive fashion. With regard to diagnosis of patients with ocular disease, P-ELISA provided a fast and sensitive VEGF assay of aqueous humor to monitor diseases such as senile cataracts, proliferative diabetic retinopathy, age-related macular degeneration, and retinal vein occlusion [17]. P-ELISA has also demonstrated the capacity for complex material collection capacity and multivalue measurement. It has, for instance, been used for outer macromolecule elimination and inner cervicovaginal fluid absorption to detect lactate concentration, glycogen concentration, and pH value in female genital diseases [19]. For patients with bullous pemphigoid, P-ELISA also delivered a simpler and faster diagnostic tool for detection of noncollagenous 16A (NC16A). By examining NC16A concentration with P-ELISA, bullous pemphigoid presence and disease state can be easily identified [20].

Previous concepts for burn depth assessment depend on measurements of tissue perfusion [24]. Laser Doppler imaging (LDI) studies are one of the most popular clinical techniques to assess burn depth. LDI is advantageous due to high accuracy and reduced invasiveness [25–27]. However, most clinical experiences using these modalities do not include examinations with intact blisters, which is a confounding factor that may skew analyzed results.

In this study, we sought to determine the burn depth by measuring angiogenin levels in burn blister fluid using the P-ELISA method. Evaluation of burn fluid contents by conventional ELISA has been successfully used to measure burn depth [9]. However, the necessity for longer operation duration severely hampered plate ELISA techniques for clinical practice. P-ELISA features operation process advantages compared to conventional plate ELISA. This P-ELISA technique required only 15 μL of reagent and an hour of processing compared to the 550 μL and 7 h–8 h required for conventional plate ELISA. Additionally, conventional plate ELISA requires a plate reader and P-ELISA results can be recorded with a camera (Table 1). Altogether, P-ELISA offers clear advantages for rapid and minimally invasive burn depth diagnosis and wound management. It may provide an easy and cost-effective method for any healthcare provider to assess burn wounds with excellent diagnostic precision and without the obstacle of a learning curve. However, P-ELISA is still conducted in a qualitative manner till now. Further refinement is needed to improve our device.

Table 1. Comparison of paper-based ELISA and conventional plate ELISA.

	Paper-Based ELISA		Conventional Plate ELISA	
antigen	angiogenin		angiogenin	
Primary antibody	Rabbit polyclonal anti-human angiogenin		Mouse monoclonal anti-human angiogenin	
Secondary antibody	Goat anti-rabbit lgG (HRP)		Goat anti-mouse lgG (HRP)	
Enzyme/substrate	HRP/TMB + H_2O_2		HRP/TMB + H_2O_2	
Detection device	camera		plate reader	
analysis	qualitative		quantitative	
Time and reagents	Volume (μL)	Time (min)	Volume (μL)	Time (min)
(1) antigen immobilization	3	10	50	120
(2) blocking	3	10	200	120
(3) primary antibody	3	10	100	120
(4) secondary antibody	3	10	100	120
(5) signal amplification	3	10	100	15
total	15	50	550	495

Wound pH may affect the healing process. A lower pH value was reported to be favorable for wound healing [28]. One study showed that healing burn wounds displayed a lower pH level (7.32) compared to unhealing burn wounds (pH 7.73) [29]. We observed an elevated alkaline pH value (8–9) in our burn fluid samples (Table S1). Aspiration of burn fluids in the early stages of injury may be responsible for this phenomenon. This finding is also consistent with a previous study showing that initial stages of healing generated a more basic pH compared to the relatively acidic environment of a repaired wound [30].

We feel that P-ELISA shows great promise for potential use in clinical practice. Although the clinical application of P-ELISA in burn wound assessment remains to be further studied, we look forward to seeing the application of this new technique in burn wounds. More cases are needed to verify our hypothesis prior to clinical adoption. Further optimization of the paper pattern and additional clinical trials will improve and advance the process and its implementation as a possible tool for healthcare.

5. Conclusions

We designed a less-invasive and faster method to assess burn depth using P-ELISA to determine angiogenin levels from burn blister fluid. This approach is cost-effective, easy to use, and potentially accurate. Despite a moderate correlation between conventional plate ELISA and P-ELISA, we demonstrated that P-ELISA is feasible to quantify blister angiogenin levels with distinct results to diagnose SPTB and DPTB wounds. We expect this novel medicine study to pave a possible path toward a simple diagnostic method for assessing burn depth without difficulty.

Author Contributions: Conceptualization, S.-C.P. and C.-M.C.; data curation, Y.-H.T. and C.-C.C.; formal analysis, Y.-H.T.; funding acquisition, S.-C.P. and C.-M.C.; investigation, Y.-H.T. and C.-C.C.; methodology, Y.-H.T.; project administration, C.-M.C.; resources, S.-C.P. and C.-M.C.; supervision, C.-M.C.; writing–original draft, S.-C.P.; Writing–review and editing, C.-M.C. All authors have read and agreed to the published version of the manuscript.

References

1. Monstrey, S.; Hoeksema, H.; Verbelen, J.; Pirayesh, A.; Blondeel, P. Assessment of burn depth and burn wound healing potential. *Burns* **2008**, *34*, 761–769. [CrossRef] [PubMed]
2. Heimbach, D.; Engrav, L.; Grube, B.; Marvin, J. Burn depth: A review. *World J. Surg.* **1992**, *16*, 10–15. [CrossRef]
3. Atiyeh, B.S.; Gunn, S.W.; Hayek, S.N. State of the art in burn treatment. *World J. Surg.* **2005**, *29*, 131–148. [CrossRef]
4. Pape, S.A.; Skouras, C.A.; Byrne, P.O. An audit of the use of laser Doppler imaging (LDI) in the assessment of burns of intermediate depth. *Burns* **2001**, *27*, 233–239. [CrossRef]
5. Droog, E.J.; Steenbergen, W.; Sjoberg, F. Measurement of depth of burns by laser Doppler perfusion imaging. *Burns* **2001**, *27*, 561–568. [CrossRef]
6. Holland, A.J.; Martin, H.C.; Cass, D.T. Laser Doppler imaging prediction of burn wound outcome in children. *Burns* **2002**, *28*, 11–17. [CrossRef]
7. Lawrence, C. Treating minor burns. *Nurs Times* **1989**, *85*, 69–73.
8. Gillitzer, R.; Goebeler, M. Chemokines in cutaneous wound healing. *J. Leukoc Biol.* **2001**, *69*, 513–521.
9. Pan, S.C.; Wu, L.W.; Chen, C.L.; Shieh, S.J.; Chiu, H.Y. Angiogenin expression in burn blister fluid: Implications for its role in burn wound neovascularization. *Wound Repair Regen.* **2012**, *20*, 731–739. [CrossRef]
10. Fett, J.W.; Strydom, D.J.; Lobb, R.R.; Alderman, E.M.; Bethune, J.L.; Riordan, J.F.; Vallee, B.L. Isolation and characterization of angiogenin, an angiogenic protein from human carcinoma cells. *Biochemistry* **1985**, *24*, 5480–5486. [CrossRef]
11. Katona, T.M.; Neubauer, B.L.; Iversen, P.W.; Zhang, S.; Baldridge, L.A.; Cheng, L. Elevated expression of angiogenin in prostate cancer and its precursors. *Clin. Cancer Res.* **2005**, *11*, 8358–8363. [CrossRef] [PubMed]
12. Pan, S.C.; Wu, L.W.; Chen, C.L.; Shieh, S.J.; Chiu, H.Y. Deep partial thickness burn blister fluid promotes neovascularization in the early stage of burn wound healing. *Wound Repair Regen.* **2010**, *18*, 311–318. [CrossRef] [PubMed]
13. Hawkes, R.; Niday, E.; Gordon, J. A dot-immunobinding assay for monoclonal and other antibodies. *Anal. Biochem.* **1982**, *119*, 142–147. [CrossRef]
14. Beyer, C.F. A 'dot-immunobinding assay' on nitrocellulose membrane for the determination of the immunoglobulin class of mouse monoclonal antibodies. *J. Immunol. Methods* **1984**, *67*, 79–87. [CrossRef]
15. Hawkes, R. The dot immunobinding assay. *Methods Enzymol.* **1986**, *121*, 484–491.
16. Cheng, C.M.; Martinez, A.W.; Gong, J.; Mace, C.R.; Phillips, S.T.; Carrilho, E.; Mirica, K.A.; Whitesides, G.M. Paper-based ELISA. *Angew. Chem. Int. Ed. Engl.* **2010**, *49*, 4771–4774. [CrossRef]
17. Hsu, M.Y.; Yang, C.Y.; Hsu, W.H.; Lin, K.H.; Wang, C.Y.; Shen, Y.C.; Chen, Y.C.; Chau, S.F.; Tsai, H.Y.; Cheng, C.M. Monitoring the VEGF level in aqueous humor of patients with ophthalmologically relevant diseases via ultrahigh sensitive paper-based ELISA. *Biomaterials* **2014**, *35*, 3729–3735. [CrossRef]
18. Wang, H.K.; Tsai, C.H.; Chen, K.H.; Tang, C.T.; Leou, J.S.; Li, P.C.; Tang, Y.L.; Hsieh, H.J.; Wu, H.C.; Cheng, C.M. Cellulose-based diagnostic devices for diagnosing serotype-2 dengue fever in human serum. *Adv. Healthc Mater* **2014**, *3*, 187–196. [CrossRef]
19. Cheng, J.Y.; Feng, M.J.; Wu, C.C.; Wang, J.; Chang, T.C.; Cheng, C.M. Development of a Sampling Collection Device with Diagnostic Procedures. *Anal. Chem.* **2016**, *88*, 7591–7596. [CrossRef]
20. Hsu, C.K.; Huang, H.Y.; Chen, W.R.; Nishie, W.; Ujiie, H.; Natsuga, K.; Fan, S.T.; Wang, H.K.; Lee, J.Y.; Tsai, W.L.; et al. Paper-based ELISA for the detection of autoimmune antibodies in body fluid-the case of bullous pemphigoid. *Anal. Chem.* **2014**, *86*, 4605–4610. [CrossRef]
21. Chan, W.C.W.; Udugama, B.; Kadhiresan, P.; Kim, J.; Mubareka, S.; Weiss, P.S.; Parak, W.J. Patients, Here Comes More Nanotechnology. *ACS Nano.* **2016**, *10*, 8139–8142. [CrossRef] [PubMed]
22. Marquez, S.; Morales-Narváez, E. Nanoplasmonics in Paper-Based Analytical Devices. *Front. Bioeng. Biotechnol.* **2019**, *7*, 69. [CrossRef] [PubMed]
23. Kishimoto, K.; Liu, S.; Tsuji, T.; Olson, K.A.; Hu, G.F. Endogenous angiogenin in endothelial cells is a general requirement for cell proliferation and angiogenesis. *Oncogene* **2005**, *24*, 445–456. [CrossRef] [PubMed]
24. Devgan, L.; Bhat, S.; Aylward, S.; Spence, R.J. Modalities for the assessment of burn wound depth. *J. Burns Wounds.* **2006**, *5*, e2.
25. Park, D.H.; Hwang, J.W.; Jang, K.S.; Han, D.G.; Ahn, K.Y.; Baik, B.S. Use of laser Doppler flowmetry for estimation of the depth of burns. *Plast Reconstr Surg.* **1998**, *101*, 1516–1523. [CrossRef]

26. O'Reilly, T.J.; Spence, R.J.; Taylor, R.M.; Scheulen, J.J. Laser Doppler flowmetry evaluation of burn wound depth. *J. Burn Care Rehabil.* **1989**, *10*, 1–6. [CrossRef]

27. Anselmo, V.J.; Zawacki, B.E. Multispectral photographic analysis. A new quantitative tool to assist in the early diagnosis of thermal burn depth. *Ann. Biomed. Eng.* **1977**, *5*, 179–193. [CrossRef]

28. Schneider, L.A.; Korber, A.; Grabbe, S.; Dissemond, J. Influence of pH on wound-healing: A new perspective for wound-therapy? *Arch. Dermatol Res.* **2007**, *298*, 413–420. [CrossRef]

29. Sharpe, J.R.; Booth, S.; Jubin, K.; Jordan, N.R.; Lawrence-Watt, D.J.; Dheansa, B.S. Progression of wound pH during the course of healing in burns. *J. Burn Care Res.* **2013**, *34*, e201–e208. [CrossRef]

30. Murphy, G.R.; Dunstan, R.H.; Macdonald, M.M.; Gottfries, J.; Roberts, T.K. Alterations in amino acid metabolism during growth by Staphylococcus aureus following exposure to H_2O_2—A multifactorial approach. *Heliyon* **2018**, *4*, e00620. [CrossRef]

15

Simulating Arbitrary Electrode Reversals in Standard 12-Lead ECG

Vessela Krasteva [1,*], **Irena Jekova** [1] **and Ramun Schmid** [2]

[1] Institute of Biophysics and Biomedical Engineering, Bulgarian Academy of Sciences, Acad. G. Bonchev Str. Bl 105, 1113 Sofia, Bulgaria; irena@biomed.bas.bg

[2] Signal Processing, Schiller AG, Altgasse 68, CH-6341 Baar, Switzerland; ramun.schmid@schiller.ch

[*] Correspondence: vessika@biomed.bas.bg

Abstract: Electrode reversal errors in standard 12-lead electrocardiograms (ECG) can produce significant ECG changes and, in turn, misleading diagnoses. Their detection is important but mostly limited to the design of criteria using ECG databases with simulated reversals, without Wilson's central terminal (WCT) potential change. This is, to the best of our knowledge, the first study that presents an algebraic transformation for simulation of all possible ECG cable reversals, including those with displaced WCT, where most of the leads appear with distorted morphology. The simulation model of ECG electrode swaps and the resultant WCT potential change is derived in the standard 12-lead ECG setup. The transformation formulas are theoretically compared to known limb lead reversals and experimentally proven for unknown limb–chest electrode swaps using a 12-lead ECG database from 25 healthy volunteers (recordings without electrode swaps and with 5 unicolor pairs swaps, including red (right arm—C1), yellow (left arm—C2), green (left leg (LL) —C3), black (right leg (RL)—C5), all unicolor pairs). Two applications of the transformation are shown to be feasible: 'Forward' (simulation of reordered leads from correct leads) and 'Inverse' (reconstruction of correct leads from an ECG recorded with known electrode reversals). Deficiencies are found only when the ground RL electrode is swapped as this case requires guessing the unknown RL electrode potential. We suggest assuming that potential to be equal to that of the LL electrode. The 'Forward' transformation is important for comprehensive training platforms of humans and machines to reliably recognize simulated electrode swaps using the available resources of correctly recorded ECG databases. The 'Inverse' transformation can save time and costs for repeated ECG recordings by reconstructing the correct lead set if a lead swap is detected after the end of the recording. In cases when the electrode reversal is unknown but a prior correct ECG recording of the same patient is available, the 'Inverse' transformation is tested to detect the exact swapping of the electrodes with an accuracy of (96% to 100%).

Keywords: ECG electrode swaps; ECG electrode potentials; WCT potential change; reconstructing correct ECG leads; MSMinv transformation; unicolor limb–chest electrodes

1. Introduction

The routine use of the standard 12-lead electrocardiogram (ECG) for noninvasive clinical investigation of acute and chronic cardiovascular diseases makes it very important to ensure the generation of diagnostically interpretable ECG leads [1]. An essential problem in the recording of multilead ECGs is the improper placing of the electrodes on the patient's body [2], reported to be as frequent as 0.8% and 7.5% for limb lead reversals in 12-lead ECG and Holter devices, respectively [3]; 0.4% and 4% for 12-lead ECG interchanges in clinical and intensive care settings, respectively [4]. Errors in electrode placement can lead to significant ECG changes that could confuse physicians and affect the clinical diagnosis. Studies and case reports dedicated to this problem are further grouped in the following three categories according to the affected ECG electrodes:

- *Reversals between limb electrodes* are reported to provoke deep QS complexes and inverted T waves in leads (II, III, aVF) that could be misdiagnosed as old myocardial infarctions (MI) involving the inferior heart wall [5]. Right arm (RA) and left arm (LA) interchange is associated with inverted T waves in leads (I, aVL) suggestive of lateral wall MI [6] as well as indicative of ECG features of dextrocardia [7]. RA and right leg (RL) swap results in low-amplitude QRS complexes in lead II [7,8] and all other frontal leads resembling scaled variations of lead III and changed QRS axes in the frontal plane [8]. LA and left leg (LL) reversal creates suspicions of inferior-wall MI [7]. RA and LL swap could be confused for the combined features of lateral wall MI and low atrial rhythm [7].

- *Reversals between chest electrodes* have been found to provoke erroneous diagnosis in 17% to 24% of cases involving wrongly placed C1 electrodes [9]. Generally, when another precordial lead is substituted for V1, the result is a tall R wave in V1, which could be taken as a sign of right bundle branch block, left ventricular ectopy, right ventricular hypertrophy, acute right ventricular dilation, Type A Wolff-Parkinson-White syndrome, posterior MI, hypertrophic cardiomyopathy, progressive muscular dystrophy or dextrocardia [10].

- *Reversals between limb and chest electrodes* are a possible scenario due to the matching colors of the two ECG cables [11] or the incorrect attachment of the cable connectors to the junction box of the ECG machine [12]. C2/LA (yellow) cable interchange is described in two case reports [13,14] to have produced right axis deviation and Q waves in (III, aVF), accompanied by an inverted T wave in both leads, together with a quick transition in V2 with qR complex and an inverted T wave. The ECGs are interpreted as an inferior MI with residual ischemia in [13] or recent inferior and a posterior MI [14]. Limb/precordial cable interchange has been observed to result in tall R waves in aVR, negative QRS complexes in the other five limb leads and inverted ST elevation/depression in some of the leads. Thus, inferior, anterior, and lateral MI could be erroneously diagnosed [12]. In another study [15], the authors suspect the same interchange to have resulted in ST-segment elevation in the inferior leads; however, their thesis has been impugned by [16], who have explained the wandering ST elevation with medical reasons.

Such studies indicate that special measures should be taken to ensure the correct placement of ECG electrodes, e.g., staff training has been reported to improve electrode placement by 50% [17], while combined training and technical improvements have succeeded to reduce the rate of electrode cable reversals from 4.8 % down to 1.2 % [18]. ECG changes induced by ECG cable reversals have been analyzed in a number of studies [19–24]. Methods for the automatic detection of ECG electrode reversals within the limb and precordial set have been proposed, such as:

- *Limb leads:* LA and LL reversal is indicated by P wave amplitude [25] and QRS, P-axes [26]; RA and RL interchange is detected when lead II presents as a flat line [27] or with peak-to-peak amplitude less than 185 μV [8]; LA-RA and RA-LL swaps are recognized by analysis of P and QRS frontal axes and clockwise vector loop rotation direction, R and T wave amplitudes in leads (I, II) [28]; various LA/RA/LL/RL combinations are detected by a number of analytical approaches based on the assessment of the QRS axis [29,30], together with P wave amplitudes [31], direction of P-loop inscription and/or frontal P-axis [32]; lead reconstruction using redundancy of information in eight independent leads [33]; morphological measurements of QRS, P-wave amplitudes, frontal axis and clockwise vector loop rotation, combined with redundancy features [34]; maximal and minimal QRS, T-wave amplitudes in leads (I, II, III) [35]; correlation coefficients of limb leads vs. V6 [36,37]; combining the features described in [26] and [33] for a more robust and accurate performance [36].

- *Chest leads:* Different reversal sets have been examined, such as five reversals of adjacent leads (V1/V2, V2/V3, V3/V4, V4/V5, V5/V6), analyzed by P, QRS and ST-T measurements [26] and PQ-RS amplitude distances [31]; nine reversals (five adjacent leads, V1/V3, V4/V6, V4/V5/V6/V1/V2/V3, V6/V5/V4/V3/V2/V1) are evaluated via correlations between measured and reconstructed leads [33]; seven reversals (five adjacent leads, V1/V3, V4/V6) are handled by processing of both morphology and redundancy features [34]; 15 reversals, including all possible pairwise V1–V6 swaps, have been tested in our previous study by applying analysis of inter-lead correlation coefficients [38].

- *Limb and chest leads:* Interchanges between limb and C2 precordial electrodes specific for a telemonitoring system are detected by correlation to a previously recorded ECG [39]. This early work, together with our recent publication on the unicolor electrode interchange detection [11], are the only studies dealing with recognition of reversals between limb and precordial leads.

The methods for the detection of ECG cable reversals should be designed/tested using dedicated databases. Only a few of the mentioned studies [7,19,27,35,39,40] use real ECG recordings with erroneous electrode placements, which are, however, small-sized and proprietary. Typically, reversal detection algorithms are trained and validated using databases with correctly recorded 12-lead ECGs and simulated reversals within the limb lead set [11,26,28–34,36,38] or the precordial lead set [11,26,31,33,34,38], where the Wilson's central terminal (WCT) is not changed. All other reversals modifying the WCT, such as swaps between the limb and precordial electrodes, have not been simulated, although they are quite possible and should be detected due to the distorted morphology of most leads [6,8,21]. For example, the interactive web-based tool [41] for the rendering of ECG leads from body surface potential maps (BSPM) separately simulates two effects—precordial lead misplacement (by linear interpolation from neighboring BSPM leads) or limb lead interchange. However, considering that this tool uses bulky BSPM data and does not allow for electrode misplacements that change WCT potential, it has restricted application for machine learning on large arrhythmia datasets with arbitrary ECG electrode reversals.

We have not found in the literature an algebraic transformation that can simulate all possible ECG electrode reversals. This paper presents the formula of such a transformation and its application in the standard 12-lead ECG setup, computing reordered leads and the WCT potential change from the correctly recorded leads. Additionally, we show the applicability of this method for reconstructing the correct leads from an ECG recorded with known electrode reversals, as well as for detection of the exact electrodes that were swapped, provided there are at least two ECGs from the same patient.

2. Methods

2.1. Derivation of the Transformation Formula

The presented transformation formula can be used to simulate reversals between arbitrary ECG electrodes in the standard 12-lead ECG, although the final transformation formula can be extended to an arbitrary number of leads.

According to the fundamental principles of electrocardiography [42], standard 12-lead ECG systems (Figure 1) use 10 electrodes on the LA, RA, LL, RL and 6 precordial positions (C1-C6), and acquire 8 independent signals (e.g. leads I, II, V1-V6):

$$\left| \begin{array}{l} I = P_E(LA) - P_E(RA) \\ II = P_E(LL) - P_E(RA) \\ V_X = P_E(C_X) - P_{WCT} = P_E(C_X) - \frac{P_E(LL) + P_E(RA) + P_E(LA)}{3} \end{array} \right. \tag{1}$$

where:

- P_E denotes the electrical potential of the respective electrodes, also referred to as the raw electrode biopotential.
- (I, II) are the bipolar leads measuring the potential differences between limbs (LA-RA, LL-RA), forming the Einthoven's triangle.

- V_X represents any of the unipolar chest leads (*V1-V6*) measuring the potential of the chest electrodes against the reference WCT potential (P_{WCT}), which is defined to be the average of the RA, LA and LL electrodes.
- Note that the ground electrode placed on the RL is used for technical reasons (driven right leg) and does not have direct influence on any ECG leads.

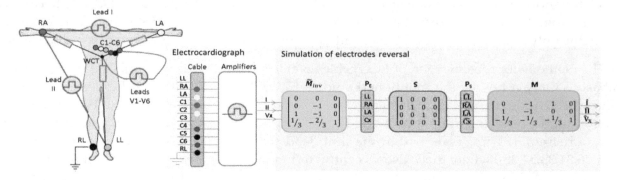

Figure 1. Acquisition of 12-lead ECG via a 10-electrode cable with standard IEC color coding, recording 8 independent leads I, II, V1-V6 (denoted as Vx) in the ECG device. The flow diagram shows the simulation of reversals between LL, RA, LA and one chest electrode (denoted as Cx) by conversion of the recorded leads (I, II, Vx) to reordered leads ($\hat{I}$, $\widehat{II}$, $\widehat{V}_X$) using the matrix transformations $\widetilde{M}_{inv}$, **S**, **M**. The specific example shows an identity **S** matrix that corresponds to the correct order of LL, RA, LA, Cx electrodes. Other estimates of the **S** matrix are presented on Figure 2 and Section 4.1 in the description of different examples for electrode reversals.

The calculations in (1) are usually performed by the input circuits in ECG devices. As soon as an electrode swap can lead to a change in the WCT potential, it becomes difficult to imagine the changes in the standard 12-lead ECG. Therefore, the derivation and handling of the electrode potentials corresponding to the nine active ECG electrodes with respect to a common reference point is the main target of further mathematical transformations.

The basic 12-lead ECG computations (1) can also be presented using the matrix notation:

$$\begin{bmatrix} I \\ II \\ V_X \end{bmatrix} = \begin{bmatrix} 0 & -1 & 1 & 0 \\ 1 & -1 & 0 & 0 \\ -\frac{1}{3} & -\frac{1}{3} & -\frac{1}{3} & 1 \end{bmatrix} \begin{bmatrix} P_E(LL) \\ P_E(RA) \\ P_E(LA) \\ P_E(C_X) \end{bmatrix} = \mathbf{M} \begin{bmatrix} 0 \\ P_E(RA) \\ P_E(LA) \\ P_E(C_X) \end{bmatrix}, \tag{2}$$

where **M** is the matrix that converts the raw electrode potentials $P_E(LL)$, $P_E(RA)$, $P_E(LA)$ and $P_E(Cx)$ into leads I, II, Vx. Formula (2) shows the setting ($P_E(LL) = 0$), which defines our choice that $P_E(LL)$ is the reference potential. This is an arbitrary choice because we can set any electrode as the reference one without changing the final outcome of our derivations. We can further simplify (2):

$$\begin{bmatrix} I \\ II \\ V_X \end{bmatrix} = \begin{bmatrix} -1 & 1 & 0 \\ -1 & 0 & 0 \\ -\frac{1}{3} & -\frac{1}{3} & 1 \end{bmatrix} \begin{bmatrix} P_E(RA) \\ P_E(LA) \\ P_E(C_X) \end{bmatrix} = \mathbf{M_F} \begin{bmatrix} P_E(RA) \\ P_E(LA) \\ P_E(C_X) \end{bmatrix}, \tag{3}$$

where $\mathbf{M_F}$ is a full-rank matrix that is further inverted ($\mathbf{M_F^{-1}}$) for solving of the opposite task for the conversion of leads into body electrode potentials:

$$\begin{bmatrix} P_E(RA) \\ P_E(LA) \\ P_E(C_X) \end{bmatrix} = \mathbf{M_F^{-1}} \begin{bmatrix} I \\ II \\ V_X \end{bmatrix} = \begin{bmatrix} 0 & -1 & 0 \\ 1 & -1 & 0 \\ \frac{1}{3} & -\frac{2}{3} & 1 \end{bmatrix} \begin{bmatrix} I \\ II \\ V_X \end{bmatrix}. \tag{4}$$

Further, $\mathbf{M}_F^{-1}$ is extended so that (4) is able to reproduce the electrical potential of the left leg, using the definition $(P_E(LL) = 0)$:

$$
\begin{bmatrix} P_E(LL) \\ P_E(RA) \\ P_E(LA) \\ P_E(C_X) \end{bmatrix} = \begin{bmatrix} & 0 & 0 & 0 & \\ & & \mathbf{M}_F^{-1} & & \end{bmatrix} \begin{bmatrix} I \\ II \\ V_X \end{bmatrix} = \begin{bmatrix} 0 & 0 & 0 \\ 0 & -1 & 0 \\ 1 & -1 & 0 \\ \frac{1}{3} & -\frac{2}{3} & 1 \end{bmatrix} \begin{bmatrix} I \\ II \\ V_X \end{bmatrix} = \tilde{\mathbf{M}}_{\text{inv}} \begin{bmatrix} I \\ II \\ V_X \end{bmatrix},
\tag{5}
$$

where $\tilde{\mathbf{M}}_{\text{inv}}$ is the matrix that allows the computation of the raw body electrode potentials in the order $\{P_E(LL), P_E(RA), P_E(LA), P_E(C_X)\}$ using the recorded leads $\{I, II, Vx\}$. Once the body electrode potentials are known, they can be reordered to simulate an arbitrary reversal between ECG electrodes. The simulated electrode order can be algebraically described by a binary swap matrix ($\mathbf{S}$), which equals an identity matrix for the correct order:

$$
\begin{bmatrix} P_S(\widehat{LL}) \\ P_S(\widehat{RA}) \\ P_S(\widehat{LA}) \\ P_S(\widehat{C_X}) \end{bmatrix} = \begin{bmatrix} 1 & 0 & 0 & 0 \\ 0 & 1 & 0 & 0 \\ 0 & 0 & 1 & 0 \\ 0 & 0 & 0 & 1 \end{bmatrix} \begin{bmatrix} P_E(LL) \\ P_E(RA) \\ P_E(LA) \\ P_E(C_X) \end{bmatrix} = \mathbf{S} \begin{bmatrix} P_E(LL) \\ P_E(RA) \\ P_E(LA) \\ P_E(C_X) \end{bmatrix}
\tag{6}
$$

where P_S denotes the simulated electrical potential at the respective electrode $\{\widehat{LL}, \widehat{RA}, \widehat{LA}, \widehat{C_X}\}$. Different examples of matrix $\mathbf{S}$ are further given in Section 4.1 upon the description of the performed theoretical simulations of electrode reversals.

The correspondence between the leads recorded by the ECG device (I, II, Vx) and the reordered leads ($\hat{I}$, $\hat{II}$, $\hat{V}_X$) after the simulation of ECG electrode reversals can be calculated by substituting successively (6) and (5) into (2):

$$
\begin{bmatrix} \hat{I} \\ \hat{II} \\ \hat{V}_X \end{bmatrix} = \mathbf{M} \begin{bmatrix} P_S(\widehat{LL}) \\ P_S(\widehat{RA}) \\ P_S(\widehat{LA}) \\ P_S(\widehat{C_X}) \end{bmatrix} = \mathbf{M}\mathbf{S}\tilde{\mathbf{M}}_{\text{inv}} \begin{bmatrix} I \\ II \\ V_X \end{bmatrix}.
\tag{7}
$$

The flow diagram of (7), further denoted as 'MSMinv' transformation, which is presented on Figure 1, clearly indicates the embedded logic of matrix operations that have a general applicability to simulate arbitrary configurations of electrode swaps. It is just necessary to adapt the values of the matrices $\mathbf{M}, \mathbf{S}, \tilde{\mathbf{M}}_{\text{inv}}$ to the specific lead configuration, assuming that the derived mathematical proof shows the full set of two independent bipolar limb leads in 12-lead ECG (can be reduced) and one unipolar lead (can be deleted or extended to multiple unipolar leads by copy of the row (C_X) in $\mathbf{M}, \tilde{\mathbf{M}}_{\text{inv}}$ and expand S accordingly).

Note that the matrices in the 'MSMinv' transformation (7) take into account only the potentials of the active input electrodes, excluding the grounded RL. The result of a swap of an arbitrary active electrode with RL can be, however, approximated by setting the potential of the swapped active electrode equal to the LL potential in the matrix $\mathbf{S}$ (6):

$$
P_S(\text{swapped electrode to RL}) = P_E(RL) \approx P_E(LL)
\tag{8}
$$

The assumption for equipotential legs can be considered from an anatomical perspective because the leg recording sites are sufficiently distant and similarly oriented to the heart, thus attaining the same electrical signal generated by the myocardium [24]. Generally, both (RL, LL) potentials are essentially very similar that is typically adopted in the known ECG lead transformations of rotated RL with other peripheral electrodes [7,8,21,22].

Another application of the derived mathematical transformations is the calculation of the WCT potential change due to ECG electrode swaps:

$$\Delta P_{WCT} = \hat{P}_{WCT} - P_{WCT}, \tag{9}$$

where P_{WCT} and $\hat{P}_{WCT}$ are the WCT potentials before and after the electrode swap, respectively. Both can be derived as a function of the recorded leads (I, II, Vx) with a reference to a zero LL potential ($P_E(LL) = 0$), as assumed in Equations (2) and (5):

$$P_{WCT} = \mathbf{W}\begin{bmatrix} P_E(LL) \\ P_E(RA) \\ P_E(LA) \\ P_E(C_X) \end{bmatrix} = \mathbf{W}\tilde{\mathbf{M}}_{inv}\begin{bmatrix} I \\ II \\ V_X \end{bmatrix} \tag{10}$$

$$\hat{P}_{WCT} = \mathbf{W}\begin{bmatrix} P_S(\widehat{LL}) \\ P_S(\widehat{RA}) \\ P_S(\widehat{LA}) \\ P_S(\widehat{C_X}) \end{bmatrix} = \mathbf{W}\mathbf{S}\tilde{\mathbf{M}}_{inv}\begin{bmatrix} I \\ II \\ V_X \end{bmatrix}, \tag{11}$$

where $\mathbf{W} = \begin{bmatrix} 1/3 & 1/3 & 1/3 & 0 \end{bmatrix}$ is the matrix that transforms electrode potentials into WCT potential, taking the potentials for the correct electrode position $\{P_E(LL), P_E(RA), P_E(LA), P_E(C_X)\}$ from (5) and for the swapped position $\{P_S(\widehat{LL}), P_S(\widehat{RA}), P_S(\widehat{LA}), P_S(\widehat{C_X})\}$ from (6) and (5). Although WCT potential is calculated only from the potentials of the three limb electrodes $(\widehat{LL}, \widehat{RA}, \widehat{LA})$, Equation (11) covers the general option for a swap between some of them and the unipolar electrode $(\widehat{C_X})$.

Substituting (10) and (11) in (9) gives the generalized notation of the 'WSMinv' transformation that is further used for estimating of the relative WCT potential change during different simulated swaps:

$$\Delta P_{WCT} = (\mathbf{W}\mathbf{S} - \mathbf{W})\tilde{\mathbf{M}}_{inv}\begin{bmatrix} I \\ II \\ V_X \end{bmatrix}. \tag{12}$$

2.2. Verification of 'MSMinv' Transformation

The correctness of the 'MSMinv' transformation (7) is verified by two approaches, depending on the kind of simulated ECG electrode reversals:

- *ECG electrode reversals with known lead transforms* are theoretically studied. For this purpose, the formula for computation of the reordered leads ($\hat{I}$, $\hat{II}$, $\hat{V}_X$) is directly compared to the published lead transformations. This simple approach is applicable only to reversals between peripheral electrodes, widely analyzed in the literature [5,7,12,21,24,36–38,43].
- *ECG electrode reversals with unknown lead transformations* (such as reversals between limb and chest electrodes) are experimentally studied with a dedicated database (described in Section 3). For this purpose, the 8 independent leads $L_R = (I_R, II_R, V1_R - V6_R)$ of 2 recordings from the same person (RC, taken with correct electrode position; RS, taken with real electrode swap) are compared in three different scenarios:

    - (L_{RC} vs. L_{RS}): *No transformation* is applied to study the lead-specific differences between recordings with correct vs. swapped electrodes.
    - ($\widehat{L_{RC}}$ vs. L_{RS}): *Forward 'MSMinv' transformation* is applied on the recording with correct lead set to simulate lead swap $(\widehat{L_{RC}} = \mathbf{M}\mathbf{S}\tilde{\mathbf{M}}_{inv}L_{RC})$ and to study the lead-specific differences of simulated vs. recorded electrode reversals (L_{RS}).

○ (L_{RC} *vs.* $\widetilde{L_{RS}}$): *Inverse 'MSMinv' transformation* is applied on the recording with reversed lead set to simulate correct electrode positions ($\widetilde{L_{RS}} = \mathbf{M\tilde{S}M}_{inv}L_{RS}$) and to study the lead-specific differences of simulated vs. recorded, correctly placed electrodes (L_{RC}).

The lead-specific differences in each of the above 3 scenarios (denoted as $\widetilde{L_{RC}}$ *vs.* $\widetilde{L_{RS}}$) are estimated for the average beat ($BEAT_i$), indexed within a window of 500ms ($i = QRS_f - 150ms$ to $QRS_f + 350ms$, where QRS_f denotes the QRS fiducial point), using three quantitative measures:

○ Root-mean-square error:

$$RMS\ Error = \sqrt{\frac{1}{500ms * Fs} \sum \left(BEAT_i\left(\widetilde{L_{RC}}\right) - BEAT_i\left(\widetilde{L_{RS}}\right)\right)^2}, \tag{13}$$

where Fs denotes the sampling frequency of the average beat.

○ Peak error:

$$Peak\ Error = \max\left(\left|BEAT_i\left(\widetilde{L_{RC}}\right) - BEAT_i\left(\widetilde{L_{RS}}\right)\right|\right). \tag{14}$$

○ Correlation coefficient:

$$CorCoef = \frac{\sum BEAT_i\left(\widetilde{L_{RC}}\right).BEAT_i\left(\widetilde{L_{RS}}\right)}{\sqrt{\sum BEAT_i^2\left(\widetilde{L_{RC}}\right). \sum BEAT_i^2\left(\widetilde{L_{RS}}\right).}} \tag{15}$$

Statistical results of all quantitative measurements over the whole ECG database are reported as a mean value and standard deviation (std). The level of significant differences between different scenarios is measured with paired Student's t-test and one-tailed p-value < 0.05.

3. Database

The database used for verification of the 'MSMinv' transformation contains 10s recordings of standard 12-lead resting ECGs taken from 25 volunteers with no history of heart diseases—gender: 28% (male), age: 49 ± 11 years (mean value ± standard deviation), 28–67 years (range). The ECGs are acquired via a 10-electrode cable with standard IEC color coding [44]. Six ECG recordings per subject are collected, applying prospective electrode cable reversals at the time of the recording, including:

- Correct positions of the electrodes (no electrode is swapped);
- Swap of red electrodes (RA-C1);
- Swap of yellow electrodes (LA-C2);
- Swap of green electrodes (LL-C3);
- Swap of black electrodes (RL-C5);
- Swap of all unicolor electrodes (RA-C1, LA-C2, LL-C3, RL-C5).

The ECG signals are recorded at 1 kHz sampling rate, 1 µV resolution, and pre-filtered in a bandwidth (0.5 to 25 Hz). Each 10s ECG recording is processed by a commercial ECG measurement and interpretation module (ETM, Schiller AG, Switzerland) for the extraction of a 12-lead average beat [45]. The average beats are commonly used for the measurement of ECG features with diagnostic precision because they provide higher signal-to-noise ratio and are more robust to respiration induced morphology changes than the single beats.

4. Results and Discussion

4.1. Theoretical Simulations of Electrode Reversals

This section simulates three major types of ECG electrode reversals (reversals of peripheral electrodes involving RL; not involving RL; reversals of peripheral and chest electrodes), applying

'WSMinv' transformation (12) for the calculation of WCT potential change (Table 1) and 'MSMinv' transformation (7) for the calculation of the reordered leads (Tables 2–4). Several general examples are shown on Figure 2. Details will be further discussed in Sections 4.1.1–4.1.3

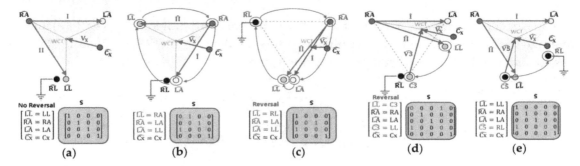

Figure 2. Classic depiction of the Einthoven's triangle, WCT and lead vectors (I, II, Vx), projected in the frontal plane for correct electrode position (**a**) and their displacement ($\hat{I}$, $\widehat{II},\hat{V}_X$) in case of four types of limb electrode reversals: (**b**) CW rotation of 3 active limb electrodes ($\widehat{RA} \rightarrow\widehat{LA}\rightarrow\widehat{LL}\rightarrow\widehat{RA}$); (**c**) CW rotation of 4 limb electrodes, including RL ($\widehat{RL}\rightarrow\widehat{RA}\rightarrow\widehat{LA}\rightarrow\widehat{LL}\rightarrow\widehat{RL}$); (**d**) swap of an active limb electrode and chest electrode, illustrated for the green couple ($\widehat{LL}\leftrightarrow\widehat{C3}$); (**e**) swap of the grounded and chest electrode, illustrated for the black couple ($\widehat{RL}\leftrightarrow\widehat{C5}$). The text with red font color highlights the electrodes in wrong geometrical positions, and the swap matrix entries different from the identity matrix in (**a**).

Table 1. Calculation of the WCT potential change from the recorded leads via the 'WSMinv' transformation (12), applying the swap matrices **S** in Tables 2–4.

Reversed Electrodes		ΔP_{WCT}
Reversals of peripheral electrodes not involving RL	■↔$\widehat{LA}$	0 *
	■↔$\widehat{LL}$	0 *
	$\widehat{LA}\leftrightarrow\widehat{LL}$	0 *
	CW rotation ■→$\widehat{LA}\rightarrow\widehat{LL}\rightarrow$■	0 *
	CCW rotation ■→$\widehat{LL}\rightarrow\widehat{LA}\rightarrow$■	0 *
Reversals of peripheral electrodes involving RL	$\widehat{RL}\leftrightarrow$■	$1/3II$
	$\widehat{RL}\leftrightarrow\widehat{LA}$	$1/3(II-I)$
	$\widehat{RL}\leftrightarrow\widehat{LL}$	0 *
	CW rotation with RL $\widehat{RL}\rightarrow$■$\rightarrow\widehat{LA}\rightarrow\widehat{LL}\rightarrow$RL	$1/3II$
	CCW rotation with RL $\widehat{RL}\rightarrow\widehat{LL}\rightarrow\widehat{LA}\rightarrow$■$\rightarrow$RL	0 *
	Bilateral arm–leg rotation $\widehat{RL}\leftrightarrow$■, $\widehat{LA}\leftrightarrow\widehat{LL}$	$1/3II$
	Cross rotation $\widehat{RL}\rightarrow$■$\rightarrow\widehat{LL}\rightarrow\widehat{LA}\rightarrow\widehat{RL}$	$1/3(II-I)$
Reversals of unicolor peripheral and chest electrodes	Red electrodes ■↔■	$1/9I + 1/9II + 1/3V_1$
	Yellow electrodes $\widehat{LA}\leftrightarrow\widehat{C2}$	$-2/9I + 1/9II + 1/3V_2$
	Green electrodes $\widehat{LL}\leftrightarrow\widehat{C3}$	$1/9I - 2/9II + 1/3V_3$
	Black electrodes $\widehat{RL}\leftrightarrow\widehat{C5}$	0 *
	All unicolor electrodes ■↔■, $\widehat{LA}\leftrightarrow\widehat{C2}$, $\widehat{LL}\leftrightarrow\widehat{C3}$, $\widehat{RL}\leftrightarrow\widehat{C5}$	$1/3(V_1 + V_2+V_3)$

Note: For comprehension purposes of various electrode combinations, the reversed electrodes are depicted with their respective colors according to the IEC color coding [44]. * $\Delta P_{WCT} = 0$ corresponds to the correct position of the active limb electrodes ($\widehat{LL}$, $\widehat{RA}$, $\widehat{LA}$).

4.1.1. Reversals of Peripheral Electrodes Not Involving RL

All 5 possible rotations of the 3 active limb electrodes ($\widehat{LL}$, $\widehat{RA}$, $\widehat{LA}$) are simulated (Table 2) and none of them is related to the displacement of WCT, as illustrated in the example of clockwise (CW) electrode rotation (Figure 2b), where the Einthoven's triangle remains geometrically unaffected. This is theoretically proven by the 'WSMinv' transformation (12), where all swap matrices **S** (Table 2) are consequently applied, and zero WCT potential differences to the correct electrode position ($\Delta P_{WCT} = 0$)

are detected (Table 1). The rearranged limb leads ($\hat{I}$, $\hat{II}$) obtained by the 'MSMinv' transformation (Table 2) match the expressions in other studies, applying geometrical perspectives between leads (I, II, III) [5,12,21,24,36–38]. Furthermore, the unipolar chest lead $\hat{V}_X$ is unchanged for all simulated swap matrices **S** that corresponds to the real case scenario of unchanged WCT (Figure 2a,b).

Table 2. Reversals of peripheral electrodes not involving RL.

Reversed Electrodes	S	MS$\tilde{\text{M}}_{\text{inv}}$	Reordered Leads
	■↔$\widehat{LA}$		
$\begin{bmatrix} \widehat{LL} = LL \\ \widehat{RA} = LA \\ \widehat{LA} = RA \\ \widehat{C_X} = C_X \end{bmatrix}$	$\begin{bmatrix} 1 & 0 & 0 & 0 \\ 0 & 0 & 1 & 0 \\ 0 & 1 & 0 & 0 \\ 0 & 0 & 0 & 1 \end{bmatrix}$	$\begin{bmatrix} -1 & 0 & 0 \\ -1 & 1 & 0 \\ 0 & 0 & 1 \end{bmatrix}$	$\hat{I} = -I$ $\hat{II} = -I + II = III$ $\hat{V}_X = V_X$
	■↔$\widehat{LL}$		
$\begin{bmatrix} \widehat{LL} = RA \\ \widehat{RA} = LL \\ \widehat{LA} = LA \\ \widehat{C_X} = C_X \end{bmatrix}$	$\begin{bmatrix} 0 & 1 & 0 & 0 \\ 1 & 0 & 0 & 0 \\ 0 & 0 & 1 & 0 \\ 0 & 0 & 0 & 1 \end{bmatrix}$	$\begin{bmatrix} 1 & -1 & 0 \\ 0 & -1 & 0 \\ 0 & 0 & 1 \end{bmatrix}$	$\hat{I} = I - II = -III$ $\hat{II} = -II$ $\hat{V}_X = V_X$
	$\widehat{LA}↔\widehat{LL}$		
$\begin{bmatrix} \widehat{LL} = LA \\ \widehat{RA} = RA \\ \widehat{LA} = LL \\ \widehat{C_X} = C_X \end{bmatrix}$	$\begin{bmatrix} 0 & 0 & 1 & 0 \\ 0 & 1 & 0 & 0 \\ 1 & 0 & 0 & 0 \\ 0 & 0 & 0 & 1 \end{bmatrix}$	$\begin{bmatrix} 0 & 1 & 0 \\ 1 & 0 & 0 \\ 0 & 0 & 1 \end{bmatrix}$	$\hat{I} = II$ $\hat{II} = I$ $\hat{V}_X = V_X$
	CW rotation ■→$\widehat{LA}$→$\widehat{LL}$→■		
$\begin{bmatrix} \widehat{LL} = RA \\ \widehat{RA} = LA \\ \widehat{LA} = LL \\ \widehat{C_X} = C_X \end{bmatrix}$	$\begin{bmatrix} 0 & 1 & 0 & 0 \\ 0 & 0 & 1 & 0 \\ 1 & 0 & 0 & 0 \\ 0 & 0 & 0 & 1 \end{bmatrix}$	$\begin{bmatrix} -1 & 1 & 0 \\ -1 & 0 & 0 \\ 0 & 0 & 1 \end{bmatrix}$	$\hat{I} = -I + II = III$ $\hat{II} = -I$ $\hat{V}_X = V_X$
	CCWrotation ■→$\widehat{LL}$→$\widehat{LA}$→■		
$\begin{bmatrix} \widehat{LL} = LA \\ \widehat{RA} = LL \\ \widehat{LA} = RA \\ \widehat{C_X} = C_X \end{bmatrix}$	$\begin{bmatrix} 0 & 0 & 1 & 0 \\ 1 & 0 & 0 & 0 \\ 0 & 1 & 0 & 0 \\ 0 & 0 & 0 & 1 \end{bmatrix}$	$\begin{bmatrix} 0 & -1 & 0 \\ 1 & -1 & 0 \\ 0 & 0 & 1 \end{bmatrix}$	$\hat{I} = -II$ $\hat{II} = I - II = -III$ $\hat{V}_X = V_X$

Note: For comprehension purposes of various electrode combinations, the reversed electrodes are depicted with their respective colors according to the IEC color coding [44], - *1st column:* The simulated placement of ECG electrodes $\{\widehat{LL}, \widehat{RA}, \widehat{LA}, \widehat{C_X}\}$ referring to their geometrical positions $\{LL, RA, LA, C_X\}$. The electrodes which are assumed to be in the wrong geometrical positions are indicated with red font color as being reversed. - *2nd column:* The values of the swap matrix **S**, where red font colored entries indicate the difference to the identity matrix as defined in (6) for the correct electrode placement. - *3rd column:* The result of matrix multiplication MS$\tilde{\text{M}}_{\text{inv}}$, considering **M** and $\tilde{\text{M}}_{\text{inv}}$ equal to their definitions in (2) and (5), respectively. - *4th column:* The formula for calculation of the reordered leads ($\hat{I}$, $\hat{II}$, $\hat{V}_X$) using the recorded leads (I, II, Vx) that is obtained after substituting MS$\tilde{\text{M}}_{\text{inv}}$ in (7). For simplification, the substitution ($III = II - I$) is applied in some formulas.

4.1.2. Reversals of Peripheral Electrodes Involving RL

Seven rotations of the 4 limb electrodes ($\widehat{LL}$, $\widehat{RA}$, $\widehat{LA}$, $\widehat{RL}$) are simulated (Table 3) and normally they should be related to the displacement of WCT, as illustrated in the example (Figure 2c), where the Einthoven's triangle is transformed to a thin 'slice'.

Table 1 shows that all electrode reversals present WCT potential change, depending only on the position of the neutral electrode RL, such that:

- RL is in the position of RA: $\Delta P_{WCT} = 1/3 II$
- RL is in the position of LA: $\Delta P_{WCT} = -1/3 I + 1/3 II$
- RL is in the position of LL: $\Delta P_{WCT} = 0$, where P_{WCT} is equal to the correct electrode placement.

Table 3. Reversals of peripheral electrodes involving RL.

Reversed Electrodes	S	MSM̃$_{inv}$	Reordered Leads
		RL↔■	
$\begin{bmatrix} \widehat{LL} = LL \\ \widehat{RA} = RL \\ \widehat{LA} = RA \\ \widehat{C_x} = C_x \end{bmatrix}$	$\begin{bmatrix} 1 & 0 & 0 & 0 \\ 1 & 0 & 0 & 0 \\ 0 & 0 & 1 & 0 \\ 0 & 0 & 0 & 1 \end{bmatrix}$	$\begin{bmatrix} 1 & -1 & 0 \\ 0 & 0 & 0 \\ 0 & -1/3 & 1 \end{bmatrix}$	$\hat{I} = I - II = -III$ $\hat{II} = 0$ $\hat{V}_X = V_X - 1/3 II$
		RL↔L̂A	
$\begin{bmatrix} \widehat{LL} = LL \\ \widehat{RA} = RA \\ \widehat{LA} = RL \\ \widehat{C_x} = C_x \end{bmatrix}$	$\begin{bmatrix} 1 & 0 & 0 & 0 \\ 0 & 1 & 0 & 0 \\ 1 & 0 & 0 & 0 \\ 0 & 0 & 0 & 1 \end{bmatrix}$	$\begin{bmatrix} 0 & 1 & 0 \\ 0 & 1 & 0 \\ 1/3 & -1/3 & 1 \end{bmatrix}$	$\hat{I} = II$ $\hat{II} = II$ $\hat{V}_X = V_X - 1/3(II - I)$
		RL↔L̂L	
$\begin{bmatrix} \widehat{LL} = RL \\ \widehat{RA} = RA \\ \widehat{LA} = LA \\ \widehat{C_x} = C_x \end{bmatrix}$	$\begin{bmatrix} 1 & 0 & 0 & 0 \\ 0 & 1 & 0 & 0 \\ 0 & 0 & 1 & 0 \\ 0 & 0 & 0 & 1 \end{bmatrix}$	$\begin{bmatrix} 1 & 0 & 0 \\ 0 & 1 & 0 \\ 0 & 0 & 1 \end{bmatrix}$	$\hat{I} = I$ $\hat{II} = II$ $\hat{V}_X = V_X$
	CW rotation with RL	R̂L→■→L̂A→L̂L→R̂L	
$\begin{bmatrix} \widehat{LL} = RL \\ \widehat{RA} = LA \\ \widehat{LA} = LL \\ \widehat{C_x} = C_x \end{bmatrix}$	$\begin{bmatrix} 1 & 0 & 0 & 0 \\ 0 & 0 & 1 & 0 \\ 1 & 0 & 0 & 0 \\ 0 & 0 & 0 & 1 \end{bmatrix}$	$\begin{bmatrix} -1 & 1 & 0 \\ -1 & 1 & 0 \\ 0 & -1/3 & 1 \end{bmatrix}$	$\hat{I} = -I + II = III$ $\hat{II} = -I + II = III$ $\hat{V}_X = V_X - 1/3 II$
	CCW rotation with RL	R̂L→L̂L→L̂A→■→R̂L	
$\begin{bmatrix} \widehat{LL} = LA \\ \widehat{RA} = RL \\ \widehat{LA} = RA \\ \widehat{C_x} = C_x \end{bmatrix}$	$\begin{bmatrix} 0 & 0 & 1 & 0 \\ 1 & 0 & 0 & 0 \\ 0 & 1 & 0 & 0 \\ 0 & 0 & 0 & 1 \end{bmatrix}$	$\begin{bmatrix} 0 & -1 & 0 \\ 1 & -1 & 0 \\ 0 & 0 & 1 \end{bmatrix}$	$\hat{I} = -II$ $\hat{II} = I - II = -III$ $\hat{V}_X = V_X$
	Bilateral arm–leg rotation	R̂L↔■, L̂A↔L̂L	
$\begin{bmatrix} \widehat{LL} = LA \\ \widehat{RA} = RL \\ \widehat{LA} = LL \\ \widehat{C_x} = C_x \end{bmatrix}$	$\begin{bmatrix} 0 & 0 & 1 & 0 \\ 1 & 0 & 0 & 0 \\ 1 & 0 & 0 & 0 \\ 0 & 0 & 0 & 1 \end{bmatrix}$	$\begin{bmatrix} 0 & 0 & 0 \\ 1 & -1 & 0 \\ 0 & -1/3 & 1 \end{bmatrix}$	$\hat{I} = 0$ $\hat{II} = I - II = -III$ $\hat{V}_X = V_X - 1/3 II$
	Cross rotation	R̂L→■→L̂L→L̂A→R̂L	
$\begin{bmatrix} \widehat{LL} = RA \\ \widehat{RA} = RL \\ \widehat{LA} = LL \\ \widehat{C_x} = C_x \end{bmatrix}$	$\begin{bmatrix} 0 & 1 & 0 & 0 \\ 1 & 0 & 0 & 0 \\ 1 & 0 & 0 & 0 \\ 0 & 0 & 0 & 1 \end{bmatrix}$	$\begin{bmatrix} 0 & 0 & 0 \\ 0 & -1 & 0 \\ 1/3 & -1/3 & 1 \end{bmatrix}$	$\hat{I} = 0$ $\hat{II} = -II$ $\hat{V}_X = V_X - 1/3(II - I)$

Note: All columns correspond to the description in the footer of Table 2.

These results and the 'MSMinv' transformation (Table 3) are obtained with the general approximation for equipotential legs that is coded in the swap matrix **S** with an entry of '1' in the position of LL (first column) for both cases: $\{\hat{X} = LL,\ \hat{X} = RL\}$, whereas $\hat{X}$ denotes an arbitrary ECG electrode. Thus, all electrode reversals leading to a 'sliced' Einthoven's triangle with two tips on both legs appear with two '1' entries in the first column of matrix **S** (Table 3), while '1' is deficient in the second (RA) or third (LA) columns (equal to '0'). Only two reversals (RL-LL and the counter-clockwise (CCW) rotation with RL) have '1' entries in each of the first three columns of matrix **S** (corresponding to the three active limb electrodes in the Einthoven's triangle tips). Just for them, the WCT potential is correctly found to be unchanged (Table 1), although the reordered limb leads ($\hat{I}$, $\hat{II}$) in CCW rotation appear to be different (Table 3). Generally, all simulated reversals show that ($\hat{I}$, $\hat{II}$) leads, resulting from the 'MSMinv' transformation, are matching the expressions in other studies that have been derived by geometrical analysis of the leads, assuming "0" [6,12,19,21,22,24,35,36] or "near zero" signal <100 μV [5,7,8,38] for the lead between the active electrodes on both legs.

Considering the chest lead V_X, we find a correspondence between 'MSMinv' and 'WSMinv' transformations so that the reordered lead $\hat{V}_X = V_X - \Delta P_{WCT}$ (Table 3) is corrected exactly with the term ΔP_{WCT} (Table 1). Generally, no chest lead V_X is considered in case of limb leads reversals, so we cannot compare the derived $\hat{V}_X$ expressions to published studies. We can justify the unchanged $\hat{V}_X$ in both aforementioned reversals with WCT not being displaced (RL-LL and CCW rotation), as well as $\hat{V}_X = V_X - 1/3 II$ for the RL-RA reversal. This reversal has been analytically described in Haisty et al. [8], who explained that WCT potential difference is equal to one third of the difference between RA and RL potentials that approximates one third of the standard lead II.

Table 4. Reversals of unicolor chest and peripheral electrodes.

Reversed Electrodes	S	$MS\widetilde{M}_{inv}$	Reordered Leads
		Red electrodes ■↔■	
$\begin{bmatrix}\widehat{LL}=LL\\\widehat{RA}=C_1\\\widehat{LA}=LA\\\widehat{C_1}=RA\\\widehat{C_x}=C_x\end{bmatrix}$	$\begin{bmatrix}1&0&0&0&0\\0&0&0&1&0\\0&0&1&0&0\\0&1&0&0&0\\0&0&0&0&1\end{bmatrix}$	$\begin{bmatrix}2/3&-1/3&-1&0\\-1/3&2/3&-1&0\\-4/9&-4/9&-1/3&0\\-1/9&-1/9&-1/3&1\end{bmatrix}$	$\hat{I}=(I-III)/3-V_1$ $\hat{II}=(II+III)/3-V_1$ $\hat{V}_1=-\frac{4}{9}(I+II)-\frac{1}{3}V_1$ $\hat{V}_x=V_x-\frac{1}{9}(I+II)-\frac{1}{3}V_1$
		Yellow electrodes $\widehat{LA}\leftrightarrow\widehat{C2}$	
$\begin{bmatrix}\widehat{LL}=LL\\\widehat{RA}=RA\\\widehat{LA}=C_2\\\widehat{C_2}=LA\\\widehat{C_x}=C_x\end{bmatrix}$	$\begin{bmatrix}1&0&0&0&0\\0&1&0&0&0\\0&0&0&1&0\\0&0&1&0&0\\0&0&0&0&1\end{bmatrix}$	$\begin{bmatrix}1/3&1/3&1&0\\0&1&0&0\\8/9&-4/9&-1/3&0\\2/9&-1/9&-1/3&1\end{bmatrix}$	$\hat{I}=\frac{1}{3}(I+II)+V_2$ $\hat{II}=II$ $\hat{V}_2=\frac{4}{9}(I-III)-\frac{1}{3}V_2$ $\hat{V}_x=V_x+\frac{1}{9}(I-III)-\frac{1}{3}V_1$
		Green electrodes $\widehat{LL}\leftrightarrow\widehat{C3}$	
$\begin{bmatrix}\widehat{LL}=C_3\\\widehat{RA}=RA\\\widehat{LA}=LA\\\widehat{C_3}=LL\\\widehat{C_x}=C_x\end{bmatrix}$	$\begin{bmatrix}0&0&0&1&0\\0&1&0&0&0\\0&0&1&0&0\\1&0&0&0&0\\0&0&0&0&1\end{bmatrix}$	$\begin{bmatrix}1&0&0&0\\1/3&1/3&1&0\\-4/9&8/9&-1/3&0\\-1/9&2/9&-1/3&1\end{bmatrix}$	$\hat{I}=I$ $\hat{II}=\frac{1}{3}(I+II)+V_3$ $\hat{V}_3=\frac{4}{9}(II+III)-\frac{1}{3}V_3$ $\hat{V}_x=V_x+\frac{1}{9}(II+III)-\frac{1}{3}V_1$
		Black electrodes $\widehat{RL}\leftrightarrow\widehat{C5}$	
$\begin{bmatrix}\widehat{LL}=LL\\\widehat{RA}=RA\\\widehat{LA}=LA\\\widehat{C_5}=RL\\\widehat{C_x}=C_x\end{bmatrix}$	$\begin{bmatrix}1&0&0&0&0\\0&1&0&0&0\\0&0&1&0&0\\1&0&0&0&0\\0&0&0&0&1\end{bmatrix}$	$\begin{bmatrix}1&0&0&0\\0&1&0&0\\-1/3&2/3&0&0\\0&0&0&1\end{bmatrix}$	$\hat{I}=I$ $\hat{II}=II$ $\hat{V}_5=(II+III)/3$ $\hat{V}_x=V_x$
		All unicolor electrode pairs ■↔■, $\widehat{LA}\leftrightarrow\widehat{C2}$, $\widehat{LL}\leftrightarrow\widehat{C3}$, $\widehat{RL}\leftrightarrow\widehat{C5}$	
$\begin{bmatrix}\widehat{LL}=C_3\\\widehat{RA}=C_1\\\widehat{LA}=C_2\\\widehat{C_1}=RA\\\widehat{C_2}=LA\\\widehat{C_3}=LL\\\widehat{C_4}=C_4\\\widehat{C_5}=RL\\\widehat{C_6}=C_6\end{bmatrix}$	$\begin{bmatrix}0&0&0&0&0&1&0&0&0\\0&0&0&1&0&0&0&0&0\\0&0&0&0&1&0&0&0&0\\0&1&0&0&0&0&0&0&0\\0&0&1&0&0&0&0&0&0\\1&0&0&0&0&0&0&0&0\\0&0&0&0&0&0&1&0&0\\1&0&0&0&0&0&0&0&0\\0&0&0&0&0&0&0&0&1\end{bmatrix}$	$\begin{bmatrix}0&0&-1&1&0&0&0&0\\0&0&-1&0&1&0&0&0\\\frac{1}{3}&-\frac{1}{3}&\frac{1}{3}&-\frac{1}{3}&-\frac{1}{3}&0&0&0\\\frac{2}{3}&-\frac{1}{3}&-\frac{1}{3}&-\frac{1}{3}&-\frac{1}{3}&0&0&0\\-\frac{1}{3}&\frac{2}{3}&-\frac{1}{3}&-\frac{1}{3}&-\frac{1}{3}&0&0&0\\0&0&-\frac{1}{3}&-\frac{1}{3}&-\frac{1}{3}&1&0&0\\-\frac{1}{3}&\frac{2}{3}&-\frac{1}{3}&-\frac{1}{3}&-\frac{1}{3}&0&0&0\\0&0&-\frac{1}{3}&-\frac{1}{3}&-\frac{1}{3}&0&0&1\end{bmatrix}$	$\hat{I}=V_2-V_1$ $\hat{II}=V_3-V_1$ $\hat{V}_1=-\frac{I+II}{3}-\frac{V_1+V_2+V_3}{3}$ $\hat{V}_2=\frac{I-III}{3}-\frac{V_1+V_2+V_3}{3}$ $\hat{V}_3=\frac{II+III}{3}-\frac{V_1+V_2+V_3}{3}$ $\hat{V}_4=V_4-\frac{V_1+V_2+V_3}{3}$ $\hat{V}_5=\frac{II+III}{3}-\frac{V_1+V_2+V_3}{3}$ $\hat{V}_6=V_6-\frac{V_1+V_2+V_3}{3}$

Note: All columns correspond to the description in the footer of Table 2. Cx represents all chest electrodes with unchanged positions, Vx denotes their unipolar leads.

4.1.3. Reversals of Chest and Peripheral Electrodes

Five swaps are simulated (Table 4) involving the matching-color electrode pairs in the peripheral and precordial cables (IEC color coding standard [44]), i.e., red (RA-C1), yellow (LA-C2), green (LL-C3), black (RL-C5) and all pairs (RA-C1, LA-C2, LL-C3, RL-C5).

Figure 2d,e illustrates the two principal types of reversals where the unipolar chest electrode is swapped either with an active limb electrode (WCT is displaced in Figure 2d) or with the grounded electrode (WCT is not displaced in Figure 2e). In both cases, we highlight two types of unipolar leads:

- $\hat{V}x$ for the precordial electrodes $\hat{C}x$, which keep their position unchanged on the chest;
- $\hat{V}n$ for the precordial electrodes $\hat{C}n$, where n = 1,2,3,5 is substituting the chest electrode number, which changes its position to some of the limbs.

The calculation of two different unipolar leads is achieved by an extension of the swap matrix **S** (4×4) to (5×5) to include 3 limb electrodes and 2 chest electrodes ($\widehat{LL}$, $\widehat{RA}$, $\widehat{LA}$, $\hat{C}n$, $\hat{C}x$), as shown in Table 4 and Figure 2d,e. The last row of Table 4 presents the most complex example for simulation of swaps between all unicolor electrode pairs, which requires the use of a swap matrix **S** (9×9), configured for the full set of electrodes ($\widehat{LL}$, $\widehat{RA}$, $\widehat{LA}$, $\hat{C}1 - \hat{C}6$). All expressions of the rearranged leads ($\hat{I}$, $\hat{II}$, $\hat{V}x$, $\hat{V}n$) in Table 4 are further verified in the experimental study of Section 4.2 because they have not been investigated in any other study. The respective WCT potential changes (Table 1) cannot be compared to examples in the literature either. We can only justify the result for the RL-C5 reversal, which corresponds to non-displaced WCT, exactly as shown in the example (Figure 2e).

4.2. Experimental Verification of Simulated Swaps Between Unicolor Chest and Peripheral Electrodes

The experimental study is used to verify the 'MSMinv' transformation for simulation of reversals between unicolor chest and peripheral electrodes (using the expressions in Table 4), according to the concept in Section 2.2 (*ECG electrode reversals with unknown lead transformations*). For this purpose, all ECG recordings in the database are analyzed and the three measurements (RMS Error, Peak Error, CorCoef) are calculated to estimate the average beat waveform differences in 3 scenarios (Table 5):

- *No transformation*, showing the largest differences between correct vs. swapped electrode recordings for all leads because WCT is considerably displaced in most chest-limb reversals (except RL-C5). We note the greatest mean value differences for the unipolar lead with a chest electrode placed on the limbs:

    - V1 (120 μV, 529 μV, 0.832) for RA-C1,
    - V2 (246 μV, 1121 μV, 0.456) for LA-C2,
    - V3 (206 μV, 868 μV, 0.512) for LL-C3,
    - V5 (131 μV, 639 μV, 0.785) for RL-C5,
    - V1-V3 (225-289 μV, 967-1235 μV, 0.365-0.652) for all unicolor pairs.

- *Forward 'MSMinv' transformation*, simulating electrode reversals which have significantly reduced differences when compared to the recordings with really swapped electrodes ($p < 0.05$). We measure mean values (RMS Error, Peak Error, CorCoef) in the range (<20 μV, <60 μV, ≥0.995), assuming they represent negligible average beat differences mainly due to rhythm variation and signal acquisition noises in the compared recordings. We have noticed one exception for both reversals involving RL (RL-C5, all unicolor pairs), where the Forward 'MSMinv' transformation introduces a slight error in the calculation of the swapped lead V5 (≤26 μV, ≤104 μV, ≥0.986), assuming the C5 potential to be equal to LL, while C5 is placed on the RL (approximation error from the equipotential legs).

- *Inverse 'MSMinv' transformation*, recovering the correct electrode order, which has significantly reduced differences when compared to the recordings with really correct electrodes ($p < 0.05$), estimated within the above outlined range of negligible errors (<20 μV, <60 μV, ≥0.995). We have again found an exception for both reversals involving RL (RL-C5, all unicolor pairs), where the Inverse 'MSMinv' transformation fails to reconstruct the correct lead V5 (<142 μV, <660 μV, ≥0.792) from a recording with RL electrode in the position of C5 electrode. As soon as RL stops being an input to the ECG device, the potential of V5 electrode is lost and not reproduced by any active electrode in the swap matrix **S** (Table 4, all **S** entries are equal to '0' for the column, corresponding to C5).

Table 5. Statistical analysis (mean value ± standard deviation) of measures (RMS Error, Peak Error, CorCoef) calculated for the average beat in 8 independent leads (I, II, V1-V6), quantifying the lead-specific differences between experimentally recorded ECGs – raw leads vs. reordered leads (based on the expressions in Table 4) for 3 different scenarios:. No transformation; Forward 'MSMinv' transformation applied on the recording with correct electrodes; Inverse 'MSMinv' transformation applied on the recording with swapped electrodes.

Unicolor Reversals		RMS Error (µV)			Peak Error (µV)			Cor. Coef. (0–1)		
		Transf. None	Transf. MSMinv Forward	Transf. MSMinv Inverse	Transf. None	Transf. MSMinv Forward	Transf. MSMinv Inverse	Transf. None	Transf. MSMinv Forward	Transf. MSMinv Inverse
(RA-LA)	I	81 ± 40	14 ± 5 *	15 ± 5 *	351 ± 162	48 ± 19 *	53 ± 20 *	0.921 ± 0.093	0.997 ± 0.004 *	0.995 ± 0.006 *
	II	81 ± 38	13 ± 5 *	13 ± 4 *	356 ± 163	48 ± 19 *	46 ± 16 *	0.909 ± 0.172	0.998 ± 0.002 *	0.996 ± 0.005 *
	V1	120 ± 52	11 ± 4 *	11 ± 4 *	529 ± 227	38 ± 15 *	38 ± 13 *	0.832 ± 0.136	0.996 ± 0.002 *	0.998 ± 0.002 *
	Vx	27 ± 13	11 ± 5 *	12 ± 5 *	116 ± 61	44 ± 9 *	42 ± 18 *	0.989 ± 0.029	0.998 ± 0.003 *	0.998 ± 0.003 *
LA-C2	I	197 ± 80	16 ± 5 *	15 ± 5 *	924 ± 336	55 ± 20 *	54 ± 20 *	0.746 ± 0.144	0.997 ± 0.004 *	0.995 ± 0.005 *
	II	18 ± 5	13 ± 3 *	13 ± 3 *	78 ± 37	44 ± 12 *	46 ± 13 *	0.994 ± 0.013	0.995 ± 0.011 *	0.995 ± 0.009 *
	V2	246 ± 102	13 ± 6 *	13 ± 5 *	1121 ± 396	50 ± 25 *	54 ± 26 *	0.456 ± 0.180	0.990 ± 0.010 *	0.998 ± 0.002 *
	Vx	58 ± 5	12 ± 4 *	12 ± 5 *	264 ± 103	41 ± 16 *	47 ± 19 *	0.956 ± 0.073	0.998 ± 0.003 *	0.997 ± 0.003 *
LL-C3	I	15 ± 5	15 ± 5	15 ± 6	56 ± 27	54 ± 23	56 ± 26	0.996 ± 0.006	0.995 ± 0.006 *	0.995 ± 0.006 *
	II	154 ± 50	18 ± 5 *	15 ± 4 *	644 ± 228	59 ± 22 *	53 ± 20 *	0.869 ± 0.146	0.998 ± 0.001 *	0.995 ± 0.008 *
	V3	206 ± 65	12 ± 5 *	14 ± 5 *	868 ± 296	47 ± 25 *	53 ± 21 *	0.512 ± 0.197	0.988 ± 0.012 *	0.997 ± 0.004 *
	Vx	52 ± 18	12 ± 5 *	13 ± 5 *	219 ± 80	45 ± 23 *	46 ± 20 *	0.970 ± 0.051	0.997 ± 0.004 *	0.997 ± 0.003*
RL-C5	I	16 ± 5	15 ± 5	15 ± 5	57 ± 24	54 ± 20	54 ± 20	0.995 ± 0.008	0.995 ± 0.008	0.995 ± 0.009
	II	14 ± 4	14 ± 4	14 ± 4	47 ± 15	48 ± 18	48 ± 17	0.995 ± 0.009	0.995 ± 0.009	0.995 ± 0.010
	V5	131 ± 60	24 ± 12 *$	136 ± 54 #	639 ± 287	102 ± 54 *$	660 ± 268 #	0.785 ± 0.210	0.957 ± 0.047 *$	0.792 ± 0.144 #
	Vx	14 ± 5	14 ± 5 *	14 ± 5 *	51 ± 25	51 ± 25	51 ± 25	0.998 ± 0.002	0.998 ± 0.002	0.997 ± 0.002
LA-C2 / LL-C3 / RL-C5	I	143 ± 72	17 ± 9 *	18 ± 8 *	726 ± 361	59 ± 33 *	69 ± 35 *	0.836 ± 0.100	0.994 ± 0.006 *	0.994 ± 0.005 *
	II	138 ± 45	19 ± 5 *	18 ± 9 *	631 ± 275	71 ± 26 *	60 ± 27 *	0.925 ± 0.062	0.997 ± 0.002 *	0.993 ± 0.009 *
	V1	225 ± 97	16 ± 5 *	14 ± 5 *	967 ± 445	50 ± 17 *	57 ± 18 *	0.652 ± 0.195	0.996 ± 0.003 *	0.997 ± 0.003 *
	V2	289 ± 125	16 ± 7 *	18 ± 8 *	1235 ± 487	62 ± 35 *	69 ± 30 *	0.365 ± 0.133	0.993 ± 0.007 *	0.996 ± 0.004 *
	V3	248 ± 92	15 ± 5 *	16 ± 4 *	1003 ± 378	55 ± 19 *	58 ± 23 *	0.494 ± 0.184	0.994 ± 0.010 *	0.997 ± 0.003 *
	V4	110 ± 56	14 ± 4 *	16 ± 4 *	443 ± 258	54 ± 20 *	58 ± 25 *	0.835 ± 0.204	0.997 ± 0.003 *	0.997 ± 0.002 *
	V5	161 ± 63	26 ± 10 *$	142 ± 75 #	615 ± 285	104 ± 50 *$	659 ± 368 #	0.705 ± 0.230	0.986 ± 0.019 *$	0.859 ± 0.106 #
	V6	113 ± 53	13 ± 5 *	13 ± 5 *	472 ± 231	50 ± 23 *	45 ± 16 *	0.886 ± 0.135	0.998 ± 0.002 *	0.996 ± 0.005 *

Note: Vx denotes the unipolar chest leads without electrode swaps; Color of electrodes follows IEC standard [44]; Gray columns highlight the baseline measurements without transformation ('None' transformation). * $p < 0.05$: Significant reduction of (RMS Error, Peak Error) and increment of (CorCoef) for the reordered leads after applying 'MSMinv' transformation (Forward or Inverse) compared to 'None' transformation. $: Approximation effect of the Forward 'MSMinv' transformation to simulate a swapped lead V5, while C5 is placed on the RL and its potential is assumed equal to the LL. #: Deficiency of the Inverse 'MSMinv' transformation to reconstruct the correct lead V5 from a recording with RL electrode in the position of C5 electrode.

Figure 3 illustrates the average ECG beats in leads (I, II, V1-V6) recorded with all types of swapped unicolor chest and peripheral electrodes. This ECG trace is almost fully overlapping with the simulated electrode reversals from the ECG raw data with correct electrode positions, applying Forward 'MSMinv' transformation. This once again validates the derived algebraic transformations in Table 4, which are able to exactly reproduce the diversity of lead-specific morphologies (amplitudes, polarities and durations) that each swap introduces to any lead via change of its electrode position and/or WCT potential.

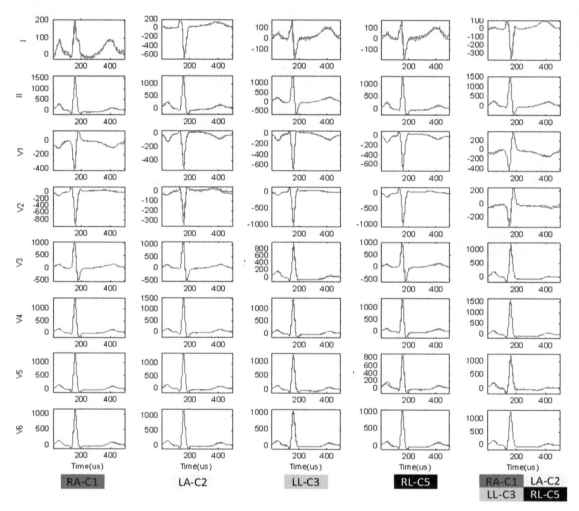

Figure 3. The average beat of 8 independent leads (I, II, V1-V6) taken from the same subject in two scenarios: (1) Red trace: Recorded ECG with swapped unicolor electrodes; (2) Blue trace: Simulated ECG with swapped unicolor electrodes, applying Forward 'MSMinv' transformation on the ECG recorded with the correct lead set.

4.3. Application of the 'MSMinv' Transformation for Automatic Detection of the Exact ECG Electrode Reversals

We further show an important practical application of the Inverse 'MSMinv' transformation for the detection of the exact reversals between ECG electrodes. This application is relevant to the case when two ECG recordings in a patient are available:

(1) an ECG recording with correct lead set (L_{RC});

(2) an ECG recording with an unknown/suspected lead swap (L_{RS}).

The 'MSMinv' transformation is applied to the swapped ECG recording, iteratively simulating all possible permutations of the nine active ECG electrodes ($i = 9! = 362\,880$):

$$\widehat{L_{RS}}(i) = \mathbf{MSi}\tilde{\mathbf{M}}_{\text{inv}}L_{RS} \qquad (16)$$

The swap matrix $\mathbf{S_i}$, which produces the lead set reconstruction $\widehat{L_{RS}}(i)$ with the minimal difference $d(\cdot)$ to the correct lead set can indicate the true lead swap (TLS):

$$TLS = \underset{1 \leq i \leq 9!}{arg\ min}\left(d\left(\widehat{L_{RS}}(i) - L_{RC}\right)\right) \tag{17}$$

We test this swap detection criterion using our ECG database under the following conditions:

- All 25 patients are considered, comparing the available pairs of recordings (L_{RC}, L_{RS}) per patient, where L_{RC} is the recording without electrode reversals, and L_{RS} represents one of the recorded 3 lead swaps (RA-C1, LA-C2, LL-C3), not involving the RL.
- The minimal difference rule (17) is applied on the average beat of each recording.
- The minimal difference rule (17) is evaluated with 3 distance metrics $d(\cdot)$ – min(RMS Error) (Equation (13)), min(Peak Error) (Equation (14)), max(CorCoef) (Equation (15)).
- The accuracy for detection of the TLS is evaluated as the true positive (TP) rate, considering the tested population of N subjects:

$$Accuracy = \sum_{p=1}^{N} \frac{TP_p}{N}, \tag{18}$$

$$where\ TP = f(x) = \begin{cases} 1, & correct\ lead\ swap\ detected \\ 0, & otherwise \end{cases}$$

Table 6 presents the experimental verification of the Inverse 'MSMinv' transformation, applied for automatic detection of the exact ECG electrode reversals. We have achieved 100% accuracy in the detection of (RA-C1) and (LL-C3) reversals, and 96% for the detection of (LA-C2) reversal when the decision rule (17) uses a minimal difference metric equal to the minimal RMS Error or the maximal correlation between the reconstructed swap and the correct recording. All false negatives are observed to present TLS with either the 2nd or the 3rd ranked minimal differences, while the decision rule (17) is presently adjusted to simply report the exact lead swap with the 1st ranked minimal difference. For example, the lowest LA-C2 accuracy is due to one case, where the true LA-C2 is 2nd ranked, while the true LA-C2 in combination with RA-C1 is 1st ranked. Obviously, the detection of the exact electrode swap among many electrodes with close geometrical positions might include a portion of uncertainty due to indistinguishable geometrical perspectives of the heart vector in neighboring leads. Further updates of the decision rule (17) could potentially improve the accuracy for TLS detection, e.g., by majority voting of many distance metrics after exclusion of those with the lowest accuracy (i.e., the peak Error with 88% to 96%).

Table 6. Accuracy for the detection of the exact lead swaps, applying the 'MSMinv' transformation on 3 swapped recordings (RA-C1), (LA-C2), (LL-C3) from 25 patients in our database. Color of electrodes follows IEC standard [44];

Unicolor Lead Swaps	Accuracy		
	RMS Error (%)	Peak Error (%)	Cor Coef (%)
■	100	96 *	100
LA-C2	96 *	88 #	96 *
LL-C3	100	88 #	100

* 1 false negative case due to TLS with the 2nd ranked minimal difference in the decision rule (17). # 3 false negative cases due to TLS with either the 2nd or the 3rd ranked minimal differences in (17).

The presented rules are easily applicable in a warning system that can alert the medical staff to check the electrodes suggested for reversal within the first seconds of 12-lead ECG acquisition.

Principally, the analysis is not fixed exactly to 10 s but can take a single beat or an average beat over ECGs with an arbitrary duration. It is important to note that the results reported in this section represent the best-case results, because they are based on resting ECG recordings that were taken within a short window of time and with exactly the same electrode positions (only the electrode cables were swapped). In a clinically relevant application, the ECGs under question will most likely have a substantially different recording date (leading to possible physiological changes in the ECG), and they will most likely be recorded with slightly different electrode positions. Although the average beat pattern of the same individual has been shown to have a long-term stability independent of recording sessions and physiological factors (age, gender, heart rate) [46,47], the reliable clinical application should always consider a final approval of the alarmed electrode reversals by the medical staff and electrode correction at the time of the recording.

5. Conclusions

This study derives a novel algebraic transformation which converts the standard 12-lead ECG leads from a correct to reordered set in case of arbitrary reversals between ECG electrodes. The formula of the 'MSMinv' transformation (7) is generalized to the calculation of all kinds of electrode reversals, giving the exact lead reordering for:

- Limb electrode swaps that have been previously drawn from anatomical perspectives (Tables 2 and 3);
- Limb–chest electrode swaps with WCT potential change which, to the best of our knowledge, have never been simulated in the literature (Table 4). The formulas are exhibited for the most probable reversals of unicolor electrode pairs in the peripheral and precordial ECG cables.

The validity of the 'MSMinv' transformation is proven in our experimental study for two bilateral applications with a certain practical significance:

- *The 'Forward' application* computing the reordered lead set from an ECG recorded with correctly placed electrodes is important for educational purposes of both humans and machines to reliably recognize and warn of electrode swaps before potentially erroneous diagnostic interpretation has been made. In this respect, 'MSMinv' transformation is applicable to the available immense databases of correctly recorded ECGs (from normal and abnormal heart conditions) for reproducing the vast diversity of distorted ECG leads that can be observed in arbitrary swaps within the limb and precordial electrode set (such as the examples in Figure 3). This is an indispensable tool for the comprehensive training platforms to visualize and study the effects of electrode swaps (e.g. online cardiology courses for physicians, researchers, and instructors) or software design platforms (training the automatic detection algorithms) on abundant ECG electrode reversals.
- *The 'Inverse' application* reconstructing the correct lead set from an ECG recorded with known electrode reversals can save time and the cost of having to repeat ECG recordings in case of follow-up detection of electrode reversals and error-screening of clinical databases. The possibility for straightforward visualization of the correct lead set and its interpretation can easily uncover diagnostic errors or answer dilemmas for suspected or mistrusted electrode swaps (such as the dispute between [15] and [16]). In the general case when the electrode reversal is unknown but a prior correct ECG recording of the same patient is available, the Inverse 'MSMinv' transformation is able to solve the non-trivial task of detecting which electrodes have been exactly swapped. For this purpose, all possible swapped reconstructions can be simulated to ultimately determine the one which yields the minimal RMS difference or the highest correlation with the known recording. We have achieved a detection accuracy of 96% to 100% for this simple criterion, which has been tested with available recordings of three electrode swaps (RA-C1, LA-C2, LL-C3, not involving the RL) from 25 healthy persons. One should consider, however, the limitations for the validation of such an application which should be tested against the functional and physiological ECG instability between the two ECG sessions (e.g., the criterion validated on a

specific population with "normal" ECG during rest could fail on cardiac patients or patients under environmental stress with lead-wise ECG morphology change). As this work is focused only on the problem of simulating all possible ECG cable reversals, the design and validation of criteria for a self-consistency check for detection of the ECG cable reversals is an extensive problem for a future study.

Another important derivation of the present study is the 'WSMinv' transformation (12), which computes WCT potential change for all kinds of electrode reversals. It quantifies the common distortion that all unipolar leads would meet while their reference potential is changed, regardless of whether or not they maintain their correct position. Table 1 shows that WCT distortion is proportional to leads I, II, and the displaced unipolar leads (V1-V3 in the simulation) with fractions, which are hardly envisaged without the derived transformation. The overall influence of WCT change on all unipolar leads is also reproduced by the 'MSMinv' transformation in Tables 3 and 4.

This study provides the means for calculation of the potentials of the ECG electrodes and WCT toward a common reference potential using Equations (5) and (10), respectively. These mathematical transformations can be applied to any standard 12-lead ECG for deriving the 'true' unipolar ECG leads and WCT measurements that have recently been experimentally acquired via special ECG machines [43,47]. The experimental studies have considered the position of the reference potential on the right leg, while this study shows the values of the matrix $\tilde{\mathbf{M}}_{inv}$ for the reference left leg leading to the same global observations (WCT measured with respect to the left leg does not have a stable voltage and is correlated to the limb leads (I, II), exhibiting all ECG waves). Although both legs have essentially insignificant potential difference, its value is the only unknown and approximated to be a zero measurement while applying our transformation equations.

Author Contributions: Conceptualization, R.S.; data curation, V.K. and I.J.; formal analysis, V.K. and I.J.; investigation, V.K. and I.J.; methodology, V.K., I.J., and R.S.; project administration, R.S.; resources, V.K. and I.J.; software, V.K. and I.J.; supervision, R.S.; validation, V.K., I.J., and R.S.; visualization, V.K.; writing – original draft, V.K.; writing – review and editing, I.J. and R.S.

References

1. Kligfield, P.; Gettes, L.S.; Bailey, J.J.; Childers, R.; Deal, B.J.; Hancock, E.W.; van Herpen, G.; Kors, J.A.; Macfarlane, P.; Mirvis, D.M.; et al. Recommendations for the standardization and interpretation of the electrocardiogram: part I: The electrocardiogram and its technology: a scientific statement from the American Heart Association Electrocardiography and Arrhythmias Committee, Council on Clinical Cardiology; the American College of Cardiology Foundation; and the Heart Rhythm Society: endorsed by the International Society for Computerized Electrocardiology. *J. Am. ColL. Cardiol.* **2007**, *115*, 1306–1324. [CrossRef]

2. Rajaganeshan, R.; Ludlam, C.L.; Francis, D.P.; Parasramka, S.V.; Sutton, R. Accuracy in ECG lead placement among technicians, nurses, general physicians and cardiologists. *Int. J. Clin. Pract.* **2008**, *62*, 65–70. [CrossRef] [PubMed]

3. Salvi, V.; Karnad, D.R.; Panicker, G.K.; Kothari, S.; Hingorani, P.; Natekar, M.; Mahajan, V.; Narula, D. Limb lead interchange in thorough QT/QTc studies. *J. Clin. Pharmacol.* **2011**, *51*, 1468–1473. [CrossRef] [PubMed]

4. Rudiger, A.; Hellermann, J.; Mukherjee, R.; Follath, F.; Turina, J. Electrocardiographic artifacts due to electrode misplacement and their frequency in different clinical settings. *Am. J. Emer. Med.* **2007**, *25*, 174–178. [CrossRef] [PubMed]

5. Amin, M.; Chowdhury, A.; Ahmed, M.; Sabah, K.; Haque, H.; Kabir, S.; Islam, K.N.; Saleh, M.A.D. Lead-Reversal ECG Simulating Myocardial Infarction—A Case Report and Literature Review. *Bangladesh Heart J.* **2016**, *31*, 104–108. [CrossRef]

6. Raut, M.; Maheshwari, A. Know the errors in ECG recording. *Curr. Med. Res. Pract.* **2015**, *5*, 81–91. [CrossRef]

7.   Vardan, S.; Mookherjee, D.; Sarkar, T.; Mehrotra, K.; Fruehan, T.; Mookherjee, S. Guidelines for the Detection of ECG Limb Lead Misplacements. *Resid. Staff* **2008**, *54*. Available online: https://www.mdmag.com/journals/resident-and-staff/2008/2008-01/2008-01_05 (accessed on 24 February 2019).

8.   Haisty, W.K.; Pahlm, O.; Edenbrandt, L.; Newman, K. Recognition of Electrocardiographic Electrode Misplacements Involving the Ground (Right Leg) Electrode. *Am. J. Cardiol.* **1993**, *71*, 1490–1495. [CrossRef]

9.   Bond, R.; Finlay, D.; Nugent, C.; Breen, C.; Guldenring, D.; Daly, M. The effects of electrode misplacement on clinicians' interpretation of the standard 12-lead electrocardiogram. *Eur. J. Int. Med.* **2012**, *23*, 610–615. [CrossRef]

10. Mattu, A.; Brady, W.; Perron, A.; Robinson, D. Prominent R Wave in Lead V1: Electrocardiographic Differential Diagnosis. *Am. J. Emerg. Med.* **2001**, *19*, 504–513. [CrossRef]

11. Jekova, I.; Leber, R.; Krasteva, V.; Schmid, R. Detection of Unicolor ECG Electrode Reversals in Standard 12-Lead ECG. *Comput. Cardiol.* **2018**, *45*. [CrossRef]

12. Lynch, R. ECG lead misplacement: A brief review of limb lead misplacement. *African J. Emerg. Med.* **2014**, *4*, 130–139. [CrossRef]

13. García-Niebla, J.; García, P.L. An unusual case of electrode misplacement: left arm and V2 electrode reversal. *J. Electrocardiol.* **2008**, *41*, 380–381. [CrossRef] [PubMed]

14. Vanninen, S.U.; Nikus, K.C. Electrocardiogram Acquisition Errors or Myocardial Infarct. *Case Rep. Cardiol.* **2011**, *2011*, 605874. [CrossRef] [PubMed]

15. Joshi, K.R.; Morris, D.L.; Figueredo, V.M. Wandering acute myocardial infarction. *Am. J. Med.* **2014**, *127*, e5–e6. [CrossRef]

16. Givens, P.M.; Goldonowicz, J.M.; Littmann, L. The electrocardiogram of chest and limb lead reversal. *Am. J. Med.* **2014**, *127*, e29–e30. [CrossRef] [PubMed]

17. Medani, S.A.; Hensey, M.; Caples, N.; Owens, P. Accuracy in precordial ECG lead placement: Improving performance through a peer-led educational intervention. *J. Electrocardiol.* **2018**, *51*, 50–54. [CrossRef]

18. Thaler, T.; Tempelmann, V.; Maggiorini, M.; Rudiger, A. The frequency of electrocardiographic errors due to electrode cable switches: A before and after study. *J. Electrocardiol.* **2010**, *43*, 676–681. [CrossRef]

19. Mond, H.G.; Garcia, J.; Visagathilagar, T. Twisted Leads: The Footprints of Malpositioned Electrocardiographic Leads. *Heart Lung Circ.* **2016**, *25*, 61–67. [CrossRef]

20. Baranchuk, A.; Shaw, C.; Alanazi, H.; Campbell, D.; Bally, K.; Redfearn, D.P.; Simpson, C.S.; Abdollah, H. Electrocardiography Pitfalls and Artifacts: The 10 Commandments. *Crit. Care Nurse* **2009**, *29*, 67–73. [CrossRef]

21. Batchvarov, V.N.; Malik, M.; Camm, A.J. Incorrect electrode cable connection during electrocardiographic recording. *Europace* **2007**, *9*, 1081–1090. [CrossRef] [PubMed]

22. Rosen, A.V.; Koppikar, S.; Shaw, C.; Baranchuk, A. Common ECG Lead Placement Errors. Part I: Limb lead Reversals. *Int. J. Med. Stud.* **2014**, *2*, 92–98.

23. Rosen, A.V.; Koppikar, S.; Shaw, C.; Baranchuk, A. Common ECG Lead Placement Errors. Part II: Precordial Misplacements. *Int. J. Med. Stud.* **2014**, *2*, 99–103.

24. Sakaguchi, S.; Sandberg, J.; Benditt, D. ECG Electrode Reversals: An Opportunity to Learn from Mistakes. *J. Cardiovasc. Electrophysiol.* **2018**, *29*, 806–815. [CrossRef] [PubMed]

25. Abdollah, H.; Milliken, J.A. Recognition of electrocardiographic left arm/left leg lead reversal. *Am. J. Cardiol.* **1997**, *80*, 1247–1249. [CrossRef]

26. Hedén, B.; Ohlsson, M.; Holst, H.; Mjöman, M.; Rittner, R.; Pahlm, O.; Peterson, C.; Edenbrandt, L. Detection of frequently overlooked electrocardiographic lead reversals using artificial neural networks. *Am. J. Cardiol.* **1996**, *78*, 600–604. [CrossRef]

27. Hoffman, I. A flatline electrocardiogram in lead II is a marker for right arm/right leg electrode switch. *J. Electrocardiol.* **2007**, *40*, 226–227. [CrossRef] [PubMed]

28. Han, C.; Gregg, R.; Babaeizadeh, S. Automatic Detection of ECG Lead-wire Interchange for Conventional and Mason-Likar Lead Systems. *Comput. Cardiol.* **2014**, *41*, 145–148.

29. Krishnan, R.; Ramesh, M. QRS axis based classification of electrode interchange in wearable ECG devices. *EAI Endorsed Trans. Future Intell. Educ. Env.* **2015**, *2*. [CrossRef]

30. Ho, R.T.; Mukherji, L.; Evans, G.T.Jr. Simple diagnosis of limb-lead reversals by predictable changes in QRS axis. *Pacing Clin. Electrophysiol.* **2006**, *29*, 272–277. [CrossRef]

31.	De Bie, J.; Mortara, D.W.; Clark, T.F. The development and validation of an early warning system to prevent the acquisition of 12-lead resting ECGs with interchanged electrode positions. *J. Electrocardiol.* **2014**, *47*, 794–797. [CrossRef] [PubMed]

32.	Ho, K.K.L.; Ho, S.K. Use of the sinus P wave in diagnosing electrocardiographic limb lead misplacement not involving the right leg (ground) lead. *J. Electrocardiol.* **2001**, *34*, 161–171. [CrossRef] [PubMed]

33.	Kors, J.A.; van Herpen, G. Accurate automatic detection of electrode interchange in the electrocardiogram. *Am. J. Cardiol.* **2001**, *88*, 396–399. [CrossRef]

34.	Han, C.; Gregg, R.E.; Field, D.Q.; Babaeizadeh, S. Automatic detection of ECG cable interchange by analyzing both morphology and interlead relations. *J. Electrocardiol.* **2014**, *47*, 781–787. [CrossRef] [PubMed]

35.	Gregg, R.; Hancock, E.W.; Babaeizadeh, S. Detecting ECG limb lead-wire interchanges involving the right leg lead-wire. *Comput. Cardiol.* **2017**, *44*. [CrossRef]

36.	Xia, H.; Garcia, G.A.; Zhao, X. Automatic detection of ECG electrode misplacement: A tale of two algorithms. *Physiol. Meas.* **2012**, *33*, 1549–1561. [CrossRef] [PubMed]

37.	Dotsinsky, I.; Daskalov, I.; Iliev, I. Detection of peripheral ECG electrodes misplacement. *Proc. 7th Int. Conf. Electronics ET'98, Sozopol, Bulgaria* **1998**, *S2*, 21–26. Available online: http://ecad.tu-sofia.bg/et/1998/Statii%20ET98-II/Detection%20of%20Peripheral%20ECG%20Electrodes%20Misplacement.pdf (accessed on 24 February 2019).

38.	Jekova, I.; Krasteva, V.; Leber, R.; Schmid, R.; Twerenbold, R.; Müller, C.; Reichlin, T.; Abächerli, R. Inter-lead correlation analysis for automated detection of cable reversals in 12/16-lead ECG. *Comput. Methods Programs Biomed.* **2016**, *134*, 31–41. [CrossRef]

39.	Végső, B.; Balázs, G.; Gaál, B.; Kozmann, G. Electrode reversal detection in ECG remote monitoring. *Meas. Sci. Rev.* **2005**, *5*, 45–48. Available online: http://www.measurement.sk/2005/S2/Vegso.pdf (accessed on 24 February 2019).

40.	Cooper, C.; Clark, E.; Macfarlane, P.W. Enhanced Detection of Electrode Placement/Connection Errors. *Comput. Cardiol.* **2008**, *35*, 89–92. [CrossRef]

41.	Bond, R.; Finlay, D.; Nugent, C.; Moore, G.; Guldenring, D. A simulation tool for visualizing and studying the effects of electrode misplacement on the 12-lead electrocardiogram. *J. Electrocardiol.* **2011**, *44*, 439–444. [CrossRef]

42.	Macfarlane, P.W.; Van Oosterom, A.; Pahlm, O.; Kligfield, P.; Janse, M.; Camm, J. *Comprehensive Electrocardiography*, 2nd ed.; Springer-Verlag: London, UK, 2010; ISBN 978-1-84882-047-0.

43.	Gargiulo, G.D. True Unipolar ECG Machine for Wilson Central Terminal Measurements. *BioMed Res. Int.* **2015**, *586397*, 1–7. [CrossRef] [PubMed]

44.	IEC 60601-2-25 International Standard. *Medical electrical equipment—Part 2–25: Particular requirements for the basic safety and essential performance of electrocardiographs*, 2nd ed.; International Electrotechnical Commission: Geneva, Switzerland, 2011.

45.	Kligfield, P.; Badilini, F.; Denjoy, I.; Babaeizadeh, S.; Clark, E.M.A.; de Bie, J.; Devine, B.; Extramiana, F.; Generali, G.; Gregg, R.; et al. Comparison of automated interval measurements by widely used algorithms in digital electrocardiographs. *Am. Heart J.* **2018**, *200*, 1–10. [CrossRef]

46.	Krasteva, V.; Jekova, I.; Schmid, R. Perspectives of human verification via binary QRS template matching of single-lead and 12-lead electrocardiogram. *Plos ONE* **2018**, *13*, e0197240. [CrossRef] [PubMed]

47.	Gargiulo, G.D.; Bifulco, P.; Cesarelli, M.; McEwan, A.; Moeinzadeh, H.; O'Loughlin, A.; Shugman, I.M.; Tapson, J.C.; Thiagalingam, A. On the Zero of Potential of the Electric Field Produced by the Heart Beat. A Machine Capable of Estimating this Underlying Persistent Error in Electrocardiography. *Machines* **2016**, *4*, 18. [CrossRef]

Permissions

The contributors of this book come from diverse backgrounds, making this book a truly international effort. This book will bring forth new frontiers with its revolutionizing research information and detailed analysis of the nascent developments around the world.

We would like to thank all the contributing authors for lending their expertise to make the book truly unique. They have played a crucial role in the development of this book. Without their invaluable contributions this book wouldn't have been possible. They have made vital efforts to compile up to date information on the varied aspects of this subject to make this book a valuable addition to the collection of many professionals and students.

This book was conceptualized with the vision of imparting up-to-date information and advanced data in this field. To ensure the same, a matchless editorial board was set up. Every individual on the board went through rigorous rounds of assessment to prove their worth. After which they invested a large part of their time researching and compiling the most relevant data for our readers.

The editorial board has been involved in producing this book since its inception. They have spent rigorous hours researching and exploring the diverse topics which have resulted in the successful publishing of this book. They have passed on their knowledge of decades through this book. To expedite this challenging task, the publisher supported the team at every step. A small team of assistant editors was also appointed to further simplify the editing procedure and attain best results for the readers.

Apart from the editorial board, the designing team has also invested a significant amount of their time in understanding the subject and creating the most relevant covers. They scrutinized every image to scout for the most suitable representation of the subject and create an appropriate cover for the book.

The publishing team has been an ardent support to the editorial, designing and production team. Their endless efforts to recruit the best for this project, has resulted in the accomplishment of this book. They are a veteran in the field of academics and their pool of knowledge is as vast as their experience in printing. Their expertise and guidance has proved useful at every step. Their uncompromising quality standards have made this book an exceptional effort. Their encouragement from time to time has been an inspiration for everyone.

The publisher and the editorial board hope that this book will prove to be a valuable piece of knowledge for researchers, students, practitioners and scholars across the globe.

List of Contributors

Hung-Chi Chang, Po-Chiun Huang, Hsi-Pin Ma and Yuan-Hao Huang
Department of Electrical Engineering, National Tsing Hua University, Hsinchu 30013, Taiwan

Hau-Tieng Wu
Department of Mathematics and Department of Statistical Science, Duke University, Durham, NC 27708, USA

Yu-Lun Lo
Department of Thoracic Medicine, Healthcare Center, Chang Gung Memorial Hospital, School of Medicine, Chang Gung University, Taipei 33302, Taiwan

Tippabattini Jayaramudu
Center for Nanocellulose Future Composites, Department of Mechanical Engineering, Inha University, 100 Inha-Ro, Nam-Gu, Incheon 22212, Korea
Laboratory of Material Sciences, Instituto de Quimica de Recursos Naturales, Universidad de Talca, Talca 747, Chile

Hyun-U Ko, Hyun Chan Kim, Jung Woong Kim, Ruth M. Muthoka and Jaehwan Kim
Center for Nanocellulose Future Composites, Department of Mechanical Engineering, Inha University, 100 Inha-Ro, Nam-Gu, Incheon 22212, Korea

Carlo Massaroni, Daniela Lo Presti, Sergio Silvestri and Emiliano Schena
Unit of Measurements and Biomedical Instrumentation, Department of Engineering, Università Campus Bio-Medico di Roma, 00128 Rome, Italy

Domenico Formica
Unit of Neurophysiology and Neuroengineering of Human-Technology Interaction, Department of Engineering, Università Campus Bio-Medico di Roma, 00128 Rome, Italy

Yida Li, Suryakanta Nayak, Yuxuan Luo, Yijie Liu, Hari Krishna Salila Vijayalal Mohan, Jieming Pan, Chun Huat Heng and Aaron Voon-Yew Thean
Department of Electrical and Computer Engineering, National University of Singapore, 4 Engineering Drive 3, Singapore 117583, Singapore

Zhuangjian Liu
Institute of High Performance Computing, A*STAR Research Entities, 1 Fusionopolis Way, #16-16 Connexis, Singapore 138632, Singapore

Rongfeng Li, Liu Wang and Lan Yin
School of Materials Science and Engineering, The Key Laboratory of Advanced Materials of Ministry of Education, State Key Laboratory of New Ceramics and Fine Processing, Tsinghua University, Beijing 100084, China

Daniela Lo Presti, Riccardo Sabbadini, Carlo Massaroni and Emiliano Schena
Unit of Measurements and Biomedical Instrumentation, Università Campus Bio-Medico di Roma, Via Alvaro del Portillo, 00128 Rome, Italy

Sofia Dall'Orso and Silvia Muceli
Division of Signal Processing and Biomedical Engineering, Department of Electrical Engineering, Chalmers University of Technology, SE-412 96 Gothenburg, Sweden
Centre for the Developing Brain, School of Biomedical Engineering and Imaging Sciences, King's College London, London WC2R 2LS, UK

Tomoki Arichi
Centre for the Developing Brain, School of Biomedical Engineering and Imaging Sciences, King's College London, London WC2R 2LS, UK
Paediatric Neurosciences, Evelina London Children's Hospital, Guy's and St Thomas' NHS Foundation Trust, London SE1 7EH, UK

Sara Neumane
Centre for the Developing Brain, School of Biomedical Engineering and Imaging Sciences, King's College London, London WC2R 2LS, UK
NeuroDiderot Unit UMR1141, Université de Paris, INSERM, F-75019 Paris, France
UNIACT, Université Paris-Saclay, CEA, NeuroSpin, F-91191 Gif-sur-Yvette, France

Anna Lukens
Paediatric Neurosciences, Evelina London Children's Hospital, Guy's and St Thomas' NHS Foundation Trust, London SE1 7EH, UK

Michele Arturo Caponero
Photonics Micro- and Nanostructures Laboratory, ENEA Research Center of Frascati, 00044 Frascati (RM), Italy

Etienne Burdet
Department of Bioengineering, Imperial College London, London SW7 2AZ, UK

Yumi Choi and Sungjin Jo
School of Architectural, Civil, Environmental, and Energy Engineering, Kyungpook National University, Daegu 41566, Korea

Chang Su Kim
Advanced Functional Thin Films Department, Korea Institute of Materials Science (KIMS), Changwon 51508, Korea

Prince Manta and Deepak N. Kapoor
School of Pharmaceutical Sciences, Shoolini University of Biotechnology and Management Sciences, Solan 173212, India

Rupak Nagraik and Avinash Sharma
School of Bioengineering and Food Technology, Shoolini University of Biotechnology and Management Sciences, Solan 173212, India

Akshay Kumar
Department of Surgery, Medanta Hospital, Gurugram 122001, India

Pritt Verma and Shravan Kumar Paswan
Departments of Pharmacology, CSIR-National Botanical Research Institute, Lucknow 226001, India

Dmitry O. Bokov
Institute of Pharmacy, Sechenov First Moscow State Medical University, 8 Trubetskaya St., Moscow 119991, Russia

Juber Dastagir Shaikh
Department of Neurology, MGM Newbombay Hospital, Vashi, Navi Mumbai 400703, India

Roopvir Kaur
Department of Anesthesiology, Government Medical College, Amritsar 143001, India

Ana Francesca Vommaro Leite and Silas Jose Braz Filho
Department of Medicine, University of Minas Gerais, Passos 37902-313, Brazil

Nimisha Shiwalkar
Department of Anesthesiology, MGM Hospital, Navi Mumbai 410209, India

Purnadeo Persaud
Department of Medicine, Kansas City University, Kansas City, MO 64106, USA

Raluca Maria Aileni, Sever Pasca and Adriana Florescu
Department of Applied Electronics and Information Engineering, Faculty of Electronics, Telecommunications and Information Technology, Politehnica University of Bucharest, 060042 Bucharest, Romania

Antonio Cobo and Elena Villalba-Mora
Centre for Biomedical Technology (CTB), Universidad Politécnica de Madrid (UPM), Pozuelo de Alarcón, 28223 Madrid, Spain
Centro de Investigación Biomédica en Red en Bioingeniería, Biomateriales y Nanomedicina (CIBER-BBN), 28029 Madrid, Spain

Rodrigo Pérez-Rodríguez
Fundación para la Investigación Biomédica, Hospital de Getafe, Getafe, 28905 Madrid, Spain

Xavier Ferre, Walter Escalante and Cristian Moral
Centre for Biomedical Technology (CTB), Universidad Politécnica de Madrid (UPM), Pozuelo de Alarcón, 28223 Madrid, Spain

Leocadio Rodriguez-Mañas
Servicio de Geriatría, Hospital de Getafe, Getafe, 28905 Madrid, Spain
Centro de Investigación Biomédica en Red en Fragilidad y Envejecimiento Saludable (CIBER-FES), 28029 Madrid, Spain

Zong-Keng Kuo and Yu-Shin Chen
Institute of Nanoengineering and Microsystems, National Tsing Hua University, Hsinchu 30013, Taiwan

Tsui-Hsuan Chang and Chao-Min Cheng
Institute of Biomedical Engineering, National Tsing Hua University, Hsinchu 30013, Taiwan

Chia-Ying Tsai
Department of Ophthalmology, Fu Jen Catholic University Hostpital, Fu Jen Catholic University, New Taipei City 24352, Taiwan
School of Medicine, College of Medicine, Fu Jen Catholic University, New Taipei City 24205, Taiwan

Su-Chun Huang and Martina Congiu
Neurorehabilitation Department and Experimental Neurophysiology Unit, INSPE-Institute of Experimental Neurology, San Raffaele Hospital, 20132 Milan, Italy

Gloria Dalla Costa, Marco Pisa, Giancarlo Comi and Letizia Leocani
Neurorehabilitation Department and Experimental Neurophysiology Unit, INSPE-Institute of Experimental Neurology, San Raffaele Hospital, 20132 Milan, Italy
Vita-Salute San Raffaele University, Via Olgettina, 58, 20132 Milan, Italy

Lorenzo Gregoris and Giulia Leccabue
Vita-Salute San Raffaele University, Via Olgettina, 58, 20132 Milan, Italy

Shin-Chen Pan
Department of Surgery, Section of Plastic and Reconstructive Surgery, National Cheng Kung University Hospital, College of Medicine, National Cheng Kung University, Tainan 704, Taiwan
International Center for Wound Repair and Regeneration, National Cheng Kung University, Tainan 704, Taiwan

Yao-Hung Tsai, Chin-Chuan Chuang and Chao-Min Cheng
Institute of Biomedical Engineering and Frontier Research Center on Fundamental and Applied Sciences of Matters, National Tsing Hua University, No. 101, Sec. 2, Kuang-Fu Rd., East Dist., Hsinchu 300, Taiwan

Vessela Krasteva and Irena Jekova
Institute of Biophysics and Biomedical Engineering, Bulgarian Academy of Sciences, Acad. G. Bonchev Str. Bl 105, 1113 Sofia, Bulgaria

Ramun Schmid
Signal Processing, Schiller AG, Altgasse 68, CH-6341 Baar, Switzerland

Index